Psychosocial Care
of the Dying Patient

Psychosocial Care of the Dying Patient

Edited by
Charles A. Garfield

Director, SHANTI Project
Volunteer Counseling for Patients and Families
  Facing Life-threatening Illness
Clinical Research Psychologist, Cancer Research Institute
Assistant Clinical Professor of Medical Psychology
Schools of Medicine and Nursing
University of California, San Francisco

McGraw-Hill Book Company

New York   St. Louis   San Francisco   Auckland   Bogotá   Düsseldorf
Johannesburg   London   Madrid   Mexico   Montreal   New Delhi   Panama
Paris   São Paulo   Singapore   Sydney   Tokyo   Toronto

NOTICE

Medicine is an ever-changing science. As new research and clinical experience broaden our knowledge, changes in treatment and drug therapy are required. The editors and the publisher of this work have made every effort to ensure that the drug dosage schedules herein are accurate and in accord with the standards accepted at the time of publication. Readers are advised, however, to check the product information sheet included in the package of each drug they plan to administer to be certain that changes have not been made in the recommended dose or in the contraindications for administration. This recommendation is of particular importance in regard to new or infrequently used drugs.

This book was set in Press Roman by Allen Wayne Technical Corp.
The editor was J. Dereck Jeffers; the cover was designed by John Hite; the production supervisor was Jeanne Selzam.
Fairfield Graphics was printer and binder.

Library of Congress Cataloging in Publication Data

Main entry under title:

Psychosocial care of the dying patient.

    1. Terminal care. 2. Death—Psychological aspects.
3. Physician and patient. I. Garfield, Charles A.
[DNLM: 1. Death. 2. Attitude to death. 3. Terminal
care. BF789.D4 P976]
R726.8.P79   610.69'6   77-8380
ISBN 0-07-022860-4

Dedication

To our patients, some living, some dead, who have taught us most of what we know about emotional support and who are quite literally leading the way.

To our medical and nursing students, the health professionals of tomorrow, who, ironically, will care for us on our deathbeds. With this thought firmly in mind, I suddenly develop an enormous passion for sensitivity and excellence in the training of our medical students.

To the medical profession, with support, concern, and the knowledge that trust and appreciation will grow in the community in direct proportion to our willingness to care as well as cure.

To all I dedicate this volume with its two basic themes, *an appreciation of the emotional realities of dying:*

> Turning again toward childish treble, pipes
> And whistles in his sound. Last scene of all,
> That ends this strange eventful history,
> Is second childishness and near oblivion,
> Sans teeth, sans eyes, sans taste, sans everything.

> William Shakespeare, *As You Like It*

and *the undeniable human need for caring:*

> Those who can sit in silence with their fellowman not knowing what to say but knowing that they should be there, can bring new life in a dying heart. Those who are not afraid to hold a hand in gratitude, to shed tears in grief, and to let a sigh of distress arise straight from the heart, can break through paralyzing boundaries and witness the birth of a new fellowship, the fellowship of the broken.

> Henri J. M. Nouwen, *Out of Solitude.*

Contents

List of
Major Contributors

Harry S. Abram, M.D., Professor of Psychiatry, Vanderbilt University Medical Center, Nashville, Tennessee.

Sandra L. Barger, SHANTI volunteer, kidney dialysis patient.

David Barton, M.D., Associate Clinical Professor of Psychiatry, Vanderbilt University Medical Center.

Jeanne Quint Benoliel, Ph.D., D.N.S.c., Doctor of Nursing Science Professor and Chairperson, Department of Community Health Health Care Systems, University of Washington School of Nursing.

Abraham B. Bergman, M.D., Director of Outpatient Services, Children's Orthopedic Hospital and Medical Center; Associate Professor of Pediatrics Health Services, University of Washington, Seattle; President, National Foundation for Sudden Infant Death, Inc., New York.

Eric J. Cassell, M.D., Associate Clinical Professor of Community Medicine and Associate Professor of Medicine at Mt. Sinai School of Medicine, New York.

Rachel Ogren Clark, Co-Director, SHANTI Project: Volunteer counseling for patients and families facing life-threatening illness.

Carolyn Driver (currently Patti Driver Scott), Co-Founder, Kairos Institute, California.

J. Fischhoff, M.D., Professor of Child Psychiatry, Wayne State University; Chief of Psychiatry, Children's Hospital of Detroit.

Michael A. Friedman, M.D., Clinical Director, Research Institute, University of California, San Francisco.

Charles A. Garfield, Ph.D., Co-Director, SHANTI Project: Volunteer counseling for patients and families facing life-threatening illness; Clinical Research Psychologist, Cancer Research Institute, and Assistant Clinical Professor of Medicine and Nursing, University of California, San Francisco.

Nancy Harjan, elementary school teacher; daughter of the late Philip H. Arnot, M.D., Professor of Obstetrics and Gynecology, University of California, San Francisco.

Milton D. Heifetz, M.D., diplomate, American Board of Neurological Surgery; Associate Clinical Professor of Neurological Surgery, University of Southern California, Los Angeles.

Howard P. Hogshead, M.D., Director Orthopaedic Surgery and Associate Professor, Department of Pediatrics, University of Florida.

Walter Hollander, Jr., M.D., Professor Emeritus, Department of Medicine, University of North Carolina School of Medicine, Chapel Hill.

Bernard Isaacs, M.D., F.R.C.P., Consultant Physician, Department of Geriatric Medicine, Glasgow Royal Infirmary Group of Hospitals.

Richard A. Kalish, Ph.D., Professor of Behavioral Sciences, Graduate Theological Union, Berkeley, and independent consultant.

David M. Kaplan, Ph.D., Director, Division of Clinical Social Work, Stanford University Medical Center.

Robert Kastenbaum, Ph.D., Professor of Psychology, University of Massachusetts, Boston.

Orville E. Kelly, Founder and Director, Make Today Count; cancer patient.

Morris D. Kerstein, M.D., Assistant Professor of Surgery, Yale University.

S. Malkin, M.D., C.C.F.P., Medical advisor to early hospital discharge home care service, Metropolitan Board of Health of Greater Vancouver.

R. Melzack, Ph.D., D., Department of Psychology, McGill University, Montreal.

G.W. Milton, M.D., Professor, Department of Surgery, University of Sydney, New South Wales, Australia.

Balfour M. Mount, F.R.C.S., Palliative Care Service, Royal Victoria Hospital, Montreal.

W. Bradford Patterson, M.D., Professor of Oncology in Surgery, Associate Director for Associated Hospital and Extramural Programs, University of Rochester Cancer Center.

E. Mansell Pattison, M.D., Professor of Psychiatry and Human Behavior, Social Science and Social Ecology; Vice-Chairman, Department of Psychiatry and Human Behavior, University of California, Irvine.

Ernest H. Rosenbaum, M.D., Associate Clinical Professor, University of California, San Francisco; Medical Director, San Francisco Regional Tumor Foundation and Associate Chief of Medicine, Mt. Zion Hospital and Medical Center.

Cicely Saunders, O.B.E., F.R.C.P., Medical Director, St. Christopher's Hospice, Sydenham, England.

Arthur H. Schmale, M.D., Professor of Psychiatry, Associate Professor of Medicine; Director, Psychosocial Group, University of Rochester Cancer Center.

Edwin S. Shneidman, Ph.D., Professor of Thanatology, University of California, Los Angeles.

Robert E. Taubman, Ph.D., M.D., Professor, Department of Family Practice and Department of Psychiatry, Uniersity of Oregon Health Sciences Center.

Lewis Thomas, M.D., President, Memorial Sloan-Kettering Cancer Center, New York.

Mona Wasow, Clinical Assistant Professor of Social Work, University of Wisconsin, Madison.

Avery D. Weisman, M.D., Associate Professor of Psychiatry at Massachusetts General Hospital and Harvard Medical School; Director, Project Omega.

T. Franklin Williams, M.D., Department of Medicine, University of Rochester School of Medicine and Dentistry, and Monroe Community Hospital, Rochester, New York.

Robert Woodson, Ph.D., Director, Santa Barbara Pain Control Clinic, Santa Barbara, California.

Ernlé W. D. Young, Ph.D., Associate Dean of Memorial Church and Chaplain to the Medical Center at Stanford University.

Preface

The purpose of this anthology is as much to inspire as to provide information. In developing the definitive (and perhaps only) resource text primarily for physicians on psychosocial care of the dying patient, I soon realized that the issues were less technical than human. As physicians, nurses, and allied professionals perfect their skill at providing care and support for the terminally ill, they must continually be aware of the enormity of the emotional trauma confronting the dying patient and his or her family. "The doctor being himself a mortal man, should be diligent and tender in relieving his suffering patients inasmuch as he himself must one day be a like sufferer."[1]

White's observation that "our current practice in caring for the dying is generally inadequate, limited and, on occasion, miserably poor,"[2] is still quite accurate. The single greatest obstacle to providing adequate emotional support to dying patients and their families is the professional distinction between "us" and "them," that is, the deeply conditioned mandate that "*we* are the professionals and *you* are the

---

[1]D. Shephard, "Terminal Care: Towards an Ideal," *Canadian Medical Association Journal,* **115**:97–8, July 17, 1976.

[2]L. White, "The Self-Image of the Physician and the Care of Dying Patients," in L. White, *Care of Patients with Fatal Illness,* Annals of the New York Academy of Sciences, **164**, Art. 3, 1969.

patients and we will help you through our technological mastery and beneficence."[3] Those physicians who provide the most effective emotional support are those who have been able to transcend this needlessly rigid distinction and relate to their patients as colleagues or advocates rather than as processors of data.

It is interesting to realize that the word *care* derives from the Gothic *kara*, which means "to lament, to grieve, to experience sorrow, to cry out with." Nouwen notes that "we tend to look at caring as an attitude of the strong toward the weak, of the powerful towards the powerless, the haves toward the have-nots."[4] We often experience great discomfort when we are invited to enter into someone's pain before we have done something about it. But, distanced concern appears strangely antithetical to the basic component of caring, namely, empathy; the more expressive German translation of which is *einfuhlung* meaning "to feel oneself into." Nouwen continues with the observation that:

> When we honestly ask ourselves which persons in our lives mean the most to us, we often find that it is those who, instead of giving much advice, solutions, or cures, have chosen rather to share our pain and touch our wounds with a gentle and tender hand. The friend who can be silent with us in a moment of despair or confusion, who can stay with us in an hour of grief and bereavement, who can tolerate not knowing, not curing, not healing and face with us the reality of our powerlessness, that is the friend who cares.[5]

Effective caring and support imply a recognition of human sameness rather than difference, an overture from those who wish not only to take our pain away but also to share it.

I would like to acknowledge the inspiration and support of a number of key individuals who were instrumental in the preparation of this volume:

Rachel Ogren Clark, my dear friend and co-director of the SHANTI Project, who has lovingly and patiently shown me the art of nurturing and learning from a hundred of the finest volunteers to be found anywhere, and for sharing in the beauty of one of the Project's essential statements. Namely, to believe in miracles can be entirely pragmatic.

Michael Friedman, M.D., Clinical Director of the Cancer Research Institute, for his much appreciated support of our efforts to meet the emotional needs of cancer patients and their families.

My friends on the nursing staff of the Cancer Research Institute, twelfth floor, Moffitt Hospital, for the dedication—often under difficult conditions—and their willingness to listen and learn from their patients.

---

[3]C. Garfield, "The Impact of Death on the Health Professional," in H. Feifel (ed.), *New Meanings of Death,* McGraw-Hill, New York, 1977.

[4]H. Nouwen, *Out of Solitude,* Ave Maria Press, Notre Dame, Indiana, 1974.

[5]Nouwen, op. cit.

Doctor Walter Alvarez, Karl Menninger, Hans Selye, and Linus Pauling, the sages and elder statesmen, whose presence and friendship at our conferences taught me much about dying.

Orville Kelly and his colleagues at Make Today Count for their efforts in establishing a nationwide network of support groups directed by patients and families facing life-threatening illness.

Elisabeth Kübler-Ross, M.D., for her courage in helping to demystify the process of communicating with dying patients and her insistence on taking a strong stand in support of human kindness and sensitivity.

Dr. Cicely Saunders, Medical Director, St. Christopher's Hospice, and Dr. Balfore Mount, Director, Palliative Care Unit, Royal Victoria Hospital, Montreal, for stressing that institutional contexts emphasizing care and compassion can become a reality and for their use of more effective and humane palliative strategies.

The many individuals working in hospitals, clinics, nursing homes, and the community who compassionately care for the dying, often with little support or appreciation.

Mrs. Carl W. Stern, Ms. Julia Bloomfield, and Mr. Martin Paley and his associates at The San Francisco Foundation for their compassionate recognition of the needs of patients and families facing life-threatening illness.

The Foundations Fund for Research in Psychiatry for supporting my postdoctoral research training in the area of psychosocial care of the dying patient.

Linda Garfield and Jonathan Garfield, who have certainly experienced a great deal of my Type A behavior during the preparation of this manuscript and Edward and Sylvia Garfield, companions since my birth; J. Dereck Jeffers, my friend and editor at McGraw-Hill for understanding the creative basis of a compelling mission and the pragmatics involved in making it happen; Ruth Veres, for her expert editorial and organizational assistance and Kathryn Brown, my friend and administrative assistant, for her dedicated allegiance to the task.

Charles A. Garfield

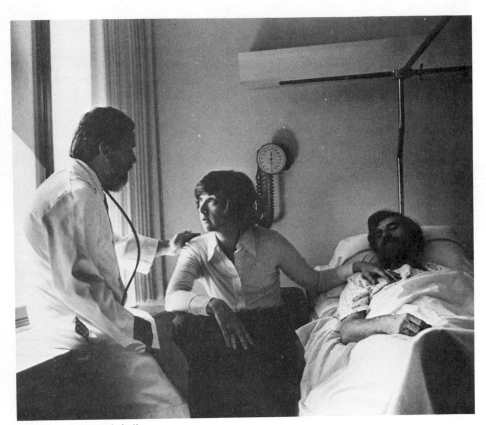

Courtesy of Katrin Achelis

Part One

Introduction

Chapter 1

On Caring, Doctors, and Death

Charles A. Garfield

A recurrent theme of this book is the <u>importance of emotional accessibility</u>, the art of <u>being fully present to another human being</u>. Present not only as an expert in the physiologic nuances of life-threatening illness and treatment, but as a willing companion. The implication is clear. To the extent that physicians restrict their interaction with patients to a certain class of "efficiency behaviors" consistent with a narrow role definition, they will delimit their effectiveness and be perceived by their patients as inflexible and uncaring. In my courses with medical students on the care of the dying patient, I frequently hear that many of the available models for students and younger physicians recommend that professionals espouse an attitude of little or no emotional involvement with patients. In as emotionally charged an environment as exists in most of our contacts with seriously ill patients and their families, attempts at decreased emotional involvement are frequently experienced by patients as painful abandonment. These attempts to remain objective are born of the notion that to become emotionally accessible to one's patients implies a loss of scientific objectivity, a compromising of rational judgment, and a decrease in the time-effective management of one's case load. When communicated to medical students and younger physicians, this bias serves to disallow authentic human communication between doctor and patient, and prevents the next generation of physicians from mastering the art as well as the science of patient care.

The battle cry of many health professionals that there is not enough time to devote to effective patient care is both true and false. That staff shortages and high admission quotas and case loads tax our emotional resources to the extreme is often painfully clear. However, how frequently have we seen a doctor or nurse argue with a patient for 10 or 15 minutes about the feasibility of waiting just 5 more minutes so that the patient might better cope with his or her anxiety prior to a frightening procedure. More importantly, we are learning that nearly two-thirds of the malpractice suits in the state of California originate in poor communication between doctor and patient, rather than in lapses or errors of medical judgment. As one patient, a lawyer, stated, "We patients will not sue doctors whom we really like, who take the time to explain to us to the best of their ability the nature of our illness and its treatment."

The simple fact remains that we health care professionals are intimately involved with our patients whether we like it or not and our attitudes and availability for emotional support will be communicated powerfully to those for whom we care. Additionally, a patient's own attitude toward his illness and its treatment will be affected considerably by the attitudes of the physicians and allied professionals with whom he has contact. The latest research in nonverbal communication indicates that 70 to 90 percent of all that we communicate to one another is through nonverbal channels and, therefore, our attitudes concerning a given patient's status will likely be communicated whether we do so verbally or not. The fundamental fact that we ourselves are not comfortable around the dying and often have little psychological understanding of the ways in which seriously ill patients and their families cope with life-threatening illness increases the strain of the patient-doctor relationship. Mastery of the psychosocial aspects of terminal patient care requires serious self-examination, some reading and study, and most of all a trust in the invaluable clinical experience that presents itself to physicians often on a daily basis. The single, 4-week crash course in psychiatry that many of our medical students receive will most certainly not provide an understanding of the emotional needs of patients. To understand the nature of effective support for patients, physicians must:

1   Realize that role models appropriate to laboratory science are largely inappropriate to the effective emotional support of patients and families facing life-threatening illness. That is, we are emotionally involved with our patients and we need to be able to discuss this involvement both with our patients and our colleagues in order to maximize the supportive nature of these basically interdependent relationships.

2   Recognize that the psychosocial aspects of patient care require a great deal more than "hand holding." Almost without exception, physicians who take the psychological and social issues surrounding life-threatening illness seriously can develop a real mastery of this increasingly important aspect of patient care.

3   Examine carefully physician attitudes concerning death and the dying patient and realize that when it comes to a subjective understanding of the nature of the dying process most patients know a great deal more than those who care for them.

As health professionals, we are often involved in situations in which we are like life-guards watching our patients flounder in the water several hundred yards offshore. Perhaps the distressed person does not know how to swim or, knowing how, simply does not have enough strength to make it to shore.

> Our professional lifeguards, it seems, do not know how to swim themselves. To be sure, they have been given extensive training in many lifesaving techniques, all of which they have tested in the children's pool. They know how to row a boat; they know how to throw out a ring buoy; they know how to give artificial respiration. But they do not know how to swim themselves. They cannot save another because, given the same circumstances, they could not save themselves (Carkhuff and Berenson, 1967).

Those physicians who have learned the art of effective patient care have learned that the flexibility of role definition is an indispensible aspect of this art. That is, in the absence of a rigidly defined role, the physician is free to select any number of appropriate roles in an effort to make any of a number of useful orientations. In other words, he or she is free to do what needs to be done, as decided upon by both physician and patient.

It is also necessary to mention the relationship between physician and nurse in the care of the dying patient. An extremely skilled and well-respected nurse, when asked to what she attributed her increased credibility and effectiveness in communicating with physicians, replied, "I realized that with some doctors I needed to first allow them their 'M.D-eity' before reestablishing a relationship built on equality." It would appear that those nurses who are most respected by their medical colleagues are those who have mastered their discipline and have exhibited at least the same level of commitment and dedication as the physicians with whom they work. More importantly, physicians and other medical personnel have the greatest respect for nurses who realize their own competence and who clearly and assertively communicate what they know rather than backing off and assuming their own inferiority—often at the expense of the patient. Finally, if we continue to insist that the medical world breaks down into physicians and ancillary personnel, we will cut off constructive dialogue and any hope of an interdisciplinary effort in the service of patients. The word *ancillary* derives from the Latin *ancilla* which means "handmaiden" and one does not frequently interact as an equal with those whom one considers to be one's handmaidens. I am continually impressed by the way some of the most respected and admired of my medical colleagues stress effective, nonpatronizing, working relationships with nurses and allied health personnel.

In an interesting and informative book entitled *When Doctors Are Patients*, physicians Max Pinner and Benjamin Miller compiled an impressive array of firsthand accounts of the experiences of physicians who were compelled to cope with serious illness. They conclude that no matter what the nature of the disease, a sick person often has strong emotional reactions to illness that may be a greater source of torment for the patient (and therefore a serious challenge to the treating physician) than the obvious somatic symptoms. Although the authors' use of the term *symptoms* to describe the strong psychological reactions of patients inaccurately implies pathology when, in fact, these emotional responses are clearly appropriate to the extreme stress of a life-threatening illness, their following point is vital.

> It remains a fact that even many physicians, both in the performance of their professional work and as patients (just like any other patients), have the impression that the distance between somatic symptoms and a lie is far greater than that between psychogenic symptoms and a lie; that psychogenic symptoms are less "real" than somatic ones—and that, in consequence, psychogenic symptoms need not be treated. All wise physicians, and many experienced physicians, throughout recorded history have known better, but the majority of physicians still need to be reminded (Pinner and Miller, 1952).

One intent of this volume is to assist the physician and allied personnel in identifying the emotional needs of the dying patient and his family and to suggest helpful ways of providing some of the necessary support. Another and admittedly more ambitious intent is to identify the entire area of basic emotional support for patients and families as a legitimate and in fact vital concern for any fully competent physician and health professional who is seriously concerned with patient care. An important, but often overlooked, corollary of this proposition is that doctors and other health care workers who spend many hours each day with patients engaged in a life-and-death struggle against disease, and who must constantly make decisions that affect the resolution of that fight, need emotional support themselves. The archaic notion that emotional expression and support are inappropriate or unprofessional derives from a model of professional comportment devised by those who have learned to view emotion as a weakness and intellect as a weapon. It is based on an inaccurate conception of the way human beings function under stress. Physicians who follow this model inevitably treat only diseases, not people, which undermines their competence and effectiveness.

Most of our attempts to understand the emotional realities of dying patients are doomed to failure because we base our approaches on a set of faulty operational assumptions:

1 We rely on summary information about the patient's emotional world, that is, notes in the chart or brief word-of-mouth explanations, and on modal or normative data.

2 Our values as health professionals are most often firmly rooted in middle-class thinking that makes it difficult to comprehend cross-cultural variation in value systems.

3 We are unable to effectively incorporate or interpret experiential and behavioral extremes in a meaningful fashion.

4 We have great difficulty dealing with emotional expression, for example, extreme anger, long-term depression, and so on; the somewhat presumptuous yet frequently

invoked assessment of the patient's chosen form of expression as *inappropriate affect* is often a signal of our inability to cope.

5 We attempt to deal reasonably with what is most often an unreasonable life situation.

Our efforts to ignore or disqualify emotional expression, make decisions on the basis of cursory and most often superficial data, and eliminate extremes from the dying patient's emotional life are usually perfectly reasonable yet superficial. Our effectiveness will increase in direct proportion to our capacity to acknowledge both the great range of quite normal emotional responses to life-threatening illness and the complexities of psychological functioning and assessment. Increased effectiveness results when we continue to be present to our patients in spite of the fact that the greater portion of their psychological functioning remains a mystery to us.

Guided mostly by our patients, we are starting to appreciate the possibilities for personal growth and maturation that can accompany the stark realization that forever does not include us. One of the more significant findings in my own research and clinical work has been that some dying patients are quite willing and able to suspend stereotypic patterns of social behavior, i.e., "the games people play," in a quest for more authentic forms of human expression. The innate power of imminent ceasing to be appears to shatter the illusion that we have all the time in the world to live our lives. I have frequently seen dying patients engage in the kind of intensive, introspective, soul-searching that the rest of us generally neglect. When the dimension of futurity, the guarantee of later, no longer exists, a kind of trivialization of trivia may manifest itself along with an insistence on honesty and clarity in human relationships. It is at these times that the individual who is incapable or unwilling to be present to the dying patient is largely excluded from being a significant part of his or her emotional world. We have already found that the living have much to learn from the dying, and I would predict that in the years ahead we will identify and clarify the existential insights offered by our dying brethren and hopefully come to understand more fully the basic realities that sustain a human being both emotionally and spiritually.

My original inspiration for this anthology came from chairing the First National Training Conference for Physicians on Psychosocial Care of the Dying Patient at the University of California Medical Center in San Francisco. After the success of that first conference and the enormous response to the following year's conference (including participation by Hans Selye, Linus Pauling, Karl Menninger, George Engel, and others), I remembered an incident that illustrates my sentiments on providing such educational experiences for physicians. My elderly grandmother who lives in a large nursing home in the East was comparing "my grandson the doctor" stories with a friend of hers. When asked what specialty her grandson represented, my grandmother enthusiastically replied, "He's a psychologist." "Why a psychologist?" her friend responded, perhaps hoping for a surgeon. "Because *someone* has to take care of the doctors, of course!" came the reply. While working on both the conferences and this volume, I have continually been reminded that given the enormous influx of new medical information appearing regularly, it would take a miracle for us to master both the physiologic and psychosocial aspects of terminal patient care. With respect for both the enormity of the task and our ability to recognize what is humane and just, I echo David Ben Gurion's observation that "anyone who doesn't believe in miracles is not a realist!"

BIBLIOGRAPHY

Carkhuff, R. and B. Berenson: *Beyond Counseling and Therapy*, Holt, Rinehart and Winston, New York, 1967.
Pinner, M. and B. Miller: *When Doctors Are Patients*, Norton, New York, 1952.

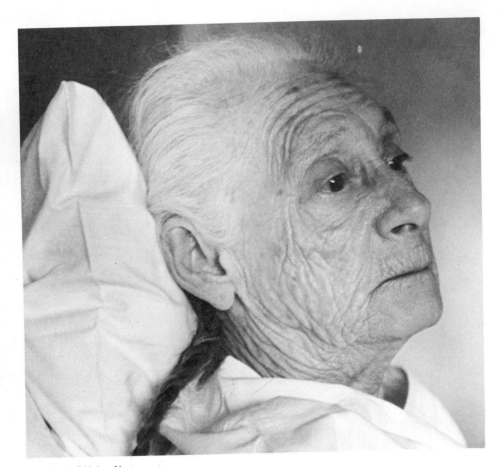

Courtesy of Helen Nestor

Part Two

Guidelines for
Terminal Patient Care

Chapter 2

Comfort Care Only—
Treatment Guidelines
for the Terminal Patient

Arthur H. Schmale
W. Bradford Patterson

Science has made us gods before we are even worthy of being man.

J. Hamburger—French physician, 1939

Modern day medicine with all its scientific and technological advances has had its effect on dying. Today the how, when, and where an individual dies are frequently determined by the instruments of medicine and the technological proficiency of the medical specialties involved. Where we used to let nature take its course, with some effort on the part of the medical professional to relieve suffering, we now try to prevent death from whatever cause as long as is possible in almost every patient. To further complicate the picture of dying we now have a host of experimental therapeutic approaches that may increase discomfort and disability and yet give only a limited chance of reversing the trajectory toward death. Finally, and particularly in this country, we have come to an awareness of the importance of informed consent,

Presented May 1, 1976 at the First National Training Conference for Physicians on Psychosocial Care of the Dying Patient, V.A. Hospital, San Francisco, Calif., UCSF Extended Programs in Medical Education.

that is, sharing with the health consumer our knowledge about his state of health, our plan for treatment, and his chances for cure. It is with this complexity of issues involving medical technology and the need for greater self-determination by all patients in mind that the First National Training Conference for Physicians on Psychosocial Care of the Dying Patient was established. Much was written and also said at that conference about the awareness, reaction, and communication of those facing death with their family and their health professionals. The following is a set of principles that, if followed, should make the dying process more meaningful for all involved.* Specific guidelines for the somatic and psychological needs of individual patients can in turn be derived from the application of these principles. Such guidelines will give the health professionals, as well as the dying patients, a more specific purpose for continuing their relationship.

PRINCIPLES

1. Patients select their physicians and agree to proposals for treatment. Physicians and their health care associates are agents employed by the patient. This role of the doctor has been accepted since the days of the writing of the Hippocratic oath. The physician as a health professional is paid for expertise in preventing, diagnosing, and treating disease.

It is the patient or, if the patient is or becomes incompetent, it is his or her legal representative or a prior agreed-upon written mandate to the physician, that should decide what should be done. The physician provides alternatives to the patient and carries out the therapy once it is accepted by the patient. (This leaves aside the emergency situation where the physician may have to proceed on the assumption that he or she is acting in the patient's best interest.) The physician is a health advisor and therapist and should not make moral or life-and-death decisions for patients.[2] (Cassell insists physicians are applied moral philosophers, however they must know their patients' values, desires, and expectations.[8]

2. Physicians make judgments as to when a therapy is ineffective in stopping the progress of disease. The physician is expected to have knowledge as to when a progressive disease such as cancer has become untreatable to the point of threatening life. How long a physician waits before he or she concedes that therapy is ineffective in halting the progress of the disease and decides there are no remaining curative or palliative courses of action available depends on the experience and judgment of the individual physician. Physicians frequently ask for a consultation at such a time to make sure that their judgment is correct. It is in the context of asking for a consultation that the patient or his designated representative is frequently informed of the ineffectiveness of the disease-oriented therapy. The patient also should feel free to ask for an independent consultation if he desires.

3. Patients are entitled to know when their disease has become unresponsive to treatment and is threatening life. The patient may come to this awareness before the

*These principles have evolved from a set of ideas discussed by Dr. Patterson in 1971.

physician.[3] The patient may be the one to initiate consideration of a change to a symptomatic approach. It is not uncommon for patients to be the first to recognize the point of no return biologically. Some physicians have difficulty in understanding this awareness on the part of the patient since the patient lacks the medical facts and figures that the physician depends on for making such a decision. (This biological awareness of patients should not be confused with expressions of panic or despair associated with a breakdown in a patient's coping mechanisms at a time of crisis.)

4. Once treatment for disease is ineffective, care should be designed for comfort rather than survival. The physician should discuss the alternatives of continuing the primarily disease-oriented treatments versus shifting to a person-oriented, comfort care approach.

The patient or his or her representative should be given an opportunity to decide to what lengths (ordinary/extraordinary means) the physician is to go in maintaining life.[4] (*Ordinary* is taken to mean all medicines, treatments, and operations that offer a reasonable hope of maintaining or increasing comfort and that can be accomplished without excessive expense, unnecessary prolongation of life, or increased disability.)

The patient may decide on a course of action in regard to his dying to which the physician may not be able to agree. If open discussion does not resolve the differences, the physician should either comply with the patient's wishes or ask to be relieved of his role as physician to the patient. Once a satisfactory replacement can be found, the physician may then turn over responsibility for the patient's care.

Once the physician agrees to a course of action the patient has selected, specific comfort care guidelines are detailed in which the patient, family, and health care team will be involved. Thus, at some point a decision is made to halt aggressive disease therapy and a plan is adopted to relieve symptoms rather than prolong the dying process. This point may come hours, days, or weeks prior to death.[5]

5. Comfort care means attention to the psychological, interpersonal, and physical needs of the dying person. The patient should be kept as comfortable as possible.[6] This requires regular, frequent contacts by all those monitoring and providing care. (If at home or in a nursing home this may be family only or family and nursing staff, plus phone calls and an occasional visit from the physician.) The specifics of comfort should be defined by the patient. The level of awareness and activity preferred versus the amount of discomfort that the patient is willing to tolerate to maintain the desired level of awareness should be determined and maintained by the use of appropriate medications. Pain is not always a problem in the terminal care phase. When pain is reported as increasing or becoming intractible in this setting it may indicate a loss of trust and fear of abandonment that have resulted from a breakdown in communication in the care-giving system. A family member or someone on the health team has failed to perform as expected by the patient. At other times it may indicate a tolerance has developed to one narcotic and another drug or combination of drugs should be substituted. Experience also has demonstrated that most dying patients are not demanding; they require a minimum of specific attention, but do like to have someone around if they have a desire to talk or need help. In general there is a narrowing of interests and concerns, with a limited attention span and long periods of quiet wakefulness or light sleep between brief periods of activity or expressed need or discomfort.

When following comfort care guidelines, emergency measures to avoid sudden death are omitted. A sudden change in the patient's condition such as cardiac arrest, heart failure, respiratory distress, intestinal obstruction, and so on, should be treated as conservatively as possible. Symptom-relieving measures are taken, but specific therapies or specific life support systems are not employed unless a new and life-saving level of care is considered appropriate. It must be recognized that any new measures for maintaining life become essential to all subsequent planning and may require continuation until the patient is legally declared dead. Such life support measures are difficult, if not impossible, to discontinue once the patient's existence becomes dependent on them. The patient should have a legally constituted representative who understands his wishes and will carry them out if he should be unable to make these wishes known, for example, if he becomes incompetent or unconscious.[7] (A strongly worded statement by the patient addressed and given to his physician that leaves no question as to the patient's wishes if he becomes unconscious and that threatens legal action if the physician does not follow his directions may be all that is needed according to Dr. Milton Heifetz, who has investigated the legal issues involved.*)

Sometimes extraordinary measures are instituted without thinking of the patient's terminal state. The house officer or physician who has these special resources available frequently will initiate their use in a reflexive or automatic way, without stopping to think of their long-term consequences. Patients receiving comfort care only should be specifically identified to all the health care team. The specific limits of intervention should be clearly spelled out in the patient's chart and understood by the patient, family, and all those participating in the patient's care.

Nutriment, electrolytes, and fluid should not be given with the goal of replacing and maintaining body stores or biochemical balance but in amounts to satisfy the patient's expressed awareness of hunger, thirst, or discomfort.

Occasionally a patient after a period of comfort care will rally, appear stronger, and ask to visit home or children; have a desire to travel; or wish to participate in an important family event, e.g., a wedding, graduation, birthday, etc. Such requests and the patient's renewed vigor may tempt the physician to reinstitute more active, palliative forms of treatment. Such a consideration should be carefully reviewed before any change in therapy is introduced. Frequently, the patient's request and the brief increase in strength that allows greater activity is related to a final, highly motivated effort to participate in a personally important event. The physician may be falsely encouraged to again direct his or her attention to the patient's disease. However, the patient should not be kept from participating in these activities in order for the physician to try a new drug or one more cycle of therapy. To delay the patient's desired activity in such circumstances may mean depriving the patient of a final opportunity to give further meaning to life and to facilitate the acceptance of approaching death.

The above discussion, including helping the patient savor a final meaningful experience, should not be taken to mean that once comfort care has been initiated there is no turning back, no possibility of reevaluating and changing to a more active and aggressive therapy. Although not a common occurrence, occasionally with additional information, new knowledge, and a patient who seems to have plateaued in his or her

*See Chapter 30, p. 308.

a bed in his hospital room so that she could remain overnight when this seemed appropriate to the two of them. The patient was more calm and alert in this final week than he had been in the previous several months. He required nasogastric suction to prevent distension. Dilaudid for pain, Dalmane and Thorazine for sleep, and vitamin K for a bleeding tendency were employed. There were periods of sadness and tears as he said his good-byes to his immediate and then his extended family. He, his wife, and his children found a closeness in his final days that they had not experienced for a long time. In fact, during the final 10 days of his life, when he made a number of difficult decisions, he was described as a changed man. His children found him patient, understanding, and pleasant to be with. Several days before he died he asked for the suction and all intravenous fluids to be discontinued. The final days of his life he required some oxygen for dyspnea, condom drainage for urinary incontinence, and frequent medication for pain, but death came with little anguish on the part of the patient or his immediate family.

4. In the following example, several courses of comfort care were separated by a 3-month period of palliative therapy and several weeks of the patient's full-time employment.

A 55-year-old executive secretary and mother of four had a period of 16 months from the time of her diagnosis of inflammatory carcinoma of the breast until she died. She was told at the time of diagnosis that she had a form of cancer that grew rapidly and was hard to control. She received radiation therapy locally and then several courses of triple drug chemotherapy and a simple mastectomy before she was found to have a mass in her abdomen—all in a period of 5 months. She was "disappointed but not surprised" when the abdominal mass was found. Within a couple of weeks she became obstructed and required a bypass colostomy because of a large bowel obstruction. At the time of surgery she was found to have tumor involvement of the omentum, peritoneum, and liver. Her physicians agreed that the palliative forms of therapy had failed. They indicated they did not favor any further treatment for her disease. She expressed a desire to go home and die peacefully. The physicians agreed to try to care for her at home and a comfort care plan was outlined. She was to receive Percodan three times a day for pain in her ileostomy site, Dalmane for sleep, and ileostomy care. Home Care, Inc., agreed to provide a health aide and a visiting nurse was scheduled to visit twice a week. A hospital bed was obtained and placed in the corner of the dining room. The patient was to be called by her surgeon once a week, to visit the cancer chemotherapy clinic every 2 weeks, and the social worker from the cancer center was to visit every 10 days.

Although weak, depressed, and bedbound the first 2 weeks at home, she gradually, with the encouragement of the health aide, began to take solid foods, tried to get up or had her bed moved to the open window, and in general became animated and interested in her surroundings. Within a month she and her physicians decided on a trial of Halotestin and in another 3 weeks she began another three cycles of chemotherapy. Over the next several months, other than losing her hair again and some pleural fluid, she appeared stabilized, hopeful, and in general physically stronger. At the end of the 3-month period she felt well enough to go back to her job. (It was the first time she had worked in over a year.)

After 2 weeks of working she had signs of GI bleeding and ulcerations were found in the duodenum. These were called stress ulcers and were thought to be caused by the chemotherapy. She was treated conservatively with transfusions and antacids. Again it was decided that she was not a candidate for further definitive treatment of the disease. She was disappointed but had the attitude that she was living on borrowed time, since she had thought she was dying once before and had outlived her expectations.

She left the hospital within 2 weeks and although in a weakened state she and her husband spent a week together at their summer place even though it was now late fall. For 5 days they managed with her husband playing nursemaid, cook, and shot-giver while she maintained a bed-to-chair existence. At the end of the time she had to be brought back and hospitalized because of intestinal obstruction. She required Dilandid every 3 hours to control her pain while she arranged to have her office and personal affairs put in order. She then called her children on the phone and told them to come home for a last good-bye. She died within 12 hours after the last of the four arrived. There was a period of excitement and loud, rapid talking before she became confused, had difficulty breathing, went into a coma, and died.

In summary, we believe that patients and the health care team would be aided if guidelines were accepted that recognized that at some point in each human life the inevitability of death is so clear that life-sustaining interventions can and should be omitted. Almost no one would disagree if the matter focused on the last few seconds or minutes of life for a patient ill with a progressive disease. However, the concept also applies to some patients weeks prior to death, and the frequency with which this is ignored in medical practice today suggests that guidelines should be formulated and put to use. Once a decision has been reached through open discussion by the physician with patient, family, and other members of the health care team, a new therapeutic approach should be started that is aimed at maintaining the patient's comfort and no more. The most important specifics that are referred to as comfort care guidelines are as follows:

1 Comfort care should be initiated whenever patient and physician agree that all reasonable measures for control of the disease have failed.
2 The purpose of this care is to minimize discomfort without specific or direct attention to the underlying disease.
3 The plan should be flexible but specific in its detail and should be known to all concerned with its implementation. It should include roles for family members or others the patient wishes to be involved in the process, with no restrictions on the frequency of personal contacts except for those set by the patient.
4 All treatment and medication will be prescribed to minimize symptoms.
   a Drugs, procedures, fluids, and so on not clearly needed to relieve symptoms will be omitted.
   b Measures to relieve pain and discomfort are provided as requested by the patient with no concern for addiction or habituation. Other measures for relieving symptoms include measures such as oxygen that may help dyspnea as may morphine; salicylate may relieve the discomfort associated with fever, and nasogastric suction should be used only as needed for distension.

    c Routines such as repeated physical examinations, measuring vital signs, and recording weight, intake, output, should be discontinued.

    d Emergency measures should not be used to prevent death, although symptoms are always treated.

5 The plan should be reviewed at regular intervals and whenever the patient desires.

6 Alternatives in types of care and in settings that are needed in order to provide for changing patient needs should be available on a standby basis. Such alternatives allow the patient to move from home to hospital to hospice or nursing home as his requirements for care fluctuate.

If patient, family, and physicians agree on these guidelines, there are no ethical or legal issues to confront. With this acceptance of death, dying may become less of a defeat, and again will come to be recognized as an inevitable consequence of living. This approach allows the family to begin anticipatory grief under medical observation and support rather than at the end when medical resources are no longer available unless the survivors declare themselves ill. Of greatest importance, however, it gives the patient a chance to say his or her good-byes.

Patients, loved ones, and health professionals who have participated in the comfort care only approach describe it as an invaluable opportunity to participate more actively in that final leave-taking called dying.

REFERENCES

1 Hamburger, J.: quoted in J. Rostand, *Pensees d'un Biologiste,* Stock, Paris, 1939, p. 7.

2 Maguire, D.C.: *Death by Choice*, Schocken, New York, 1975, pp. 177–184.

3 Weisman, A. and T. Hackett: "Prediliction to Death," *Psychosomatic Medicine*, 23:232–256, 1961.

4 Sullivan, M.T.: "The Dying Person—His Plight and His Right," *New England Law Review*, 8:197–216, 1973.

5 Lach, J.: "Humane Treatment and the Treatment of Humans," *New England Journal of Medicine*, 294:838–840, 1976.

6 "Towards Standards of Care for the Terminally Ill," Notes from International Convocation of Leaders in the Field of Death and Dying, *Ars Moriendi News-Letter*, 2:5–7, 1975.

7 *Euthanasia Rights and Realities*, a compilation of material from papers and discussion at the Fifth Euthanasia Conference, New York Academy of Medicine, December 2, 1972, Euthanasia Educational Council, New York.

8 Cassell, E.J.: "Healing," *Hospital Physician*, 4:28–29, 1976.

Chapter 3

Terminal Care

Cicely Saunders

I think I have gained a small insight into the use of both drugs and of oneself to help the dying patient, and the whole patient rather than just the diseased body.

A letter from a student after a teaching round

DEFINITION

The time for terminal care is reached when all active treatment of a patient's disease becomes ineffective and irrelevant to his real needs. It is not always easy to recognize this moment but it is important that we should do so for there is still much to be done that *is* relevant and which should claim our attention and enthusiasm. Sir Stanford Cade's question, "what is the relative value of the various available methods of treatment in this particular patient?" (Cade, 1966) is just as pertinent now as at any other stage of a patient's illness.

Sadly, the terminal stage could also be defined as beginning at the moment when someone says "There is nothing more to be done," and then begins to withdraw from

Reprinted from K. D. Bagshawe (ed.), *Medical Oncology: Medical Aspects of Malignant Disease*, Blackwell Scientific Publications, Oxford, England, 1975, chap. 28.

the patient. The feelings of hopelessness and isolation which may be the worst suffering a patient has to bear can be overcome if those treating him could either see terminal care as a challenging and rewarding part of the total care of their patients with
cancer or be more prepared to enlist other help for them.

Terminal care includes the control of pain and other physical distress but we owe
more than this to our patients. We have to try to understand and ameliorate his mental
pain and so are inevitably made aware of many social and also environmental factors.
The doctor is one partner of a team whose help may be needed if a patient is to live
on until he dies and his family are to go on living afterwards.

THE NEEDS AT HOME

Someone with terminal cancer desires above all to be in an environment where his individuality and integrity as a person can be maintained. Most people would choose to
remain in their own homes, at least as long as their physical condition and the strength
of their families make this possible. The number of cancer patients dying in their own
homes is decreasing (in 1965 37.5 percent of total cancer deaths occurred at home, in
1970 33 percent) but many of those who died in hospital would have liked to have returned home and many families would gladly have tried to manage if they could only
have received more support there.

Ideally the family doctor is the coordinator of a team which includes social workers
as well as nurses and a number of ancillary workers. The ideal is not always achieved
and patients suffer and families become exhausted because services or supplies are not
available or because they do not know of their existence until it is too late. Information is a primary need of everyone in this situation. The family doctor needs immediate reports from the hospital concerning plans and any drugs prescribed. The family
needs to know what financial supplements are available and how to apply for them.
They need to know how to obtain equipment without delay when the need arises.
Above all they need to have confidence that any new problems that emerge will be
appreciated quickly and tackled efficiently. Good though care can be, in all too many
cases lack of communication means that a family feels totally abandoned when a crisis
comes. Some doctors are too busy to pay more than a quick visit, at times it is difficult to contact the member of a group practice who knows the dying person and (especially in cities) evening or weekend calls may reach no further than an answering
service or the emergency doctor. If care at home is to be maintained there needs to be
a twenty-four-hour call service which will reach people who already know the family.
Even when we have the proposed improvements in community services and their better coordination it seems likely that there will still at times be a need for a special service to fill gaps. An experimental project has already shown how much can be done by
specially trained nurses operating a domiciliary service based on a unit where beds are
available for admission should it become necessary. These nurses visit on referral by
the doctors (and nurses) in the community but with the unit doctors available for consultation and they are able to bring special skills and confidence into the stresses of
the situation.

THE NEED FOR IN-PATIENT TREATMENT

Some patients will reach the stage when adequate relief can no longer be given at home in spite of all available material and emotional help. Severe pain which needs regular injections for its control, incontinence, night restlessness and the consequent physical and mental exhaustion of the family make admission necessary. It is much easier for all concerned if it can be admission to a place which is already known and trusted.

Many people, especially those who have had frequent admissions for treatment, are anxious to return once more to the wards they know. If the ward team can see this final visit as being as important as all the admissions for active treatment and are able to accept a new role in caring for a person rather than for a disease, this may well be the best. But it is not always so—the dying person may be an embarrassment to a staff completely orientated to cure and can feel deserted in the midst of activity which is rightly concentrated upon those who are getting better. Patients admitted to single rooms need extra staff if they are not to be rather too easily forgotten. Hinton's study of 102 patients who died in a general hospital showed how difficult it was in the sometimes hectic activity of the busy ward for the staff to give the dying patient the understanding of his emotional problems and the discriminating handling of drugs that he needs to control his symptoms (Hinton, 1963). These patients and their problems may also have a sad effect on ward morale, both patients and staff finding them hard to watch. Those around find that there are many ways of disengagement and a patient may easily retreat into an apathy that is considered to be peaceful because no one has time to discover that in fact he is depressed.

Many years of experience in terminal care have served to strengthen the belief that those patients who do not need the manifold resources of a large hospital are frequently better cared for, happier and more active in a smaller, specialized unit. Such a unit must have flexible liaison with both the doctors at the treating hospital and those in the community. It should have more than one group of patients in its care, perhaps including those needing long-term nursing, those temporarily admitted for the control of pain, possibly some who need half-way house, or hostel accommodation. But, most important of all, it should also include some form of domiciliary service. This enables people to remain at home longer and also increases the number who can be discharged under supervision.

Much of this could be based on a special ward of a general hospital. But the self-contained unit will usually be better able to maintain its own enthusiasm and tempo and to attract and sustain a staff community who have chosen the work and are therefore able to build up the relationships that support first each other and then the patients and their families.

THE RELIEF OF PHYSICAL DISTRESS

There appear to be no studies in the community to compare with Hinton's work. Retrospective studies based on the memories of the families show that there is still much suffering which can and should be relieved (Aitken-Swan, 1959; Cartwright, 1973; Parkes, 1973).

Statistics may show us the size of the problem but eventually our attention must be concentrated on the individual patient who is in our care. How are we to relieve him?

Two units concentrating on this problem have found that over 70 percent of their patients, mainly referred because of distress, had pain severe enough to need narcotics for its control. They were often admitted after weeks or months of inadequate relief. They made such remarks as "Pain? It was all pain," thus summing up all the fear and despair of long pain as well as the accumulation of other symptoms common to this phase of illness.

We can and should be able to approach these patients with confidence, our aim being that a person should go on living as himself and not just as an "uncomplaining residue" (Weisman & Hackett, 1962). This part of care is demanding and important in its own right. Only a few patients will achieve an unexpected remission but with imagination and attention to detail we will see practically all respond positively. We sometimes fail to understand what it is they really expect at this stage. They are commonly too realistic to expect us to cure them but they do ask for attention and the concern which makes us keep coming back to try some other way to help them.

Not all pain calls for the use of analgesics nor is it always due directly to the malignant process. Pain can be controlled by treating infection, by immobilizing fractures, by paracentesis, by reducing oedema, to name but a few specific measures. Painful bone metastases may still call for DXT or respond to the judicious use of chemotherapy, of steroids or phenylbutazone. Toothache, haemorrhoids and indigestion will still afflict and also still respond to the usual treatment. Even when the pain is due to malignancy there are ways of helping dyspnoea, anorexia and nausea, bowel disturbances and all the other common trials of terminal illness. The doctor who is prepared to give attention to detail will continue to transmit a positive attitude to his patients. Symptomatic treatment is now mandatory and calls for the modern equivalent of the elegant prescriptions of a former generation of physicians.

Only a minority of patients have pain which will call for nerve blocking procedures but these are sometimes needed even now. They should be carefully planned and followed up. But by this time patients are often intolerant of residual numbness and discomfort and seem to be more likely to suffer the loss of bowel and bladder control which are often precarious already.

The diagnosis of terminal cancer is not in itself a reason for using powerful analgesics. Weaker drugs are often adequate, especially if pain is treated specifically wherever possible. Nearly all patients resent being made sleepy by drugs which are too strong and if this happens some people then refuse all medication. Not all are wrong who say "all pills upset me, doctor." Many people elect to have some discomfort in order to feel fully alert. They are able to relax once they are confident that pain will never be allowed to become severe. They do not have to concentrate on it continually in an attempt to arrest our attention.

But by one means or another we must give adequate relief. Terminal pain *can* be controlled and there is no excuse for inept medication. Pain and the relief of pain are both self-perpetuating. Patients with the constant pain that is so typical of terminal cancer require their analgesics regularly and should neither suffer pain nor have to ask for relief. Analgesics should now be used to prevent pain from occurring rather than to

control it once it appears, exacerbated by anxiety and tension. Drugs should be ti-
trated to the patient's need so that pain is controlled adequately for a period slightly
longer than the elected routine time. This with a somewhat relaxed time schedule
should prevent clock watching. If patients have to ask continually for analgesics they
are reminded each time of their dependence upon them and also upon the person who
gives them. As their physical dependence increases we should aim to give them all the
independence we can in other spheres.

Those who work constantly with these patients find that narcotics are still the
drugs of choice for the relief of severe terminal pain and that, if they are properly
managed, they will maintain their value over long periods. We have found that with
a regimen such as the above, coupled with the constant use of adjuvants and symptomatic treatment most patients could be relieved of pain by comparatively small doses
of narcotics and that the majority need little increase. Most doses can be given orally
and will be effective for weeks on end (Drug and Therapeutics Bulletin, 1965;
Saunders, 1964; Twycross, 1974).

Tolerance and drug dependence are too often due to faulty management. This can
happen with any strong analgesic, it is no prerogative of the opiates. Physiological
dependence is not a matter of great concern at this stage but emotional dependence
is an intolerable burden to the patient and all around him, even if it only lasts for a
few days. We need continual research into the control of chronic pain if we are to give
rational teaching about this subject and ensure that these patients, wherever they may
be, are neither swamped by distress nor smothered by treatment or the miseries of
dependence.

There is no space to discuss all the drugs which have so transformed the treatment
of terminal distress over the past years. Analgesics should be used now in combination
with adjuvants, particularly the drugs of the phenothiazine group, but we need to balance the dose carefully to the individual's personality and need, lest we oversedate
him. These drugs should be used to help anxiety, for example that almost inevitably
induced by dyspnoea. If we recognize the first signs of confusion, so often incipient
paranoia, we can usually avert a crisis.

There is also a definite place for glucocorticosteroids. Not only do they reduce
intra-cerebral pressure but they will ease bronchial constriction, correct hypercal-
caemic states and help as a nonspecific tonic and restorer of appetite.

Finally, let us not forget alcohol. It is often the best sedative for the elderly; it
makes people feel better and presents splendid opportunities for social exchange. Man
is a social being and will still find gratification in being convivial or in a relaxed or
special occasion with family or friends. Diversion may be the best pain reliever of all.

THE UNDERSTANDING OF MENTAL DISTRESS

What is essential is invisible to the eye.

Antoine de Saint Exupéry: *The Little Prince*

It is rare to find among all the results of investigations, x-rays and examinations with
which a patient's case papers are filled any comment on his feelings or estimation of

his insight into what is happening. Yet these may well be his main problems. Feelings of failure and an obscure sense of guilt are part of any deteriorating illness whether or not someone knows that he is dying. People who have had a protracted illness are inevitably worried about job and family, finances and other responsibilities and are apprehensive about the future. Too often they are left alone with these fears and only receive reassurances which they strongly suspect to be false. Silence and avoidance build up a barrier between them and everyone else. They are not stupid just because they are ill but they cannot break through the barrier alone and they too join the conspiracy of silence.

This emotional suffering will be bound up with and exacerbated by physical distress and so will be helped to some degree as this is successfully treated. But this is no reason for ignoring it and for concentrating exclusively upon the physical. Drugs such as the phenothiazines, diazepam and the tricyclics may help but do not relieve us of our responsibility for listening. We must make some effort to understand what it feels like to be mortally ill if we are to care for the person who happens to have terminal cancer. Those who stay away from these people because they feel they can bring nothing but a lack of comprehension perhaps do not realize that it is the desire to *try* to understand and not our success in doing so that eases the loneliness which is so hard to bear. The only visitor who helped the dying Iván Ilých was the one who came with simple goodwill (Tolstoy, 1886). We do not have to feel 'like' our patient (that could well destroy our capacity to help him) but rather 'with' him, with empathy rather than with sympathy. In the same way, willingness to be aware of the anguish of the family will help them to feel less alone and have less need to express this isolation in angry and demanding behaviour towards nurses and other members of staff.

Those who have had opportunity to listen constantly to dying people recognized a variety of reactions among them. Ross (1970) has described these as stages in realization and Murray Parkes (1973) has compared them to the progress through bereavement and other forms of loss. Both these writers emphasize that some of these stages may be omitted, that they may not occur in clear-cut order, may overlap or be gone through more than once. Many of us have seen our patients' progress as some sort of journey.

STAGES OF REALIZATION

Anyone who is faced with disaster or bad news tends to react initially with disbelief or denial. So patients will at first avoid truth and do not ask questions. They may even make statements such as "If I knew I had cancer I'd do something to myself" which is an attempt to prevent us from facing them with knowledge they are not yet ready to contemplate. Successful denial is difficult to sustain and a fuller realization overtakes most people whether or not information is given to them in words. Unfortunately, this initial feeling is often the only approach that those around can themselves contemplate. They continue to bolster denial of the illness and so the patient, who has left this behind, has then to travel the rest of the journey alone (Weisman, 1972).

A visitor was talking with a widow about her husband's death from cancer. The widow said firmly that he had never known that he was dying, she "had kept it from him." When she went outside to make a cup of tea for the visitor her daughter, who had been listening in silence, said "He knew. I remember him sitting, crying, in that chair and saying 'I'm dying and I can't talk to your mother about it'."

As the denial begins to waver, a patient may display yearning and protest similar to the restless pining of early bereavement (Parkes, 1972). They may feel very angry about what is happening to them and project this on to their treatment and those who give it, to their families, their circumstances and to fate. "I was all right until I had radiotherapy," "The operation went wrong," "It's your pills, doctor." The family, facing bereavement, suffer the same feelings and may also defend themselves by projecting their anger on to the staff. But these are all feelings which can be worked through if they can be expressed, if possible to those who will understand the pain that causes them and not react by offended silence and withdrawal.

The next "stage" is reached when a patient appears to give up hope, stops fighting and lapses into depression or despair. Family and staff often support denial in an attempt to protect the patient from this reaction but in so doing may well leave him alone with the very truth from which they persuade themselves they have protected him. He then has no one to support him in his attempt to come through this phase. People only rarely contemplate suicide but they may become withdrawn and sometimes become confused. They are frequently given antidepressant drugs. These can be helpful but often they seem to exacerbate the confusion. This phase is perhaps best regarded as sadness, a natural reaction, rather than as clinical depression. Certainly it responds best to the listener who understands but is not overwhelmed by the situation.

Many people can and do work their own way through all these reactions. Hinton (1963), Parkes (1972), Ross (1970), and Weisman (1972) all describe a "last stage" of acceptance and our experience would endorse this. People can accept death as inevitable although a faint hope of an unexpected recovery against all expectations is common—"I may yet walk out of this hospital and fool you, doctor." Hope can exist in different ways all through such an illness, gradually changing in context. It helps the patient to accept the responsibility of living the life that remains to them.

Mr. P's comments as recorded in his notes

19.4.72. "My arthritis is more painful than the cancer."   (Ward Sister)

27.4.72. "I'm not worried about dying. I have no regrets. I've had 47 fights and lost every one of them."

> This was overheard during a conversation between Mr. P and Mr. K—they were apparently discussing funeral arrangements. There seemed to be a certain amount of bravado about it all.   (Nurse)

4.5.72. "Before I came here I couldn't care less about anything but I have come back to life again now. I am going to give trouble to my insurance company in living another couple of years: I'm a rough man! I'll live with my daughter as soon as she'll find a flat. I'll come back to that marvellous hospital when I'll be too much of a burden for her. I used to drink, drink and drink

after my wife's death seven years ago but now beer or brandy don't excite
me any more." (Student)

23.6.72. *Mr. P's views on cancer.*

"No relationship to smoking—its either in you or not in you."
"Smoking actually helps because coughing helps to bring up the phlegm."

At the same time Mr. P states he is cutting down on smoking and wouldn't
begin if he had the choice again. (Nurse)

10.8.72. "I've had enough—I want to get out of here. My daughter isn't going to get
this flat." (Nurse)

17.8.72. "You really mean I've had it, don't you?"
"I was a fighter—I don't want to be dopey."

He emphatically doesn't want injections to "finish him off." (Doctor)

22.8.72. While having his breakfast Mr. P said "My time is really up," I said "We all
have to go sometime." "Yes," he replied, "but it's painful." (Student)

2.9.72. Told him that ENT consultant had said it was glands pressing on throat—
a.m. from lung trouble—and our treatment should continue, including injection.
He said "You won't give me that strong one, will you?" I said, "You're in
charge, Mr. P. You tell us if you need it." He just thanked me. (Doctor)

p.m. Mr. P indicated in several small ways that he knew the end was near. He
asked me to take the phone numbers of his sons so that I could get in touch.
Said to night nurse "I may give you trouble tonight." (Ward Sister)

He died at 6:15 a.m. 3.9.72.

Mrs. B—a week before she died

"It doesn't hurt ... my husband ... obviously he does know but we can relax and
take it as one of those things that happen in life and feel naturally instead of being full
of strain and stress. ..."

Mr. P fought until his last day. Mrs. B let go earlier much more easily, being more
able to trust herself to others. Acceptance is an active and creative attitude, quite distinct from the negatives of despair and resignation. Perhaps the main difference is in
the outlook towards the life that remains; those who accept are able to live rather than
merely endure and their happiness is often surprising to those around who sometimes
wrongly interpret it as a resumption of denial.

WHAT AND WHO TO TELL?

The continuing and often heated discussions on this subject are frequently wide of the
mark. A patient's knowledge is not confined to what he has been told and he will go

through something like the journey described above whether or not anyone has spoken to him about his illness. We cannot assume that because someone asks no questions he has none to ask. He is afraid; we convey to him that the whole subject is too dangerous to discuss and so he keeps silent.

So often our debates on this theme are irrelevant because the wrong questions are being asked. "How do you tell your patients?" is more important than "What do you tell them?" and "What do you let your patients tell you?" is more important than either. On the whole the different ways in which this question is discussed reveal more about the attitudes of the doctors than of the patients. This is hardly surprising for no one can discuss this nor try to deal helpfully with it in a manner which is at variance with his character and convictions. But we all need to remember that the alternatives are not only stark and hopeless truth or a bland and obviously false reassurance. The whole process is more subtle than that and frequently lies in a relationship rather than in words. Indeed, one might question whether those who have no relationship to offer should use words at all. The patient needs people who will try to be aware of what he is thinking and time their help to his need. This may not be the doctor. We should be ready to recognize that another member of the caring team—nurse, social worker, priest or minister—may be the one who is best fitted to help here.

A PATIENT'S CONTRIBUTION

"The problem is posed: when should a patient be told that he (she) is suffering from an incurable illness?

"In general terms this is unanswerable, thus it is necessary to draw on one's own experience and this I will endeavour to do.

"I had always had a subconscious dread of surgery and operations so that when I went for the first consultation I was apprehensive to say the least. But, the surgeon was so forthright that when an operation was discussed I felt such complete confidence in him that this banished all sense of fear. I knew I was going to be safe in his hands.

"I was admitted to hospital and very soon had the 'exploratory' operation. The following day I was told of the tumour in the oesophagus and that a major operation was essential. Again, because I was given the details of what was to be done I felt no fear.

"After the immediate post-operation discomforts I had difficulty in still not being able to swallow and this caused me some depression. However, eventually I began to manage to swallow small quantities of soft food and by the time I was discharged my confidence had returned.

"In the following weeks I appeared to make 'remarkable' strides towards recovery and I began to plan the early activities in which I should be able to re-engage. But I began to feel my strength failing and my ambitions seemed less attractive—depression returned.

"Then came the Sister's visits and the invitation to attend the clinic. Soon I began to feel a new interest and visits to the clinic became something to anticipate with real pleasure and the treatment soon brought about improvement. Meantime, a germ of suspicion had been forming in my mind that there might be something more than the weakness following a major operation and I made some probing observations in the family to see if they were keeping something from me. I learned nothing!

"Eventually I made up my mind—I would ask the direct question of the doctor. Doctor had apparently come to a similar conclusion—I was now ready to be told.

"I felt no sense of shock nor any fear—doctor had crystallized my own thoughts and a feeling of calm and relief took the place of doubt.

"And so I have been able to analyse the situation.

"I am sure that in my weak and confused condition just after the operation and the depression of the ensuing months it would have been quite wrong to burden my mind with the knowledge that I could not be cured.

"Each individual patient needs to be treated according to his particular personality and the doctor, by his frequent contacts with the patient, will be able to decide when the time seems right to tell him the truth."

His wife wrote:

"My husband was operated on for a tumour in the oesophagus and he had been told by the surgeon that this was a major operation. After the operation I was told that he had been through a severe trial and that I should not hope for too much—indeed it was probable that he might live only for two months.

"I asked that my husband should not be told at this stage as I knew he was in too weak a condition to withstand any further strain after what he had endured.

"The news gave me a great shock—my whole body seemed to freeze and I seemed incapable of understanding fully what this meant. I had this feeling for quite a week or two until I slowly recovered from the shock.

"When my husband came home I had made up my mind that as far as possible life should go on as near normal as could be expected. I had come to grips with myself, determined to do everything within my power to help him back to health. His condition improved, he put on some weight and seemed to be getting better all the time. Now the two months had passed and my spirits rose—perhaps we could go on for even a year or two. However, he slowly began to lose his strength and by this time we had begun our visits to the clinic and to receive the Sister's visits. This proved to be a great tonic and when he began to hint at his suspicions I felt that with the help of the clinic the time had arrived for him to be told the truth. He took it very well—as I knew he would—and I now consider it was right to wait until he regained his composure before revealing the facts. We are now able to discuss the future without difficulty and to make arrangements accordingly."

Many people are able to make this kind of achievement especially if they have the same kind of support that helped this couple. It is good to feel proud of a dignity that makes those around forget their physical weakness and many are comforted by a chance to say goodbye and to discuss the continuation of the hitherto shared life and responsibilities. Awareness of the needs of the bereaved family is part of terminal care (Parkes, 1972).

The emotional needs of a dying patient are really those of all of us. We all need the affirmation of ourselves as persons and as members of our families, the freedom to react spontaneously and to communicate with those around us, the recognition of our responsibilities. These can all be maintained albeit in a diminishing compass (MacMurray, 1932).

THE PLACE OF FAITH

Hinton (1967) noticed that his patients with a strong religious faith were the least anxious but those with tepid faith were more anxious than those with none. Those who think of religion as a sort of insurance against trouble do not find such a belief sustaining in adversity. They sometimes find a more mature faith when they are dying although they may not express it in orthodox terms.

Liaison with the priest or minister of the patient's own choice may have an important part to play. The ward sister is often the person with whom the hospital chaplain has the most to do but contact with the doctor here and at home may be the more important. It is consultation concerned with the patient's needs that is wanted rather than medical information. Such liaison is most effective when it is personal, informal and continuing. It would be unwarranted intrusion to suggest such a contact when there is no understanding or willingness on the part of the patient but in spite of the gap that may seem to exist between families and this kind of help we will often be surprised how welcome such a visit can be when it is introduced with care and courtesy and proper timing.

Our regard for our patient will never allow us to impose our own faith or philosophy or lack of it upon him. But unspoken confidence and conviction can help to create a climate in which the patient finds his own key and can reach out trustfully beyond himself to what he sees as true.

The religious attitude is one of trust in a transcendent reality in whose presence questions become irrelevant and not a dogmatic answer to a question. In his recent book *The Go Between God* John Taylor quotes the following lines from a poem of Daniel Berrigan:

Lover, child, in the immense dignity of birth or death refuse an answer
There is no answer
The genius of the gospel is in the name of man to refuse an answer.

As he says:

"Job never found an answer to the problem of unmerited suffering. The problem remained insoluble, but in it he met God. That is where man always meets God. That is where man most frequently meets his fellows."

REFERENCES

Aitken-Swan J. (1959) Nursing the late cancer patient at home—the family's impressions. *Practitioner* **183**, 64.
Cade S. (1966) Cancer: the patient's viewpoint and the clinician's problems. *Proc. R. Soc. Med.* **56**, 1.

Cartwright A. (1973) Personal communication.

Drug and Therapeutics Bulletin (1965) Drugs in the treatment of the dying. *Drug. Ther. Bull.* **2**, 101.

Hinton J.M. (1963) The physical and mental distress of the dying. *Q. J. Med. N.S.* **32**, 1.

Hinton J.M. (1967) *Dying,* Chapter 8. Penguin Books, Harmondsworth.

MacMurray J. (1932) *Freedom in the Modern World.* Faber & Faber Ltd, London.

Parkes C.M. (1972) *Bereavement.* Tavistock Publications Ltd, London.

Parkes C.M. (1973) Personal communication.

Ross E. Kübler (1970) *On Death and Dying.* Tavistock Publications Ltd, London.

Saunders C.M. (1964) The symptomatic treatment of incurable malignant disease. *Prescribers' J.* **4**, 68.

Taylor J.V. (1972) *The Go Between God.* SCM Press, London.

Tolstoy L. (1886–1935) *Iván Ilých and Hadji Murad and Other Stories,* Section VIII. The World's Classics, Oxford University Press.

Twycross R.G. (1974) Clinical experience with diamorphine in advanced malignant disease. *Int. J. Clin. Pharm. Therapy & Toxicol,* 1974.

Weisman A.D. (1972) *On Dying and Denying.* Behavioural Publications Inc., New York.

Weisman A.D. & Hackett T.P. (1962) The dying patient. *Curr. Psychiat. Ther.* **2**, 121.

Chapter 4

Care, Communication, and Human Dignity

Jeanne Quint Benoliel

INTRODUCTION

In recent years much has been written about the problematic nature of providing humane services to patients with fatal illnesses and to their families during these stressful periods of time. Relatively less attention has been directed toward clarifying the conditions necessary and sufficient for making terminal illness a dignified human experience for the person whose life is moving toward a close. As a step toward that goal, I offer for your consideration some thoughts about the fundamental needs for assistance faced by dying people and their families and the kinds of helping services required to assist them in living through the psychosocial transition known as dying.

My thinking of dying as a psychosocial transition is in keeping with the ideas developed by Murray Parkes (1971), who uses that phrase to refer to those major changes in state that cause an individual to restructure his or her ways of looking at the world and his or her plans for living in it. In his view these changes include a variety of disruptive events such as childbirth, disaster, retirement, migration, bereavement, and

Prepared for presentation at the First National Training Conference for Physicians on Psychosocial Care of the Dying Patient, University of California School of Medicine Extended Medical Care Programs, San Francisco, California, on April 30, 1976. Reference is made to research supported by grant awards M-5495 from the National Institute of Mental Health and NU00024 from the Division of Nursing, DHEW.

many others. In addition to change per se, being given a diagnosis of life-threatening disease has an added property of introducing the concept of one's own death as an explicit part of the individual's personal reality. At the same time, the introduction of this change in state serves as the beginning of a psychosocial transition for all the other people who have an important relationship with the diagnosed person.

NEEDS FOR ASSISTANCE

It is clear that many patients have death-related fears and concerns long before they reach the point of being defined by someone as terminal. As I learned in studying the processes by which women adjust during the first postoperative year to having had a mastectomy, the diagnosis for them meant learning to live with an uncertain future and an underlying concern as to whether and when the cancer might return (Quint, 1963, 1964, 1965). In this presentation I have chosen to focus my remarks primarily on the needs for assistance that come into being when the ravages of prolonged illness or progressive disease cause the person to move into a state of physical and social dependency. At this point in time, one often observes a tendency on the part of well-intentioned people in the person's social network to take over some of his or her decision-making power and to initiate protective maneuvers to keep certain information from him or her. My major point here is that terminal illness places the dying person at the mercy of other people, and his opportunities to participate in decisions affecting the remainder of his life are dependent upon the choices and decisions of these other people.

Physicians, nurses, and other health care personnel are heavily socialized into the primary life-saving values of Western society. As a result, they have learned very well to treat consumers as patients and to define their own roles as practitioners primarily in terms of initiating and implementing the cure goals of practice. The problem of what to do and how to behave become somewhat more difficult when the patient becomes a person for whom there is no more workable life-saving activity to use. Yet it is at this point in time that the patient needs, perhaps more so than ever, health care providers who are able to implement the goal of care.

Care and Cure

I am using the terms *cure* and *care* to differentiate two distinct goals that health care providers amalgamate in their practices. As I define these terms, cure refers to the diagnosis and treatment of disease whereas care refers to the assessments and interventions used to make judgments about the welfare and well-being of the person. Cure deals with the objective aspects of the case; care is concerned with the subjective meanings of the disease/treatment experience to the person. Cure is often implemented by the practitioner "doing things to" the patient; care is fundamentally offered by "doing with" the person (Benoliel, 1972; Benoliel, 1976a).

A first question to be asked is: What are the basic needs for care that people have when the cure goal can no longer be met? Cancer is perhaps the prototype of death-related disease since so many people appear to equate dying with the experience of having cancer. Using what I have observed about advanced malignancy and its impact,

I first want to identify for you some fundamental problems that I have observed to be relatively common for people with advanced disease and for their families.

Problems Faced by the Person with Cancer

From the perspective of the person with malignancy, cancer can be viewed as catastrophic in nature because it produces major changes in living for him. In a very real sense, *dying* begins at that point in time when the diagnosis is first made. Often, however, the full impact of its meaning does not appear until the period of metastatic progression or progressive disease requiring movement into physical and social dependency on other people (Abrams, 1974). A major turning point for people with cancer comes with the loss of significant roles and role relationships created by the results of the disease. Having to give up one's work to move into the role of sick person is hard to do in a society that places a high value on independence and self-reliance. Having to watch another woman take over the management of one's home is far from easy for any woman in her own home.

Physical changes associated with progressive illness create another loss for the individual, and these physical changes often are associated with a need to depend increasingly on other people for assistance. Such assistance may be of little import when it involves transportation to the doctor or assistance with preparation of meals. This dependency can assume mammoth proportions when the inability to provide self-care reaches a point where intimate personal tasks must be performed by another. It seems reasonably clear to me that finding oneself in the role of infant again does not do very much for the self-esteem of any adult, but this change in status is precisely what happens to many people as the cancer worsens.

A related problem associated with progressive disease is physical discomfort or troublesome symptoms that interfere with ordinary activities of living and create the need for modifying an established living style to accommodate to the imposing demands of these physical changes. Progressive involvement of the lungs, for instance, can interfere with an individual's capacity to breathe and his concomitant ability to engage in such ordinary, taken-for-granted activities as going for a walk or climbing the stairs. Intestinal involvement can bring vomiting, diarrhea, or other unpredictable experiences that may not be easy to control and can readily lead to social isolation. Pain is a particularly difficult and disturbing problem for many people with advanced cancer, in part because of a commonly held fear that pain in advanced malignant disease cannot be controlled, thereby leading easily to loss of emotional control (Donovan and Pierce, 1976, p. 45). Regardless of whether the pain is actually due to the cancer or from another cause, regardless of whether the offending symptom is dyspnea or loss of bowel control, the person with the progressive illness once again finds himself in a state of reliance on other people for finding relief and some sense of comfort.

A fourth problem that the dying person experiences with movement into physical and social dependency is a reactivation of all kinds of unresolved problems in living and the emergence of unfinished personal business, often involving relationships with other people. Tensions between husband and wife can increase, leading to frequent quarrels and unpleasant interactions. At the other extreme, people can withdraw from one another, contributing in this way to an atmosphere of unspoken tension. Thus, it is not surprising that with advanced malignancies come breakdowns in communication patterns with significant other people. Conversations with patients confirm what others have reported; they experience a good deal of social isolation and often a personal sense of abandonment by other people. With a breakdown in communication often comes loss of personal control over many decisions affecting how each day will be lived and how dying will be managed. In a profound way, institutionalization is the extreme form of loss of control, especially when the individual concerned has not been consulted.

Problems Faced by Families of Cancer Patients

Just as the diagnosed person faces the loss of significant roles and role relationships, so too do the key people in his or her network of family and social relationships. The task of coping with major changes in roles and role relationships associated with the terminal stage of illness is compounded by a lack of preparation for knowing how to behave in the presence of someone who is dying. Modern Western society is organized in such a way that little opportunity is available for learning how to communicate with one another about the personal meanings of death. Young people today have little opportunity to develop the art of standing by and with a dying person instead of running away to avoid their feelings of helplessness and hopelessness.

As Aries (1974) has recently described, people today are poorly prepared for the personal suffering and concrete problems that the dying of a family member brings into being. The adaptation of the family as a complex system of social relationships to the demands imposed by the dying transition requires modifications in ordinary social roles, often thereby placing new strains on already existing points of tension in interpersonal relationships. Someone, for example, must move into the care-giving role if the dying person is to remain at home, regardless of whether or not the people involved are prepared for the change. May (1974) makes the point that the crisis of death becomes problematic for the dying person and those closest to him precisely because the crisis interferes with the very basis of their relationship. He offers the example of the dependent wife who built her life around a domineering husband and now finds herself in a completely new situation with a man totally helpless and dependent on her for everything. The dying transition for a woman in this position means living with a stranger: the old established rituals of their relationship no longer exist as markers of social reality and personal confirmation.

A family's capabilities of adapting to the demands of progressive illness also vary, and many do not have well-developed social support systems on which they can rely. Hoffman and Futterman (1971), in describing the impact of fatal illness on leukemic children and their families, cogently described three developmental tasks that challenge the basic resources of these families. First, the parents face the problem of maintaining some investment in the future of the sick child while at the same time preparing for his death through anticipatory mourning. Secondly, the parents face the difficult problem of maintaining a sense of mastery and control while at the same time coming to terms with the terminal nature of the illness itself. Finally, the child faces the task of integrating the losses and physical changes produced by his illness into a new definition of self while at the same time fulfilling his potentialities for life during the period of time remaining. The conflicting pulls of these difficult tasks create a situation of maximum stress on any family's system of social relationships. In my judgment, they apply equally well to situations in which the dying person is an adult.

Unresolved and unspoken fears about death can also directly affect social relationships within the family. Bermann (1973) studied one family in which the father's cardiac condition was such that he lived continuously on the brink of death; in this family unspoken death fears lead to scapegoating as a way of coping with the stress. Bermann's sensitively written description of that family's adaptation style showed how one boy suffered personal and social consequences because he was the focal point for unresolved tensions. In a more general sense, families as well as the person who is dying suffer from problems in communication associated with the threat of death.

It is also clear that prolonged illness can make *excessive demands* on financial and social resources of any social group. A report by Cancer Care, Inc. (1973) showed that even the best put-together families were apt to be thrown off balance by having a relative with cancer in the home. These difficulties appeared to coalesce around the problem of imminent death and the potential disintegration of personal and familial goals. Fatal illness was disruptive of vocational plans, educational ambitions, established marital and parent-child adjustments, financial stability, and lifestyle itself. In a word, prolonged illness put extreme pressure on existing social support systems within and around the family, including depletion of financial and social resources and breakdowns in patient-family relationships.

HELPING SERVICES AND THE DYING TRANSITION

Given the death-denying and death-controlling nature of American society, the much-reported practice of withholding information about forthcoming death from the dying person is not very surprising. Among the reasons frequently offered for not talking with cancer patients about their condition is the opinion that patients will thereby become depressed and unduly concerned (McIntosh, 1974, p. 174). Yet, according to Feder (1966), Rothenberg (1961), and Wahl (1973), not talking with these people about the meanings of their experiences and their understanding of what is happening only adds to their sense of helplessness, psychological tension, and concern about abandonment.

A major problem for people with life-threatening disease comes from the tendency for families and health care providers to deny or withhold information about the disease, treatment, and related information. These practices are often supported by the rationale of protecting the dying person from unwanted news about his future, yet as May (1974, p. 28) points out, these practices do a gross disservice to the person by placing him in a child's position and maintaining control over the decisions to be made. The outcomes for the person facing death are far from pleasant.

Helping services that foster and encourage respect for human dignity during the process of dying can only be developed when the purposes of these services explicitly incorporate *Care* rather than *Cure* as the major goal to be achieved (Benoliel, 1972). As it functions at present, our health care system with its intense focus on cure and cure-related activities has not been well organized to provide care-centered services to dying people. This has especially been the case in hospitals where resources are clearly mobilized to implement the life-saving goals that our society so clearly values.

Alternatives of Hospitalization

Proposed alternatives to hospitalization for dying patients include the availability of hospice-type institutions and/or home care programs, but these alternatives have always had to struggle for survival in this country for sheer lack of financial support. It seems clear to me that development of alternatives to hospitalization requires that some of the resources now allocated for cure activities of necessity must be redirected to other purposes. Redirection of such resources in the field of health care services means that physicians in particular must be willing to give up some of their present privileges (in the form of readily available resources and activities) so that these differently oriented programs can be encouraged.

More than that, the development of such programs requires a willingness for physicians to move into collaborative working relationships with other health care providers and to learn new patterns of communication with patients, families, and other professional and nonprofessional health care members. Indeed, the provision of personalized services can only come about when collaboration among providers replaces professional control of alternatives as an established working relationship among health care providers and when the person who is dying is encouraged to play a central role in the decision-making processes about his or her final days, weeks, and months of living.

Dignity and Dying

The delivery of personalized care to people who are dying has implications for the concept and value of moral worth; that is, people who are dying have a right to be treated with dignity on the basis of their membership in the human community. Assuming this idea to be accepted, the achievement of dignity in dying depends on the willingness of other people to treat the dying person as a fully competent social being capable of participating in decisions about his or her forthcoming death. Under such conditions, a central aim of personalized services is to facilitate the dying person's opportunities to maintain social control over his living and his dying. Such a system of services would be designed to help him in achieving three personal goals not easily obtainable in our present society: (1) the opportunity to be informed about what is happening to and around him and to be able to talk about it with someone who will listen, (2) the opportunity to participate in decisions affecting his final days of living and the setting for his death, and (3) the opportunity to experience the many and conflicting reactions to forthcoming death in the presence of a caring individual instead of maintaining a tight control over emotional reactions to protect other people from their own emotional distresses.

The provision of personalized care also requires that the purposes of the proposed service be clearly stated in operational terms. One home care program attached to a community hospital in the eastern part of the United States has identified five such purposes as follows: (1) to provide continuity of patient care, (2) to decrease health care costs, (3) to promote the dignity of the patient and his family, (4) to extend health care services and teaching by the hospital into the home, and (5) to assist physicians in caring for long-term patients (Dancull, 1973).

The delivery of personalized home care services for dying patients and their families depends heavily on the availability of nursing skills and nursing resources of various types. In my judgment, insufficient public attention has been given to acknowledging the contributions that nurses make to the successful implementation of home care programs. Neither have the social interventions used by nurses been clearly recognized in the literature as contributing importantly to continuity of care for the dying patient and his family.

Clearly nurses alone cannot provide the broad range of services needed for coping with the multiple problems introduced by prolonged dying. Yet, by virtue of their middle position in the health care system and their particular background of health care and medical knowledge, professional nurses are uniquely equipped to assist dying patients and their families in coping constructively with the energy-depleting demands of terminal illness. The competencies utilized by nurses for implementing the caregiving role consist of a combination of public health, mental health, and physical assessment skills and the ability to accept responsibility for *continuity of care* through coordination of essential activities and resources on behalf of the dying person and by facilitation of the flow of communication among the principal persons involved. The provision by nurses of support, instruction, coordination, and care can perhaps best be clarified by using specific incidents to illustrate some psychosocial problems encountered by nurses in practice and the strategies chosen by them for responding to these problems (Benoliel, 1975; Dancull, 1973, pp. 16–18).

PSYCHOSOCIAL PROBLEMS ASSOCIATED WITH DYING

These incidents are drawn from personal experiences in clinical practice, from verbal reports of experiences by colleagues in nursing, and from written records describing nursing interventions and patient/family outcomes. The first incident was chosen as an illustration of communication strategies used by a nurse to assist the patient and members of the family in facing and dealing with the strong feelings and conflicting demands they experienced during the final month of the dying transition.

Incident One: Rapid Dying

In case number one, the nurse began contact with the patient and her family when they were referred for home care services following a postsurgical diagnosis of pancreatic malignancy with a poor prognosis (Dancull, 1973, pp. 19-31). The patient and her husband had been told by the physician about the nature of her illness and the shortness of her future. Two weeks after discharge she was suffering from nausea and moderate pain and was essentially bedfast except for trips to the bathroom. Referral for home care services was done because of the patient's wish to remain at home and her husband's request for guidance in the provision of care. The nurse's first meeting with the husband took place in the offices of the home care services department, and in this initial conversation he talked freely about his reactions of helplessness whenever his wife became nauseated or experienced severe pain.

On the following day the nurse made her first home visit, allowing ample time for an initial history and assessment of the patient's physical and emotional well-being. Although initially somewhat reluctant to discuss herself, the woman responded readily to the nurse's verbal indications of interest and concern. During the course of this first conversation, the nurse also conveyed an explicit message that strong feelings such as sadness or anger could be expected to occur as normal responses to the transition of dying, and she encouraged the woman to acknowledge these feelings rather than to keep them under control. Recognizing the woman as quite depressed and anxious, the nurse made a second home visit on the following day, at which time the patient was able to express many feelings of anger and frustration in addition to talking further about the meaning of her life. The husband called the nurse on the following day to indicate that his wife had finally had a tranquil night, and he expressed appreciation for the help she had provided to bring about this change.

During subsequent visits to the household, the nurse encouraged the husband and wife to share their experiences of grief together. She also listened while the patient talked in great detail about a long-standing conflict with her oldest daughter. The nurse subsequently encouraged the patient to arrange for a tête-à-tête with her daughter to resolve these long-time difficulties as part of the process of bringing closure to her life. On another occasion the nurse was available as a supportive listener while the younger daughter struggled with her feelings of anguish and pain at seeing the change in her mother's physical state.

During the nurse's next to last home visit the patient was taking no fluids and was fluctuating between states of alertness and delirium. Yet she spoke clearly to the nurse about the importance of being able to die in the company of her family and her feelings of regret that her dying took so long and was so hard on them. At the end of the final visit, the woman was in a comatose state; and the nurse took the occasion to spend time with the husband, who spoke at some length about their readiness for death to come at any time. Subsequently the nurse maintained daily telephone contact with the husband until the time of death, and she encouraged him to call her again whenever he wished to talk.

Although the nurse provided other kinds of assistance during her contact with this family, I have chosen to emphasize only two kinds of strategies: those used for encouraging the various members to identify and cope with their emotional reactions to the dying transition; and those used for facilitating open communication among the family members and shared responsibility in matters of decision making.

Over a period of 1 month the nurse made eight home visits to this family, each lasting on the average 1½ hours. Approximately half of this time was devoted to offering support to various members of the family in terms of their needs of the moment. The term *support* as used here is based on the writings of Robert S. Weiss (1976) and refers to the communication, verbal and nonverbal, extended by a helping person to a patient that indicates that the helper's background, knowledge, special expertise, experience, and understanding are available to the distressed individual as he or she struggles to come to terms with a personally disorganizing psychosocial crisis.

Incident Two: Inadequate Communication

The second incident illustrates nursing interventions that were part of a collaborative endeavor to help a dying woman achieve her own goals for a personalized dying. This woman was referred to a medical center hospital for treatment of a leiomyoma with extensive metastatic spread that caused considerable amounts of pain and the continuing possibility of bowel obstruction. While recovering from a cordotomy for pain relief, she and her husband asked the cancer coordinator if someone were available with whom they could talk about some of their problems. The nurse was invited by the coordinator to serve in this capacity, and she met with the couple on the day that the referral was made.

This woman had received extensive chemotherapy, but at this point in time the treatments were no longer of value. The medical treatments being offered were palliative in nature and designed to facilitate comfort as much as possible. The nurse began the introductory meeting by asking the couple to describe what was happening to them. Immediately the woman began to talk about the shortness of time remaining to her, of her sadness at not being able to see her 5-year-old daughter as an adult, and mostly of her sense of being cut off from other people because they would not let her talk about the cancer. The problem of feeling cut off was especially acute in her relationship with her mother, who changed the subject whenever efforts were made to talk openly about cancer. The nurse then suggested that the woman's mother was probably caught up in her own deep feelings and perhaps was unable to be open because of her reactions to the forthcoming loss of her child. The couple then began to talk about their own children, and the nurse inquired as to whether the children had been informed about their mother's imminent death. The parents indicated that the children had been informed about the disease and the treatment, but death itself had not been discussed. The nurse then suggested that they might want to consider together some ways of preparing their children for their mother's death.

The woman returned again to talking about her feelings of isolation, adding that she sometimes felt cut off from her husband. At this point the husband indicated that although he did not break down, he also was experiencing pain and a strong sense of being alone. Almost as though the words served as a trigger, he began to cry, and they shared several moments of grieving together. Ten minutes or so later the husband spontaneously commented that he felt tremendously better and, in fact, no longer had the pain he had been experiencing in his chest. As a final comment, the nurse suggested that they might want to look among their friends and relatives for those people who could truly provide them with supportive relationships during the difficult weeks that lay ahead.

A second contact took place 1 week later when the woman was hospitalized for pain and possible obstruction of the bowel. The woman indicated in conversation with the nurse that she was not interested in surgery if it only meant prolonging her life for something like 2 more months. She also said she wanted to stay home as long as possible, and if hospitalization were necessary, to be sent to a local hospital close to her home.

Later that day the nurse met with the attending physicians to review the woman's present condition and treatment plan and to discuss various alternative courses of action. All were in agreement that curative efforts were of little value and every effort should be made to help her and her family achieve their wishes for her dying at home.

The next contact occurred approximately 1 month later when the woman once again was admitted for possible surgery. She was feeling very angry at this time and indicated to the staff that she had not been given complete information about the limitations of the surgery. Following a conversation with the patient to verify the patient's perspective, the nurse met with the surgeon involved in the case to discuss the situation. Following that meeting he made arrangements to meet with the patient to explain clearly that the surgery available could offer only temporary relief and the possibility of living for only a month longer or thereabouts. A day or so later she decided against the surgery, and followed that decision by pulling out the intravenous infusion and indicating to the staff that she was ready to die. A hurried call was sent to members of her family, who arrived at the hospital in time to share the final experience of her dying. The family accepted her decision to stop the treatment and did not want another one started.

Although this woman was not able to achieve her goal of dying at home, she was supported in her decision to stop active treatment. All of the providers who participated in this team operation believed that the woman had been able to bring things to a close in her own way, and they experienced a positive feeling about the part they had played together in assisting her toward achievement of her own goals for living and dying. The nurse in this case had played an important role in the ongoing coordination of activities and care by serving as an active communication link between the woman and her family and the several physicians involved in medical care.

Transition Services and Nursing Care

The incidents just described were selected to illustrate the ongoing and stressful nature of the problems and pressures imposed by the process of dying. They also indicate some specific communication strategies used by nurses to facilitate the dying person's opportunities for achievement of personal goals, to assist the major participants in dealing with changing demands and new experiences, and to facilitate collaboration of effort and coordination of the multiple services being offered. In addition, nurses are often in a position to provide assistance in the following general ways: (1) to maximize a family's coping capacities by supplementing their social support system and/or by guiding them in effective utilization of the resources already available; (2) to provide guidance in the management of physical changes associated with progressive illness and direction for the wise use of medications and medical treatments; and (3) to socialize the dying person and the members of social network in anticipation of the expected and unexpected elements of the dying transition. As I have indicated elsewhere, nurses are uniquely qualified to serve a key function in the delivery of transition services to dying patients and their families (Benoliel, 1976b). This presentation has attempted to make explicit several specific ways by which nurses make contributions to the welfare and well-being of these people, but one additional comment would appear to be in order.

Nurses whose work brings them into frequent contact with dying patients and their families know from experience that work of this nature takes a great deal of energy and can be emotionally draining—sometimes to the point of having detrimental effects on the provider. If the delivery of *personalized* services is seriously to be considered, the program needs to provide for a backup support system by which the health care providers themselves have access to assistance in coping with their own reactions to problems encountered in practice. Such a support system is necessary to provide health care providers with opportunities for validation of their own expectations and consideration of alternative approaches to the problems they are attempting to solve. . In this regard, I have come to agree with Caplan (1974) that people whose experience of living brings them into frequent contact with emotional stresses and strains are able to function more effectively when they receive emotional support and task-oriented assistance from a social network that makes available consistent communication, appropriate rewards, and feedback about their performance.

SUMMARY

As I have tried to suggest, the delivery of person-centered services to people who are dying depends on a shift in priorities away from an emphasis on cure-centered activities toward a primary focus on care-centered goals. Such a shift in orientation is not a matter to be taken lightly, for the delivery of care requires that providers of health care services be involved with and concerned about the subjective and personal meanings that the dying experience carries for consumers as well as for themselves. The achievement of person-centered outcomes for dying patients depends on practitioners who are committed to the preservation of human rights and human dignity in the face of many institutionalized pressures toward dehumanization of patient care. The creation of person-centered services probably can only come about when the stressful nature of practitioner problems in the face of dying are fully recognized and ways can be found for building ongoing systems of social support into the organized institutions through which health care services are made available.

BIBLIOGRAPHY

Abrams, Ruth: *Not Alone with Cancer*, Thomas, Springfield, Ill., 1974.
Aries, Philippe: "Death Inside Out," *The Hastings Center Studies*, 2:3–18, May 1974.
Benoliel, Jeanne Quint: "Nursing Care for the Terminal Patient: A Psychosocial Approach," in Bernard Schoenberg et al. (eds.), *Psychosocial Aspects of Terminal Care*, Columbia, New York, 1972, pp. 145–161.
———: "The Terminally Ill Child," in Gladys Scipien et al. (eds.), *Comprehensive Pediatric Nursing*, McGraw-Hill, New York, 1975, pp. 423–440.

———: "Care, Cure, and the Challenge of Choice," in Anne Earle et al. (eds.), *The Nurse as Caregiver for the Terminal Patient and His Family*, Columbia, New York, 1976a, pp. 9–30.

———: "Dying Is a Family Affair," unpublished paper given as the Third Alexander Ming Fisher Memorial Lecture on Death and Dying on April 21, 1976, at the College of Physicians and Surgeons, Columbia University, New York City, 1976b.

Bermann, Eric: *The Impact of Death-Fear on an American Family*, University of Michigan, Ann Arbor, 1973.

Cancer Care, Inc.: *The Impact, Costs, and Consequences of Catastrophic Illness on Patients and Families*, University of Michigan, Ann Arbor, 1973.

Caplan, Gerald: *Support Systems and Community Mental Health*, Behavioral Publications, New York, 1974.

Dancull, Mary Veitch: "The Role of the Nurse in the Care of the Terminal Patient Through a Home Care Program," unpublished master's thesis, University of Maryland, 1973.

Donovan, Marilee Ivers and Sandra Girton Pierce: *Cancer Care Nursing*, Appleton-Century-Crofts, New York, 1976.

Feder, Samuel L.: "Psychological Considerations in the Care of Patients with Cancer," *Annals of the New York Academy of Sciences*, 25:1020–1027, 1966.

Hoffman, Irwin and Edward H. Futterman: "Coping with Waiting: Psychiatric Intervention and Study in the Waiting Room of a Pediatric Oncology Clinic," *Comprehensive Psychiatry*, 12:67–81, January 1971.

May, William: "The Metaphysical Plight of the Family," *The Hastings Center Studies*, 2:19–30, May 1974.

McIntosh, Jim: "Processes of Communication, Information-Seeking and Control Associated with Cancer," *Social Science and Medicine*, 8:167–187, 1974.

Parkes, Murray M.: "Psycho-social Transitions," *Social Science and Medicine*, 5:101–115, 1971.

Quint, Jeanne C.: "The Impact of Mastectomy," *American Journal of Nursing*, 63:88–91, November 1963.

———: "Mastectomy: Symbol of Cure or Warning Sign?," *GP*, 29:119–124, March 1964.

———: "Institutionalized Practices of Information Control," *Psychiatry*, 28:119–132, May 1965.

Rothenberg, Albert: "Psychological Problems in Terminal Cancer Management," *Cancer*, 14:1063–1073, September–October 1961.

Wahl, Charles W.: "Psychological Treatment of the Dying Patient," in Richard H. Davis (ed.), *Dealing with Death*, University of Southern California, Los Angeles, 1973, pp. 9–23.

Weiss, Robert S.: "Transition States and Other Stressful Situations: Their Nature and Programs for Their Management," in Caplan and Killilea (eds.), *Support Systems and Mutual Help: A Multidisciplinary Approach*, Grune and Stratton, New York, 1976.

Chapter 5

Care of the Terminally Ill at Home

S. Malkin

Care of the terminally ill at home demands the attention of the medical and paramedical community. Patients who choose to remain at home while death approaches must be given full physical, emotional and psychological support by the attending physician and home care services personnel. In 1974 the Vancouver early hospital discharge home care service provided such care to 47 patients. A few families were unable to cope for more than a few days but most continued the care almost to the end, a large number (14) keeping the patient at home until death occurred. Added benefits are the lower costs and the freeing of hospital beds.

The need for the dying patient to be cared for in his own home is being recognized increasingly, both by the general population and by health professionals.[1] This care has been given successfully, to the mutual advantage of patient and family. The latter feel a need to be intimately involved in the care of their loved one, and the emotional, psychological and physical support that the patient requires can be extended by his family 24 hours a day.[2]

There are certain requirements for the home care of the patient with terminal illness. Diagnosis and definitive treatment must already have been completed, and the

Reprinted from *Canadian Medical Association Journal*, **115**:129–130, July 17, 1976.

patient must be at the stage where nursing care is the only remaining therapeutic support.[3,4] The health professionals can now supervise and assist with the care at home. Certain equipment, such as dressings, catheters, irrigation solutions, hospital beds, mattresses and wheelchairs are available, as are physiotherapists and homemakers, when needed.

Below is a brief report of the experience with one such group of patients.

PATIENTS

In 1974, 47 terminally ill patients were cared for at home under the early hospital discharge home care service of the metropolitan board of health of Greater Vancouver. Most were referred from hospital, but a few were referred directly from the community. Although the service is available throughout the metropolitan area, these 47 patients all lived in Vancouver or Richmond, BC.

Ages ranged from 15 to 87 years, with 37 patients being between 51 and 81. Sexes were about evenly divided: there were 22 males and 25 females. Thirty-one were married and living with a spouse; of the other 16, 14 were cared for satisfactorily by a relative or friend. The remaining two lived alone, but their situation rapidly became unsatisfactory, for they required some attention 24 hours a day; consequently, they were readmitted to hospital.

In 42 instances the terminal illness was malignant disease (lung, 9; breast, 4; gastrointestinal, 18; genitourinary, 6; brain, 2; primary unknown, 3). In the remainder it was a nonmalignant medical condition (cirrhosis of the liver, 2; cardiorenal disease, 1; gastric ulcer, 1; diverticulitis, 1).

In 32 instances both family and patient knew the diagnosis and prognosis and accepted the situation, in 6 instances only the family had this information, and in the remaining 9 instances the family denied and did not accept the prognosis.

ASPECTS OF HOME CARE

Duration

For 18 patients the duration was up to 10 days; for 15, up to 20 days; and for 7, up to 30 days. The remainder received the service for longer periods, one patient for over 100 days.

All 33 patients readmitted to hospital died within a few days of admission. The other 14 were cared for to the end and died at home.

Team Approach

Throughout the treatment it is essential that the family practitioner be closely involved with both patient and family.[5-7] His knowledge of the family and his expertise in caring for patients at home should make him the leader in this care. He must be attentive to the physical and emotional needs of the patient and to the psychological needs of the family. He must be aware of the changing equipment requirements and be available to the nurses for advice and support. Doctor and nurse must be prepared to discuss dying with sympathy and sensitivity.[6]

The main burden of care falls on the nursing service. The total number of nursing visits was 1,436, with an average of 30.5 visits per patient. Most patients required only one visit daily. On two occasions patients required five visits in 1 day. Repeated daily visits were necessary for patients suffering intractable pain and requiring hypodermic injections and for those with discharging wounds requiring frequent changes of dressings. Sometimes visits were made to the family chiefly to provide the almost constant emotional support required.

Physiotherapists made 56 visits. This was generally to clear a chest or to assist a family in mobilizing a patient and instructing them in use of equipment such as Hoyer lifts.

Homemaker services consisted of 221 "units" of 4 hours' service. The homemaker took care of household chores so that the family was free either to provide nursing care to the patient or to take a much needed rest. At times the homemaker also gave emotional support to various family members.

An important requirement was that the patient be amongst family or friends 24 hours a day. The home care program could not accept those who lived alone because it could not provide care or presence for a full day.

Intractable Pain

Twenty patients suffered intractable pain and required hypodermic injections of various analgesics, usually morphine or meperidine. Generally one or more members of the family were taught to give the injections. When this was not possible the nurses gave them. The remaining patients were kept comfortable with various oral tranquillizers and analgesics, singly or in combination.

Complications

Almost any complication could be handled at home. Two patients were paraplegic because of metastatic disease. The visiting nurses educated the families in the procedures required for proper care of these patients, who were then able to remain at home.

DISCUSSION

The patient with a terminal illness should be allowed to choose his environment as death approaches. At home with his family he is in familiar surroundings and does not feel abandoned. The close, loving bond amongst family members envelops him. No hospital staff, no matter how attentive, can substitute for this. The psychological needs in this trying time for both family and patient are answered in the home. For families who are able to cope with the many difficulties, the emotional trauma is eased and the satisfactions are great. Some people are unable to cope with the emotional strain of seeing a loved one deteriorate and prefer to have the patient in hospital. Their wishes should be respected.

The health professionals must support those who wish to have the dying patient at home, providing home visits by family physician, nurse, physiotherapist and home-maker, and the necessary equipment and medication. Care at home should be continued as long as possible. If the burden on the family becomes too great the patient may be readmitted to hospital. For the group reported, generally both patient and family were happy with the program. A few families were unable to cope for more than a few days but most continued care almost to the end.

This service is less expensive than treatment provided in an acute-care hospital and at the same time releases a bed for an acutely ill patient.

The home care service has been able to provide this small but important aspect of nursing care to patients in the terminal stages of their lives because of the recognition of its importance by the British Columbia Department of Health, which funds the program (no charge is made to patient or family) and the coordination of existing community resources by the metropolitan board of health of Greater Vancouver. Local health departments have provided the community health nurses and consultants necessary for original patient assessment. The visiting nurse organization (in metropolitan Vancouver this was the Victorian Order of Nurses) also employs rehabilitation therapists. The Greater Vancouver Area Homemaker Association, Meals-on-Wheels and Red Cross Loan Supplies were also actively engaged in services to these patients.

REFERENCES

1 Strauss A.: *Chronic Illness and the Quality of Life*, St. Louis, Mosby, 1975, p. 119.
2 Care of the dying. *Br Med J* **1**:29, 1973.
3 Keywood O.: Care of the dying in their own home. *Nurs Times* **70**:1516, 1974.
4 Kobrzycki R.: Dying with dignity at home. *Am J Nurs* **75**:1312, 1975.
5 Kyle D.: Terminal care. *J R Coll Gen Pract* **21**:382, 1971.
6 Wilkes E.: How to provide effective home care for the terminally ill. *Geriatrics* **28**:93, 1973.
7 Gilmore A.J.J.: The care and management of the dying patient in general practice. *Practitioner* **213**:833, 1974.

Chapter 6

Treatment of the "Irremediable" Elderly Patient

Bernard Isaacs

Here is a title as full of questions as a pomegranate is full of seeds. How does one treat the irremediable? If the irremediable is treated, is it irremediable? Is "to treat" less than "to remedy?" And why the contiguity of "irremediable" and "elderly?" Are all elderly irremediable? Are all irremediable elderly? These questions concern attitudes. They are important because attitudes rather than expertise determine the outcome of treatment.

ATTITUDES

There was a time, before I entered on that state of grace peculiar to the geriatrician, when the phrase "treatment of the irremediable elderly patient" would have concisely defined geriatrics for me. Later, when I began to work in geriatric medicine, I would have indignantly rebutted the implication that anyone or anything old was irremediable; for did we not profess our faith in the liturgical phrase: "an ill old person is ill because he is ill and not because he is old?" Now, after years of the pragmatic practice of my art, I welcome the recognition that we geriatricians, and not we alone, devote much of our activities to the treatment of the irremediable. Few diseases at any age

Reprinted from *British Medical Journal*, 3:526–528, September 8, 1973.

are cured; most whisper to the patient of their continuing presence, long after the ink is dry on the discharge letter. The treatment of the irremediable is both a worthy objective and an accurate description of much modern medicine.

WHO ARE THE "IRREMEDIABLE?"

First who are they not? They are not, and must not be confounded with, the undiagnosed. They are not the confused, the incontinent, the senile. Confusion and incontinence are symptoms of impaired function of the nervous system and bladder. The words give no information on cause or cure. The term "senility" offends the geriatrician; it requires an effort of will even to write it. In my mind's eye I see the word garbed in a cloak of black, with the blood of ill old people dripping from its lanky fingers. A melodramatic image perhaps; but how often has the attachment of this label to an ill old patient spelt the end of diagnostic and therapeutic endeavour, and condemned him to a slow death by stewing in his own urine?

Every ill person of whatever age has a right to a diagnosis; and only when this has been established is it possible to talk about remediability or irremediability. "Senility" is not a diagnosis; it spells relegation for the patient and abdication by the doctor. I look forward to the day when the word "senility" will have disappeared from acceptable medical terminology, as the word "insanity" has done.

IRREVERSIBLE DISEASE

Many pathological processes which are common in old age are at present irreversible. These include neoplasm, atherosclerosis, and neuronal degeneration—one or more of which accompany most old people on their last long journey to the grave. It is among these sadly disabled people that the doctor seeks opportunities for effective intervention; and opportunities abound.

TREATING THE IRREMEDIABLE

A man of 69 was seen for the first time 2 months after the onset of a right hemiplegia, and after failure of a trial of rehabilitation. The patient was bedfast, there was no return of movement to the affected side, he had a catheter in his bladder, and he was unable to speak or to comprehend. He had been found picking faeces from his rectum and smearing them on his locker. He disturbed other patients by shouting. He had struck out at the nurses, and given his wife a black eye.

First the wife was interviewed. Who was this man? What kind of person was he? He had been a good husband, a loving father, abstemious, a steady and conscientious worker, a keen amateur gardener, a fit man, proud of his good health and work record, inclined to disparage those less healthy than himself. What did she know of his illness? What did she say to him when she visited? She talked to him; sometimes, she thought, he understood her; sometimes he pushed her away and turned his head away from her. Once he lifted his hand to her, a thing he never did in his life. Did she ever cry? She had gone home and wept to herself every night since his illness began, but hadn't told anyone. Did she think he was going to die? She didn't know, but sometimes she found herself half-wishing that he would, and that made her feel wicked. Had she told this to anyone? Not a soul. Had anyone told her what was likely to happen to her husband? No one.

Next the patient was examined. His tongue was dry, his rectum packed with hard dry faeces. There was a pressure sore on his heel; his urine was infected; his haemoglobin level had dropped. He couldn't speak or understand language, but he could pick up situational clues. He could sing "Tipperary" with the words matching the tune; he could count up to ten if he was started off; he could correctly identify "bottle," "tumbler," "spectacles." He could build toy blocks one on top of the other. He could match dominoes. He had no movement in his arm or leg, but he could sit up in bed with minimal support. Suddenly, out of this irremediable situation, all kinds of opportunities of effective intervention were appearing, like crocuses piercing the wintry soil.

The nurses began first. They put him on a fluid chart, gave him adequate nourishing drinks, talking to him as they did so, telling him what they were trying to do, encouraging him to take the cup and drink himself, trying to find out what he would like— orange juice, milk, tea, beer, perhaps even a glass of whisky. They found his pipe, his false teeth, his razor and comb. They emptied his bowel, they gave him fruit. They put him in the bath twice a day, gave him a support to take pressure off his painful heel. They spigoted his catheter, emptied his bladder every two or three hours for a day or two, then tried him without the catheter, carefully showing him how to use a bottle, and ensuring that there was one where he could reach it on his left side. They sent for his clothes and shoes. They got him up, dressed, shaved, hair brushed, and showed him his image in the mirror. With the help of the physiotherapist they put him in a self-propelled wheelchair and taught him how to use his good foot to drive himself about.

The physiotherapist mobilized his limbs and trunk, stood him up with support to give him the feel of the ground under his feet. The occupational therapist trained him to assist in his own dressing. The speech therapist discovered routes of communication by gesture and situational clues, and taught the relatives and the nurses how to exploit these. The doctor treated the accompanying urinary infection and anaemia, relieved pain, ensured sleep, conferred with relatives and with the therapeutic team. In the end the patient did not fully "recover"—but he regained self-respect and a limited degree of independence. He became much less demanding and frustrated. He was able to go on outings, and could spend an occasional weekend at home. He took up indoor gardening and filled the dayroom with pot plants. We did not "cure" him of the irremediable disease, but we were privileged to watch the tide of his personality begin to flow again over the dry sand of his disability.

PRINCIPLES

All this required the full geriatric team. In the more usual setting of the patient's home or a general hospital ward the same basic principles apply. These are:

1   Listen carefully to the patient. He will tell you what needs to be done.
2   Make yourself available to talk to relatives in privacy. They too have needs.

3 Information is the fuel of opinion. So do not hesitate to investigate, but keep the investigation relevant to possible treatment.

4 No form of treatment should be rejected dogmatically; always the benefits should be weighed against the hazards. To secure comfort in the last days of life risks are justified.

INVESTIGATION AND SURGICAL TREATMENT

The undiagnosed are often the unremedied; so no patient should be denied investigation. Evaluation of the haemoglobin, blood urea, electrolytes, and blood sugar is a minimum. A chest x-ray film may show unsuspected cancer, tuberculosis, or osteomalacia. Sternal marrow examination is well tolerated and should not be withheld on grounds of age alone. Barium meals seldom lead to useful treatment. Barium enemas are more often helpful, but may be frustrated by nonretention or by faecal accumulations. Urine cultures often yield organisms, but their eradication less often relieves symptoms.

Surgery and anaesthesia are well tolerated, and should not be withheld if they offer hope of improvement in the quality of life. Postoperative rehabilitation may be very successful, and old people can learn to use colostomies or artificial limbs.

RELIEF OF SYMPTOMS

Intractable pain is mercifully rare in the elderly. Its adequate control requires timely relief with nonnarcotizing doses of potent drugs, a technique which needs organization, but which yields benefits by relieving the fear of having to endure pain.

Dyspnoea is more common and more difficult to control. Good posture is best obtained at home by nursing the patient in a chair. Adequate diuresis is sometimes resisted, because the patient and his relatives become exhausted by frequent potting. A catheter should be used without hesitation. Oxygen usually causes more anxiety and tension than it relieves.

Anorexia is treated by indulgence. Favourite foods and beverages are prescribed; and a glass of whisky or sherry acquires a new and glorious flavour through having been prescribed by the doctor.

Treating dehydration is important, since ill old people do not experience thirst. Their fluid intake should be charted, aiming at an intake of 1,500 ml a day. If they have difficulty in swallowing they should use a straw or a child's feeding cup. Their fluids can be given in the form of jelly or liquidized foods.

Constipation is compounded by lack of roughage in the diet, lack of physical exercise, poor somatic muscle tone and evacuating power, inadequate opportunity, and fear of discomfort, quite apart from any autonomic dysfunction. The provision of a commode which the patient trusts and is prepared to use is as important as the prescription of the correct laxative or suppository. Regular enemas are required; regular rectal examinations are even more important.

Sleep disturbances send the doctor off on a prescription odyssey, sailing from drug to drug in an endeavour to secure sleep by night and wakefulness by day. From time to time one stops all drugs and starts again at the beginning with one aspirin at 9 p.m. —and sometimes this works. The hot milky drink may secure sleep at night, but the full bladder may alert early waking.

PSYCHOLOGICAL FEATURES

Doctors are often urged to allow old people to die with dignity. I find this very difficult to do, since I associate dignity with black silk hats, the measured tread, the grave nod of the head—at very least with ambulation, continence, and mental clarity—features which are lacking as death approaches. Near the end of life some old people become undignified, remove their clothing in public, and revile their dear ones with obscenities. Others lose self-control and become irritable, demanding, and selfish; refuse to be left alone; moan repetitively; ceaselessly ask for drinks; or demand to be taken to the lavatory, do nothing, then wet themselves. These anxiety symptoms are hard for relatives to bear; and many have confided to me that the last months of a loved parent's life were the worst they had ever experienced.

These situations test to the utmost the doctor's capacity to treat the irremediable. He must listen, sympathize, reassure, explain. The relatives require our ears and our time, but the doctor can also give practical help by arranging day hospital care or short-term admission.

CONCLUSION

Much of medical work is concentrated on the final months or year of life. The curative role of the doctor is being attenuated. But equal or greater professional satisfaction can be found by the skilled and perceptive treatment of "the irremediable."

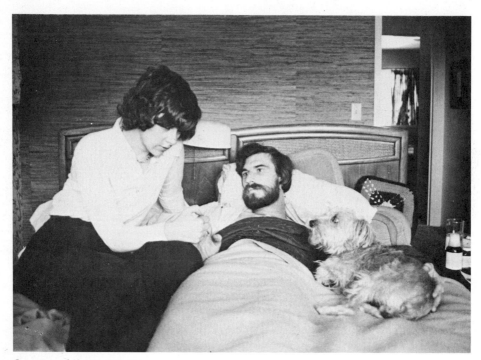

Courtesy of Katrin Achelis

Patients and Families Facing Life-Threatening Illness

Chapter 7

Living with a Life-Threatening Illness

Orville Eugene Kelly

It is Sunday afternoon in Iowa, as I write these words. The sky is overcast this February day and more snow is forecast. My wife, Wanda, and three of our four children, Mark, 16, Lori, 11, and Britton, 7, are shopping. Tammy, 15, stayed home to finish cleaning house. Tonight, we will grill steaks and then light the firewood in the fireplace so we can share an evening together.

It sounds as if I am describing the normal weekend activities of a typical American family.

There is a difference. I am a cancer patient. I was diagnosed in June 1973. The type of cancer I have is called lymphocytic lymphoma. It is advanced, which means it is incurable. In other words, I know I will die of cancer within a limited time, unless I die of something else first.

How much time? I do not know; neither do my physicians, who tell me my remission is almost certain to end sometime during the next year or two. The relapse will spell serious problems. Since I always seem to be bargaining for more time, I hope I can live at least 2 more years. But if death comes sooner, there will be nothing I can do to prevent it.

I remember June 15, 1973 and the scene in the operating room at the hospital. The physician was forced to go to a depth of 3 inches under my arm to reach the tumor for diagnosis. The tumors had appeared in April, two under my arm and one in my groin. For nearly a year, I had been ill, but no one had diagnosed my problem as cancer, until the tumors appeared.

Even before the diagnosis of the tumor came back from the pathology department, I suspected the worst. When the surgeon confirmed my fears by telling me it was malignant, I still didn't feel the full impact until I heard the answer to my question:

"I guess that means I have cancer, right?"

"I'm afraid so."

There it was. My death sentence. Just the word *cancer* meant death to me. My own death. I looked around me, at the nurses in the operating room and outside in the corridor. Suddenly, they were different. They weren't dying, but I felt fear closing in on me because I was.

The surgeon spoke again: "Do you want to tell your wife, or do you want me to do it? She's waiting in the emergency room."

How could I look Wanda in the eye without breaking down completely? Our world had been destroyed by a diagnosis of the most dreaded disease in America. She would be able to see the fear in my eyes. I had always been healthy until the past year, and we had never anticipated anything like this.

"Please tell her for me."

I could see Wanda walking down the corridor as I glanced through the glass wall panels, but I refused to look directly at her. I knew the surgeon was talking with her. One of the nurses helped me from the operating table and I walked out to the corridor where Wanda took me by the arm.

"How are you feeling, Honey?" she asked.

"Fine."

"Can you walk all right?"

"Yes."

Together, Wanda and I walked to the waiting room to join my oldest son, Mark, and my mother-in-law, Lora.

"Oh, Kelly! What are we going to do?" Wanda asked me, in a soft tone of voice.

"I don't want to talk about it. Everything will be all right. Don't worry about it," I replied.

The surgeon had applied a sling to my arm and told me I could go home for a day or two, before being admitted again as a patient. No one spoke during the ride home. It was a gloomy day and I felt more depressed than ever before in my life.

Oh, God! How could you do this to me? I kept thinking. I would never see my oldest son graduate, nor my youngest son enter kindergarten. What would happen to my family? I had been forced to quit my job when I became too ill to work. Now my wife was working to support our family. I had no life insurance.

How much is one man supposed to take? I thought to myself. *How much pain is there going to be?* I felt fear every time I thought about death. I had always been afraid of dying and now I had joined the ranks of other cancer patients I had known, most of whom were dead.

The two days I spent at home were depressing ones. Sometimes I dared to wonder if a mistake had been made; maybe I didn't have cancer at all. But in more realistic moments, I knew better. I didn't talk to Wanda very much. I didn't want to worry her any more than she already seemed to be. I never told my four children I had cancer.

I couldn't sleep very much at night. I would awaken from a nightmare and then start thinking about dying. I envisioned what my funeral would be like and I thought about being in a casket, underground. I couldn't imagine the world going on without me. Every time I looked at my wife and children, I started thinking about having to leave them, forever.

I spent a week at the community hospital in my home city of Burlington, where initial tests were carried out. After a series of scans and blood counts, I was sent to the University of Iowa Hospitals and Clinics at Iowa City, Iowa.

I was allowed to go home some weekends to be with my family. There was a new world awaiting me there. Friends and relatives were uneasy around me. They were afraid they might say the wrong thing. It was very depressing. I think I reminded many of them of their own mortality.

One young visitor exclaimed, "I've just been *dying* to meet you!" Then she realized what she had said and was very embarrassed.

People were very careful not to mention words like *cancer*, *death*, or *funeral* when they were around me. My disease became known as my *problem*.

An old friend of the family came to visit one day while I was home from the hospital. Wanda and I greeted her at the door.

"How's he feeling?" she asked Wanda.

Why didn't she ask me? I was standing right there.

Many people think that cancer might be contagious. I remember attending a small party one evening while on a pass from the hospital. Everything seemed to be going all right until I noticed that I was being served my drinks in a paper cup, while everyone else had glasses! The hostess obviously believed cancer might be contagious. However, if it were, we would have had quite an epidemic on our hands, instead of a *major problem*.

I was very depressed. I began to isolate myself from everyone. Much of the time I spent in bed, although I was physically able to walk and drive a car. Since I didn't want to worry Wanda, we still hadn't talked about it. I worried about what would happen to my family when I was gone.

I even began to imagine that something would happen to Wanda or the children. After all, since I was dying of cancer, maybe my family was being haunted by bad luck.

My family was falling apart. Communications had nearly stopped. The children knew something was wrong because I was in the hospital most of the time, but they didn't know I had cancer. Our home atmosphere became depressing. It was as if we were observing my funeral every day before it actually occurred. Wanda had been sleeping in another bedroom. Later I found out that she didn't want me to hear her crying at night.

As a hospital patient in Iowa City, I had asked for a prognosis. The doctors didn't tell me everything at once, but they did tell me what they knew as the weeks went by. When I asked one doctor how long I had to live, he told me, "Perhaps 6 months to 3 years." He went on to tell me that this was just a guess, based on statistics.

"However, we don't know how *you* will respond to treatment," he added.

There it was. This official prognosis confirmed my fears. It was over. Not only did I have to face the prospect of dying, but I had to endure the endless tests.

In September 1973, I considered suicide, but I wanted to spend one more Christmas season with my family.

Since I couldn't talk with Wanda about my feelings, I wrote a poem to express how I felt about life and her:

Spring, and the land lies fresh green
Beneath a yellow sun.
We walked the land together, you and I
And never knew what future days would bring.
Will you often think of me,
When flowers burst forth each year?
When the earth begins to grow again?
Some say death is so final,
But my love for you can never die.
Just as the sun once warmed our hearts,
Let this love touch you some night,
When I am gone,
And loneliness comes—
Before the dawn begins to scatter
Your dreams away.

Summer, and I never knew a bird
Could sing so sweet and clear,
Until they told me I must leave you
For a while.
I never knew the sky could be so deep a blue,
Until I knew I could not grow old with you.
But better to be loved by you,
Than to have lived a million summers,
And never known your love.
Together, let us, you and I
Remember the days and nights,
For eternity.

Fall, and the earth begins to die,
And leaves turn golden brown upon the trees.
Remember me, too, in autumn, for I will walk with you,
As of old, along a city sidewalk at eveningtime;
Though I cannot hold you by the hand.

Winter, and perhaps someday there may be
Another fireplace, another room,
With crackling fire and fragrant smoke,

And turning, suddenly, we will be together,
And I will hear your laughter and touch your face,
And hold you close to me again.
But, until then, if loneliness should seek you out,
Some winter night, when snow is falling down,
Remember, though death has come to me,
Love will never go away!

I was dismissed from the hospital in the late fall of 1973. I went home to await my first chemotherapy treatment. The doctor explained some of the possible side effects from the drugs used in this treatment—lowered white cell counts (which meant a lower resistance to infections), bone marrow depression, possible loss of hair, fatigue, and nausea. It appeared to me that the treatment might be almost as bad as the cancer itself.

I considered not returning to the hospital for medical treatment. I had heard about the toxicity of the drugs from some other patients and I dreaded it.

However, I decided that chemotherapy treatment might be my only hope. The day of my first treatment, blood was taken from my arm and the counts were found suitable for injecting the drugs. I received dosages of Cytoxan and Vincristine Sulfate intravenously and was given Prednisone tablets to take orally for 5 days.

I was driving home from the treatment. Wanda and my youngest son, Britt, were with me. I looked toward Wanda. Words can't really describe the look on her face—depression, dejection, hopelessness. I decided then that I couldn't stand it any longer.

"Wanda," I began, "I want to talk about it. I have cancer and I will probably die of it. I don't want to die. I'm afraid. But I'm not dead yet! I can't change what has happened, but I can do something about the future. I've got to tell you how I feel. When I look at the children, I realize how terrible it is that I am dying. When I see healthy people around me, I resent their good health. But I'm going to try to live with it. I've reached the bottom emotionally. Things can't get any worse. We can't continue to live this way any longer—lying and pretending that everything is all right. I have cancer, and I want the children to know about it. Tonight I want to barbecue ribs like we used to."

"This is what I've been waiting to hear," Wanda told me. "I've been wanting to tell you how *I* feel. You know it hasn't been easy for me either. I feel so helpless, just watching what's happening to you."

We had our barbecue that night. Although the night was cool, the stars had never looked brighter. Later, I told our three older children. My youngest son was asleep. Of course, it wasn't easy then. It still isn't. The children cried, but at least everything was out in the open. No more pretending. There wasn't anything to hide. Now we could begin to cope with the problem. There is no substitute for the truth, even when death is the subject.

The death rate for any generation is 100 percent. We *all* die. However, I know what will probably kill me, while most people do not. We have no guarantee of how long we will live. But I believe it is truly the quality of life, not the quantity, that is most important.

The prospect of death made me more aware of life. I noticed things around me that I had never noticed before. Things seemed a little brighter.

I wrote an article for the local newspaper in January 1974, describing my experience as a terminal cancer patient. I stated in the article that there should be an organization enabling seriously ill patients, family members, and other interested persons to meet informally to discuss some of the emotional problems created by cancer. Other patients and family members began calling me after the article appeared. I discovered that we shared common anxieties and fears. I identified with them. I knew they were people who understood my own problems.

I also discovered there are worse things than death.

A young man told me, "My wife left me after she found she couldn't live with a terminal cancer patient. I thought I could never live with the thought of death, but now I find living without my family is worse."

One lady pleaded, "Will you please help me? I'm living in the same house with a man who has become a stranger. He doesn't mistreat me. He just ignores me. He's never admitted I have cancer. I try to talk to him, but he refuses to discuss my problems with me."

One middle-aged man remarked, "My family doesn't want me to know that I have cancer. I know I have it, though. They think I don't know my wife has a separate plate, cup, and silverware for me. We were happy before the cancer, but now I feel lost. I guess my wife thinks it is contagious because she doesn't even kiss me anymore."

"I tried to pretend everything was still all right," a lady wrote. "But it isn't. I have cancer. I just can't live this way any longer. I need to talk to someone who cares about what is happening to me."

Apparently, just when a seriously ill patient needs understanding and support more than ever before, friends and relatives often isolate themselves from him or her because they can't cope with the many problems connected with terminal illness. Although terminal illness sometimes causes a family to become closer than ever before, too often the attendant problems destroy family life, as when divorce follows the death of a child from cancer.

I feel that physicians, even if they can't spend more time with their patients, can through certain words and actions either cause a patient to become more depressed or help him or her immensely. When I was in the hospital, the five physicians making rounds would sometimes congregate outside my hospital room door and converse. They may have only been talking about the next patient they were going to visit, but I always thought they were talking about me and didn't want me to hear what they were saying.

Some patients who are told not to come back to the hospital for 3 months, after they have been coming every 30 days for treatment, feel "They are giving up on me." Actually, the fact may be that the patient is doing well and perhaps is even in remission. However, unless this is explained, the patient often assumes the worst. Therefore, it is important to open up excellent communications between physician and patient.

As a consequence of my article, eighteen of us held a meeting to determine if there was a need for the type of organization I had envisioned. The group included patients, family members of seriously ill patients, and professional persons. We decided to call the group Make Today Count. After all, that was what we were trying to do—make time count.

Most of us had become more aware of life. None of us had planned to have cancer, nor were any of us happy about the prospect of death. But we did have someone to share our problems with, and that is what we did. We did not promise miracles at our meeting—only understanding and support. From my own experience with cancer, I know how important it is to know someone cares about you. We didn't compare medical treatments or find out who was suffering the most pain, but we brought our emotional problems out in the open where we could try to cope with them.

United Press International and Associated Press carried the story about our meeting over their wire services. Soon the calls began to pour in from persons who wanted information about our group, and I received invitations to appear at universities and hospitals and on television and radio. I had never imagined that there was a universal need for an organization such as Make Today Count.

More MTC chapters were organized throughout the United States. Today, there are approximately eighty chapters in thirty states. Some of the chapters have been started by cancer patients—others by ministers, physicians, nurses, and families of patients.

Often, cancer patients are bombarded with advertising about all types of "miracle" cures. Most patients, however, seem able to reject quack treatments until they become desperate. Then, many seem willing to try anything in the event that it might work. For them, false hope is better than no hope at all. False hope, however, is usually costly and time-consuming. I found that since I was responding to chemotherapy, my advice helped to convince many desperate patients that legitimate medical treatment is the wisest course of action.

Many patients experience deep emotional problems centering on loss of sex appeal and rejection after a scarring operation for certain types of cancer, or on loss of hair or disfigurement from radiation therapy.

It isn't possible to solve all of these problems, but bringing them out in the open and discussing them seems to help. Just knowing that others face some of the same problems relieves the anxieties of many patients and family members.

One patient remarked, "I no longer feel alone. I used to have the feeling I was the only cancer patient in the world suffering from emotional problems."

Meanwhile, I appeared at several universities to discuss how a patient copes with a life-threatening illness. Although I was receiving chemotherapy, I only had to cancel a few appearances.

As a result of my activities, I was contacted by Dell Publishing Company of New York, and I agreed to write my first book, Make Today Count. In it I describe my earlier years and my experiences as a cancer patient.

I thus became busier as an advanced cancer patient than I had ever been before. I didn't have much time to think about dying. Although I still had periods of depression, staying active helped me cope with these moods.

Each day became another day of life, instead of another day closer to death. I had reason to stay alive; I had a job to do. I received great satisfaction from helping other patients cope with their problems.

A lady from Wisconsin wrote, "Please be alive when you get this letter. If *you* can make it, I can too."

I have learned much from my association with thousands of seriously ill patients and their families. I have learned that if you love someone, you should let him or her know it before it's too late. Don't wait until the funeral to send flowers. Survivors have too many guilty feelings after the death of a friend or relative occurs. "Why didn't I tell my husband how much I loved him before it was too late?" "I think my wife wanted to talk to me about her feelings, but she died before we could communicate."

I have also learned that we hide from unpleasant things. But evading the problems only makes them worse. Sooner or later, we must face reality.

Much has happened in my life since that day in June 1973 when I learned I had cancer. Once I became involved in helping others, my life changed completely. As a matter of fact, I would not return to the lifestyle of the past. I will take cancer. I know things will never be normal again, and I still do not want to die. But neither do I want to live as I did before, when I did not appreciate life.

Each day is a gift for me. It is another day I never thought I would have to enjoy.

Because of my way of living during the past 3 years, it will be easier to say goodbye.

Chapter 8

Personal-Professional Support: From a Patient's Point of View

Sandra L. Barger

I have had diabetes for 25 years. In the past 5 years I have been the wife of a terminally ill patient with heart disease and have lived through chronic renal failure, hemodialysis, and a successful kidney transplant. It is on my relationships with many different doctors and on my discussions with other patients and the families of patients that I base the following reflections about the support doctors can provide for patients and their families, especially for those involved in a terminal illness.

Probably the most important factor affecting the support doctors provide for their patients is their ability to separate the need to help a patient from the role of healer (that is, the need to prolong life). Maximal prolongation of life may not be the patient's priority.

It is understandably difficult for doctors who treat terminally ill patients to reconcile the need to heal (this wish to prolong life) with the desire of some patients to let the disease take its natural course with no efforts at treatment, or conversely, with the desire of others to curtail anticipated suffering by taking their own lives at the time of their own choosing. Doctors who wish to be truly supportive of their patients should be able to acknowledge these feelings in their patients, if they occur, and discuss them rationally.

A friend who was having extremely negative feelings about going on dialysis and seriously considering death rather than accepting a kidney transplant finally found a doctor who was willing to discuss these feelings with her. It was partly because of the support given to her by this doctor that she finally decided to submit to dialysis for the short time before arrangements could be completed for transplant from a sibling donor.

Doctors should realize, however, that most terminally ill people occasionally desire to escape suffering. If a patient only once (or occasionally) expresses such sentiments, and if the doctor acknowledges these sentiments nonjudgmentally, the doctor can be fairly confident that the patient really desires to prolong his or her life.

One question about the prolongation of life concerns the quality of that life. For most diseases there are a variety of possible treatments or treatment combinations doctors can use, with varying degrees of effectiveness and with varying side effects. The doctor's knowledge of the possibilities is extensive; usually the patient's knowledge is slight and may be colored by stories he or she has heard—some true, some untrue. A doctor who is attempting to allow his or her patients to live out their lives in the manner that is most acceptable to them, must explain as clearly as possible the various alternative treatments, their expected side effects, and their expected effectiveness. I have greatly appreciated the use of this approach by my doctors on more than one occasion.

With some patients, one explanation is enough to allow a decision to be made and the selected treatment to be carried through to the end. Most patients, however, will probably vacillate, making it necessary for the doctor to repeat essentially the same information many times before it becomes at all meaningful to the patient. A person who is diagnosed as terminally ill, especially if the news is unexpected, will almost always react with some degree of shock and fear, emotions that will block out to some extent whatever else the doctor may wish to discuss (including the diagnosis), sometimes for months after the diagnosis is originally explained.

I recently met a man who had had a malignant brain tumor partially removed. He had been told repeatedly by doctors and by his wife that the tumor was malignant, and he had begun chemotherapy but kept saying the doctors were talking double-talk, they didn't seem to know what it was and what to do for it. This went on for about 3 months before he finally said to his wife, "The doctor said the tumor *might* be malignant."

A doctor's patience in allowing a person to face facts at his or her own pace can be most helpful. Almost every patient needs some time to make life-and-death decisions, and many change their minds once or several times during the course of the disease, opting for cure, or management, or death. Family members should also be allowed time to make decisions. There have been several occasions when I felt I could have made wiser decisions for myself and for my husband had I been allowed a little time to consider the choices.

It is perhaps most difficult for physicians specializing in such fields as nephrology and cardiology, where long-term management has become more usual than short-term death, to acknowledge that some patients may prefer death to the restrictions imposed by dialysis, organ transplant, open heart surgery, and the special diets, exercise plans, medications, related surgeries, and repeated, sometimes painful, examination procedures involved. Even those patients who choose treatment aimed at long-term management, will occasionally question their choice; they may at some point decide that imminent death is preferable to continued long-term management, or, recognizing the risks involved in the procedures imposed to sustain life, they may ask to be prepared "in case I die on the operating table."

When I started on dialysis while waiting for a kidney transplant, I wanted to make sure all my affairs were in order so that if I did not make it through the surgery, my death would not create undue hardship for my family. When I asked my doctor if arranging to donate my body for research would be helpful for anyone, he brushed me off with, "You're not going to die. Maybe you could donate your corneas. I'll look into it." That was the end of it. In fact, I did stop breathing after the surgery. Had I not been revived, I would have died with my affairs out of order.

Doctors seeking to be helpful to their patients can acknowledge the feelings and requests of those they care for and be willing to discuss questions and support patients in their decisions.

Our society has not resolved the moral issues generated by organ transplantation and the various related techniques of keeping bodies alive through mechanical devices. Patients faced with the necessity of a transplant and the doctors and families who care for them have extremely divergent reactions to their dilemma, which can create both intra- and interpersonal conflicts. These reactions may focus more on the donor than on the recipient.

I received my new kidney from a cadaver donor. The hardest things for me to deal with were the idea that someone had to die so that I might live, and the fact that the donor would be kept biologically alive until the doctors were ready to remove his kidneys, at which time the machines would be turned off. Friends who were to receive kidneys from sibling donors, and their families, were concerned about the siblings who would be giving up one of their kidneys, the hardship of the nephrectomy, and especially, the possible danger in leaving the sibling with only one kidney. A doctor should acknowledge (to both himself and others) his own feelings as well as those of his patients. He will find that it is helpful to some patients if he avows his own feeling of ambiguity, and to most patients if he expresses his sorrow over unsuccessful treatment and his joy over treatment that provides relief.

An important consideration alluded to above is time and timing. Most doctors prefer to start treatment immediately after making a diagnosis. However, many patients are unable to handle too many important decisions too soon and require time to consider the various alternatives. A patient may wish to spend a great deal of time discussing the alternatives with the doctor, who may find it difficult to find time in his schedule for several long sessions with each of his terminally ill patients while still meeting the needs of his other patients and also attending to his own needs. As far as possible, however, a doctor should attempt to give each patient the feeling that there is plenty of time to discuss the patient's concerns. The doctor should also be sensitive to the best timing in presenting the facts concerning the nature and treatment of each patient's disease. Some patients may want to know as few details as possible, preferring to let the doctor do whatever he thinks best without asking the patient to contribute

to the decision-making process. Doctors should, however, be alert to the difference between this kind of patient and the one who, like myself, wants to know more but does
not know what questions to ask.

Much of what doctors can do to show their support for chronically and terminally
ill patients consists of things that most doctors do for their patients anyway. However,
little things can become extremely important to the patient—for example, expression
and follow-up of interest in some of the patient's activities that are not directly related
to his or her state of health, or remembering medical facts without having to obviously
check the chart (the patient will never know if you check the chart *before* you see him
or her). Such medically insignificant indications of personal interest can help make patients feel they are real people in the eyes of the doctor, and not just "osteogenic sar-
comas metastasized to lungs and liver."

Listening to the observations and opinions of patients and their families can both
provide support for the patient and provide the doctor with information he or she
might not be able to gain from a physical examination alone. Because of their familiarity with the normal responses of the patient, family members may notice variations
that the doctor might not otherwise be aware of. With semiconscious patients, close
family members may elicit a much greater response than the less familiar doctors and
nurses.

A series of images from the last few weeks of my husband's life pass through my
mind. His heart stopped four times within a 12-hour period. Because he was in the
hospital emergency room and intensive care unit when these crises occurred, he was
revived each time. However, he was left in a deep coma which gradually lessened to
a state of semiconsciousness during the 7 weeks before his death by miocardial infarction unattended in his room in an extended-care facility. I recollect: (1) (in the
intensive care unit) a nurse saying to me, "He always seems to know when you are
here. He is more active"; (2) (in the hospital after he was moved from the intensive
care unit) a nurse rushing out of the room to excitedly tell her colleagues, "He smiled
at her!" (which resulted in increased and successful efforts on their parts to get him
to respond to them); (3) the look of incredulity on the doctor's face as he left the
room after telling me he was having my husband transferred to an extended-care
facility, when my husband raised up and waved good-bye to him; (4) the doctor to
whom he was assigned at the extended-care facility telling me when I called to protest
about the heavy sedation he had prescribed, "I think you are fooling yourself to think
that he is more than a vegetable. He only lies there on the bed"; and (5) the tone of
utter amazement in which a nurse who had slipped in behind us as we arrived a few
days later said, "He *does* know you!" They were getting very little response; we were
getting a great deal.

It is also very helpful for a doctor to express confidence and admiration for the
other doctors and health care professionals responsible for a patient's care. If a doctor
can say, as mine once did, "This is the gynecologist who recently did a hysterectomy
on my wife," or can mention something that reflects on a doctor's competence in his
field, such as his thoroughness in researching all possible alternative treatments, the
patient will usually be more confident that he or she is getting the best treatment
available.

Doctors, because they are individuals, must find their own methods for best meeting the psychosocial needs of their patients, methods that will vary from patient to patient, because patients are individuals too, requiring individualized care. Methods may vary, but those doctors who truly desire to be of maximal help to their patients will find that this desire will communicate itself, becoming the basis for the personal-professional support that is an integral part of medical care.

Chapter 9

What a Dying Man Taught Doctors About Caring

Caroline Driver

I smelled an incident coming the moment the young doctor turned from the corridor into our room. He brandished his stethoscope in the accepted fashion as he approached the bed, but his eyes and his heart were planets away. I say "our room" because I had moved into the hospital to be with Bob, my husband, during what proved to be his last illness, a case of acute myeloblastic leukemia.

That doctor didn't even say "Hello." He just glanced at the chart and proceeded to check Bob over. When Bob winced out some jocular remark during a rectal probe, the physician ignored him. If he realized that his hands were touching a human being, he certainly didn't show it.

His wall of detachment was all the more remarkable because my husband was the easiest person in the world to get to know. He was an incredibly vital, joyous young man with visions of a more human world for everybody, including himself and myself and our five children. He'd been a moving force behind Kairos—a group-encounter movement aimed at breaking down walls between people. He and I had dedicated our lives to that concept.

Reprinted from *Medical Economics*, **50**:81–86, January 22, 1973.

Now, at 34, Bob was dying. Even though he was to make comeback after comeback and neither of us ever really gave up hope, he knew the odds. What's more, the staff knew he knew. Yet he might have been a piece of protoplasm with a serial number; the young doctor simply marked the chart and started to leave. But at this point Bob stopped him.

"Just a moment, Doctor . . ."

The physician turned in surprise at the directness of Bob's tone.

"Doctor," Bob continued evenly, "I don't . . . like you."

The startled physician reacted with arrogance. "Mr. Driver," he snapped back, "I'm a doctor here. What's more, I'm *your* doctor."

"Then you know I'm fighting for my life," Bob said. "So why do you come in with negativeness and coldness. Why?"

Shaken, the young M.D. sat down. "I'm sorry," he said, "I don't like to be that way with people. I just find it hard to reach out the way you do. Sometimes I wonder why I'm this way myself."

With that the two men talked for nearly an hour. When the doctor finally departed they had begun a genuine friendship.

Unfortunately the outcome of this incident is far from typical, some of my doctor-friends tell me, especially in our bigger institutions. There, my friends say, a lessened awareness of human needs is often the price a patient pays for bigness and technical excellence. I can vouch for that. Because we'd traveled from California, I slept in as Bob's almost constant roommate during all 15 months of his confinement as a private-paying patient at a medical center in a nearby Western state, and what I observed about impersonalized medical care proved depressing indeed.

It is only fair to point out that the hospital is a respected teaching institution with an excellent record in leukemia cases. The doctors there achieved near-miraculous results with Bob in the early stages of his illness. And many of the doctors and nurses we met went out of their way to show Bob kindness and concern and to do favors for both of us that can never be forgotten.

What bothered us then and bothers me still, though, is that *we* had to make most of the initial human contacts. Few patients have Bob Driver's capacity for reaching out to a fellow human being or his courage in demanding a human response. In a hospital environment most patients instinctively look to doctors and nurses to do the reaching out, to take the risk of caring. Instead, too many ill, bewildered, bedridden people find themselves ground down by detachment, by grim adherence to antiquated rules and procedures. Perhaps this account of how Bob and I tried to cope with our situation will make doctors everywhere more aware of their patients as human beings and help bring an end to this seeming callousness.

The whole idea of my "living in" with Bob came about as a result of an early encounter with institutional indifference. There were no private vacancies when Bob was first admitted, so he was assigned to a ward for a few days. On his first night, despite a confirmed diagnosis of leukemia, Bob was placed next to a patient with pneumonia. I protested, only to meet blank stares and shrugs. Finally I sought out the resident.

Yes, he said, the low white count could make my husband highly susceptible to pneumonia. I asked whether something couldn't be done. Then—and only then—did they move Bob to a safer bed.

We decided right there that once Bob got his own room I'd stay in it with him, day and night. But when that time came, the floor nurse had other ideas. After visiting hours were over, there was a good deal of palaver at the nursing station before—finally—a cot appeared.

I was to occupy that cot for much of the next two and a half years because the 15 months of hospitalization were actually spread over four visits. The first, lasting seven weeks, resulted in a full remission. Bob and I returned home to a normal life for a blessed nine months. Then Bob relapsed. He returned to the hospital three times for stays of four to five months each before he died.

None of this could be foretold when we settled into that first private room. We knew only that a thunderbolt had struck Bob in the prime of life, that death could come in a matter of weeks. That's why, when we looked around at that cold, sterile, antiseptically white room, we decided to do a little humanizing on our own. Step No. 1, it seemed obvious, would be some brightly colored pillowcases. And that threw down another gauntlet.

"Oh, no, Mrs. Driver," said the floor nurse. "We couldn't allow colored pillowcases. They couldn't be sterilized."

"I'll wash them myself," I answered.

"But it's just not allowed!"

"Is there a specific rule here against colored pillowcases?"

"Well . . ."

It was great to see that room come alive. The color was a kind of declaration. Bob and I weren't out to make unreasonable demands or to challenge rules. But we weren't afraid to make the best of our situation and to show our love openly, and our choice was to live in a loving, warm environment. That room soon became an extension of our home.

I kept colorful bedspreads on both our beds and I brought in four thick throw rugs for the floor. We lined one wall with photographs of the children playing, singing, being alive and free as we had taught them to be. Books began to pile up on the windowsill. The scratchy hospital radio gave way to our own FM stereo from home. We even laid in some good white wine, keeping it cool on top of the air-conditioner and drinking it from heirloom blue wine glasses from home. And on one wall we tacked an arresting poster: "You are a child of the universe. You have a right to be here." Bob loved it.

The rest of that first visit went pretty smoothly. Innovative chemotherapy, injections of cytosine arabinoside, proved spectacularly successful. Bob's strength began to flow back. I can't begin to describe the sheer joy we felt when the doctor in charge at the hospital said Bob could go home, that the leukemia might not return for a considerable time. They could have painted our room black for all we cared.

Then came one of the unforgettable incidents of needless dehumanization. We packed to leave, and I sailed around on Cloud Nine saying thank-yous and good-bys. We had become friends with most of the nurses by then. But in the kitchen one of the older hands—a woman we'd always trusted because we'd never seen her make a mistake—looked at me and said flatly: "Don't worry, sweetie. You'll be back." That wiped me out.

Maybe she was trying to be helpful. Or maybe she was simply of the old school, speaking frankly to spare me from later disillusionment. But she might as well have used a knife. It was all I could do to keep a smile on my face so Bob wouldn't suspect what she'd said.

We did come back nine months later. Bob's successive relapses and partial recoveries, their direction ever more predictable, intensified our search for getting the most out of every moment. This made staff mistakes and detachment all the harder to take. I recall the time an intern made three unsuccessful and painful attempts at a spinal tap. We tried to sympathize with his obvious discomfiture, and I'll give him credit for confessing that this wasn't any easier on him than on us. I've heard it said that three unsuccessful taps aren't all that many—but on a man who's *dying*? At this point Bob refused to continue; he insisted that a resident be called to give the spinal.

Bob never forgot another intern who started to give an intravenous injection of a powerful new medication. I recalled the chief of medicine's saying that it would be injected into Bob's muscle. I questioned the intern about this, and he brushed me off. But Bob pricked up his ears. He wouldn't let the doctor proceed without first going out and checking the medical orders. That intern was a thankful, humble young man when he came back, for the medication indeed wasn't to have been given intravenously.

Impersonal care contributed to other goofs and near-misses. With the blood transfusions, for instance, you'd think they were putting a charger on an automobile battery, not extending the life of a human being. On one transfusion they got the wrong speed. One doctor started the procedure and left. A second doctor came in and speeded it up. Then they had to stop it, and Bob went into a bad reaction. I can't believe this could have happened if somebody had only cared enough, in the first place, about the patient as a person.

I could go on. There were the interminable queues at the x-ray department, with sick people lined up in the hall and being wheeled through like so many cattle, with never a kind word, a pat of the hand, even a friendly eye contact. Those things don't cost a cent, but they can mean the world to a person who is seriously ill. Above all, there was the suspense after tests. We waited and wondered, on the razor's edge, for results that might tell whether Bob would live or die. Sometimes we prayed through the night that the results would be good this time. *And then we wouldn't hear!* Five or six hours would go by, and we wouldn't hear. We'd ask somebody to check, and still we wouldn't hear. Later, maybe, we'd learn that the tests hadn't been sent to the lab that day or that the machine had broken down. Think of the heartaches we could have been spared if only *we'd* known about it as soon as *they* did!

It wasn't that the staff were "bad" people. They were simply afraid to break conventions, afraid to reach out to others on a human-to-human level. But Bob and I weren't afraid. The more we realized that time was closing in, the more we worked to live every day for itself.

I had long since refused to let the nurses bathe Bob if he had to be awakened or to let the maid clean the room if we didn't want to be disturbed. And don't think stopping them was easy. I did those jobs myself when necessary. But there wasn't much we could do about the stream of doctors and other clinical personnel who swept in and out of the room whenever it suited their convenience. One day, Bob took the bull by the horns and posted *our* schedule on the door. "This is the Drivers' Kairos West Schedule," the notice read, and it spelled out the hours when Bob would receive hospital personnel and when we would be "at home." The rest of the time the door was closed. We were still a young, very alive couple, and we intended to maintain our intimacy.

Next we broke the rule against children's visits. I put masks on my five, and we just walked on past the front desk. In my view it is totally inhuman to allow a man to die in a hospital room while his children wait outside in the corridor. All that most children remember is Mommy coming out crying. Well, that didn't happen with our children. We moved them to a temporary home near the hospital just so they could see Bob. There was no way we were going to be separated as a family at a time like this. As a man lives, so should he die!

We humanized the meal program, too. The hospital food was adequate, but the dishes were usually cold by the time they reached us. And there was none of the excitement that could be so important to a sick person—things like a different sauce occasionally, a flower on the tray, or even a happy face on a napkin. So we did our own cooking. I brought in an electric frying pan and assorted cookware and began turning out omelettes, veal cutlets parmigiana, and steak teriyaki.

A few of the uptight nurses complained about the cooking. They told the administrators we were "living like hippies" and made comments about Bob being the only patient in the hospital who had wine with meals. Bob's standard reply was that if the other patients wanted the same cooking privilege, let them have it. Gradually, people came over to our side. Eventually, most of the nurses let us store our food in their refrigerator and wash our dishes in their sink.

Before long some of the other leukemia patients began putting up posters and things. Sometimes they would come to our room to talk because Bob was the kind of man who always held out his hand to help. As our room became a sort of refuge for survival, Bob's way of opening up to people began attracting doctors and nurses too.

I've already mentioned the doctor whose cold bedside manner Bob questioned with such warm results. Later on there was a nurse we thought was unfriendly till we found out it was because Bob resembled a brother who had died. She had to fight back the tears every time she came near us. Bob encouraged her to sit down and let the tears flow. That broke the tension, and she relaxed with us from then on. Another nurse happened to like us but feared being accused of playing favorites if she got too chummy. After Bob got her to laughing at herself a bit, she said, "Oh to hell with what people think!" and sat down too.

Sometimes the doctors would drop in between rounds to recharge their batteries with good talk. Or they would sniff the cooking aromas in the corridor and help us finish off the teriyaki or whatever. Often there would be as many as 20 doctors and nurses or friends in the room. We even had a couple of parties, with somebody bringing in cheese, salami, a barrel of ice, and more wine.

One doctor turned his home over to us at Christmas. Another used his own time to accompany Bob back to San Diego on one of our remission trips home. One head nurse made her car available when needed. Other nurses brought in extra kitchen equipment and records for our hi-fi. With it all, though, the nagging thought persisted: What of the other terminal patients who didn't have Bob's gift of making contact or the financial resources to sustain this kind of environment? From where in the institution would *their* human contact come?

Some doctors were quick to reply that there simply wasn't time enough for the staff to give *all* the patients in the hospital the same personal attention Bob had managed to win for himself. And some doctors defended their detachment as a shield, developed to preserve their sanity in the constant presence of oncoming death. But others, both then and later, decried these rationales as forms of "ethical cop-outs," as one man put it. This, of course, was Bob's main point. It was his feeling and mine that nobody has the right to deny his own awareness of another's pain and suffering, least of all a doctor whose mission is to heal that pain. Who but the doctor can significantly develop the sense of humanity that medicine needs so badly? The change has to come from within.

Appropriately enough, the case of Robert Driver has already generated momentum in this direction. Money gifts to the hospital in lieu of flowers have honored Bob's memory with a fund of about $3,000. The university is planning a teaching program called "The Robert J. Driver Program for Humanistic Medicine." The planned course will help doctors become aware of just what they do to patients.

It would be heartening to conclude this report by saying that Bob completely won his personal campaign for more humanization of the hospital environment. Unfortunately, that isn't true. In fact, he was forced to endure one final affront that epitomized the whole institutional callousness that troubled him so deeply.

When the end was near, the doctor in charge understandingly permitted Bob to come home for a few days to our temporary quarters. So the family did have some precious last hours together, away from what my husband had come to consider "that terrible inhuman place." But when Bob took the final turn for the worse, we arranged for readmission.

By this time he was incredibly fragile, his once-strapping 190-pound body down to less than 90 pounds, spasms of pain racking him despite massive doses of morphine. At the hospital he asked to be spared the admitting physical. In the circumstances, he said, what difference did it make how much he weighed? I agreed, but the admitting office didn't. The rules say that patients must be weighed and measured on admittance. The system was satisfied—through a cruel, senseless, farewell indignity to a pain-ridden, dying man.

Chapter 10

One Family's Experience with Death

Nancy Harjan

My son Michael passed away early on the evening of December 6, 1973 following a 5-month long battle with acute leukemia.

Michael's leukemic condition was first noticed in late June 1973. There were little pin-point-size red marks under his skin and larger bruise marks on his body that indicated unusual bleeding. He had had similar symptoms 10 years before when, following a strange virus, his platelet count had dropped dangerously low. Ten years before the lowering of his platelet count was treatable with cortisone and, after 3 months, the count was back to normal. This time, at age 16, it was not only the platelet count, but also the white cell count, that had begun to climb abnormally. Mike's illness was diagnosed as leukemia. Initially it was difficult to determine whether Mike's kind of leukemia was *chronic* (more typical of children and easier to control) or *acute* (more typical of adults and harder to control). The doctors at Kaiser Hospital in Redwood City where Mike was a patient had the advice of the doctors at Stanford Hospital where much research in leukemia has recently been done. At first Mike was treated for chronic leukemia but, when his body failed to respond to treatment, it was realized that he had a more serious form of leukemia, an acute kind that demanded more radical medication. A relatively new drug, Donnamycin, that was not readily available and that had been used experimentally for only the past 5 years or so, was administered to Mike. It had the desired effect and within 24 hours Mike's white count began to go down. We all had been praying or hoping mightily for this to happen, so of course we felt great joy at this first triumph. However, Mike spent another 3 weeks in the hospital during which time he was quite nauseated, could not eat very much, and hence lost 20 pounds. He also went through a few battles with infection of his gums and bleeding of his lips. His glands underneath his jaws alongside his neck were swollen and he was quite pale. He was given three different kinds of medication, two of them intravenously. He had just two dosages of the Donnamycin; they were administered a week apart in order to minimize toxic effects. During this first stay in the hospital (from June 26 till July 28), he used 58 units, or pints, of blood.

SUPPORT OF FAMILY AND FRIENDS

Throughout Mike's illness, he had the constant, loving support and care of his dear friend, Nancy Siegel, also 16. Michael and Nancy had met 1½ years earlier and had been constant companions since February 1973.

Although going from one crisis to another, Mike nevertheless won the first round against leukemia. He had the love and encouragement of his family and friends and especially that of "Little Nancy" as she came to be called by Michael's father, Yuri, in order to distinguish her from me, whom Yuri dubbed, "Big Nancy." Yuri flew out from Toronto in mid-July and spent 10 days here visiting with Mike in the hospital and with Tanya (Mike's sister) and me, my father, and my friends.

From the beginning the specter of death hovered in the background since Mike's form of acute leukemia was particularly dangerous and did not warrant much optimism. In spite of that, all of us, including Michael, fought hard with determination and faith to win this life-and-death struggle. Mike's physician, Dr. Barkin, and I would couch whatever we told him about his illness in as optimistic terms as possible, but at the same time, we could not lie to him. However, Mike never asked too many questions that were difficult or painful to answer. He seemed to know, however, just how serious his illness was. It was to Little Nancy that Mike confided his deepest concerns and feelings. To her he could say that he felt like he was dying when, during the first week in the hospital, his white count skyrocketed to 100,000 (a normal white count is from 4,000 to 10,000). In the midst of this crisis, while we were anxiously waiting for the shot of Donnamycin to bring the white count down, Michael and Little Nancy remained cool and calm. I remember feeling worried and depressed as I went to the hospital to visit the two of them and, after seeing them playing cards together, deeply engrossed in their game, coming away feeling relieved and encouraged. During the day, every day of that month, from the start of visiting hours at 10:00 a.m. until 8:30 in the evening, Little Nancy was at Michael's bedside. She nursed him, read to him, played cards and games with him, and encouraged him to keep going. And, indeed he did; his own courage and morale were equally amazing. Michael and Nancy became an inspiration to all of us and won the respect and love of the doctors and nurses as well. During a later crisis after the white count had come down when Mike was still quite weak, I spent three nights with him in the hospital; Little Nancy's mother, Myrna, spent another and my friend, Sheila Spaulding, likewise stayed with him a night.

When Mike was discharged from the hospital on July 28, it seemed quite natural for Little Nancy to move in with us and so she did. What a help she was in caring for Michael and in providing companionship for him. Mike made a remarkable recovery, gaining weight and approaching total remission as his blood returned to a near-normal count. However, as the doctor later put it, "Leukemic cells remained somewhere in his body" even though none were detected in the bone marrow. By early September Mike was well enough to go to school and so began classes at Ravenswood High School as a junior. The doctor scheduled a splenectomy for Mike (since the spleen frequently harbors leukemic cells). The day before the operation, Mike's blood count suddenly took a wrong turn, causing the doctor to cancel the operation. Anticipating a relapse, the doctor scheduled a series of radiation treatments on the spleen instead. These went on for 3 weeks during which time Mike continued to look and feel well. The relapse was slow in getting started. By the end of October, Mike's white count was up sufficiently to warrant putting him in the hospital for medication as before. Again, although she was now going to school, Little Nancy spent every available minute at Mike's bedside. I had been granted a sabbatical that school year and thus did not have to teach. I had started going to California State University at San Francisco for an administrative credential. My classes didn't begin till either 4:00 or 7:00 p.m. so my days were free. As soon as Little Nancy was through with school, I would pick her up and take her to the hospital where she'd spend the rest of the day with Michael. Later in the day on my way to class, I would take some food to Michael and Nancy. This time Michael was not nauseated and was able to eat. Since he didn't like hospital food, I would prepare or buy something he did like and take it to him and Nancy. Later in the evening, Nancy's mother would pick Nancy up from the hospital. Again, Mike was in the hospital about a month, this time getting three dosages of the experimental drug that had worked so well the first time to bring his white count down. However, it seemed that this time Mike was building up a tolerance to the medication and that each time his white count went down in response to the drug, it would nevertheless start to climb back up again. Finally, the white count was pushed down quite low and Michael came home in time for Thanksgiving at Myrna's house, which we all enjoyed so much. During his second stay in the hospital Mike had used a total of 83 units of blood, all replaced by donations.

However, about a week after Thanksgiving Mike's white count suddenly went from a low of 700 to 7,000 in just one day. Michael, who was home just for the day, was feeling both nauseated and depressed. He talked to Little Nancy about being "tired of being sick" and said, "he wanted to go away someplace." That same day he took Nancy for a ride on his motorcycle, and showed her how to ride it. The next morning Mike returned to the hospital. His white count had gone up to 100,000, as high as it had been the summer before. That Tuesday evening the doctor gave Mike another dose of Donnamycin. If it were to take effect, it would do so by Thursday. Mike asked if Little Nancy could stay with him all night in the hospital. By this time Nancy had gained the respect of the hospital staff, and she was allowed to stay.

The next morning, Wednesday, Mike's vision was slightly blurred, causing him to see double images in the distance. For all that he was still in remarkably good spirits. And even Little Nancy decided to go to class so I picked her up at the hospital and took her to school. Later, I picked her up again at school and took her back to the hospital. By Wednesday evening, Mike's white count was up to 230,000. Again, at Michael's request, Nancy stayed at the hospital all night with him. Even though we all had the foreboding thought that the end was near, we still hoped for some miracle to happen, that the medication would work again as it had the first time.

Thursday morning the nurse called me to say that Michael had had a bad night and was having trouble breathing. I went right over to the hospital and from there called my family and friends who soon joined us at the hospital. I also called Michael's father, Yuri, who was in Toronto. He decided not to come right away but to keep in touch by phone. A clear plastic respiratory device was put over Mike's nose to give him more oxygen. The bed was also propped up to aid his breathing. Mike's sense of humor was still in evidence: at one point, when the respiratory device irritated him, he picked the device up, put it on his ear, and smiled at us. We all cracked up. By mid-morning there were eleven of us who had gathered together to keep a vigil. Little Nancy kept her constant watch and hardly ever left Michael's side. The rest of us took turns being with Michael, usually four to six of us at a time, just quietly watching, standing, or sitting close together, feeling certainly the awe of death but also sensing the energy and love that flowed to and from Michael and among all of us. By early afternoon Michael slipped into unconsciousness. He had been given sedatives as well as 4 units of blood to make him more comfortable. By this time the white count was up to 360,000. Since Mike's pajama top had been removed because of his fever, we could literally see his heart pounding quite fast and strongly; likewise he was breathing fast and deeply. The doctor assured me he was not in pain—he was so heavily sedated. But even while in such a deep state of unconsciousness, Little Nancy could feel Michael's hand squeezing hers from time to time. In addition to Little Nancy, Myrna, and me, the watchers included Tanya, my good friend, Sheila Spaulding, my brother, Phil, and his wife, Randi, my father, Michael's aunt, Jeanne Larkin, and two young friends of Michael, Jeff Miller and Tara Bonner. When we were not gathered at Mike's bedside, we would visit with each other in the hall around a couch and a coffee table. Here I first thought of the idea of doing our own memorial service for Mike at Peninsula School.

At about 5:30 in the evening my father, thinking that Michael might live another 24 hours or more, left the hospital. And later in the evening, at around 7:30, I decided to go home for a few hours rest. Tanya and Myrna also left the hospital at about the same time with the intention of returning again soon. As I left the hospital and walked toward my car, I said aloud, "All right, so be it. Now let it come quickly, peacefully, and painlessly." And so it seemed to be. After I'd been home for 20 minutes, my phone rang. It was Sheila telling me that Michael's breathing and heartbeat were both slowing down, that the end was probably near, and that I should come back to the hospital. So I went to get Tanya and Myrna and all three of us returned. When we reached the hospital, Sheila and the nurses were in the hall telling us that Michael had just passed away and that he'd gone very peacefully. I went in to say good-bye to Michael and remember thinking to myself how beautiful he looked, that his dead body was neither frightening nor repulsive. I thought to myself, *Death isn't so bad.* Most of us I guess are indeed afraid of death. I certainly have been. I've been very possessive of my own life. But seeing Michael go so beautifully and knowing that he'd lived such a full, well-loved life in his 16 years, I felt more courage to face my own death.

It was only after Michael passed away that Little Nancy gave in to her grief and wept. We let her have 15 or so minutes alone with Michael. Then, very gently, Myrna and I led Little Nancy from the hospital room. For a while Tanya and Myrna sat with her in the hall while we all comforted each other. Finally, we all went home. Little Nancy went home to her mother's house where, after taking a tranquillizer, she finally fell asleep. My brother, Phil, and his wife, Randi, came home with me.

The next day, Friday, December 7, Tanya, Sheila, Little Nancy, and Myrna gathered at my house to make plans for Mike's funeral. Although drained and low in spirits, Little Nancy was all right; she was holding together. Kaiser Hospital agreed to hold Michael's body till the following Monday. In the meantime, an autopsy was performed that showed that it was the leukemia alone that had killed Michael. He showed no signs of major infection nor internal bleeding—a fact that amazed the doctors. His body was essentially strong and in good health; it was the leukemia alone that was responsible for his death.

On Monday, December 10, a lovely day, eighteen of us gathered in the afternoon and went to the hospital to get Michael. From the hospital we took Michael in his beautiful handmade casket to the cemetary in the hills of Palo Alto. It was the loveliest route lined with many trees bearing autumn leaves. Again, we all felt so close to each other, united by our love for Michael. Little Nancy found much comfort in her relationship with Tanya, a relationship that was now becoming closer. Phil's young wife, Randi, was a wonderful source of comfort also, especially to the young people. Leaving Michael at the cemetary, we all returned to my house for supper together. Michael's aunt had prepared a wonderful lentil soup and bread for us that we shared. Although feeling our sorrow over Mike, again our love for each other seemed enhanced and we spent the evening eating, talking, and even had moments of gentle gaiety together. Never, in all of this was there a moment of morbidity or hysteria. We cried together to be sure and felt much pain in our loss. But, as I've tried to tell my friends, I would never have believed that death could be so beautiful. The awareness that Michael's life had been so full of love was a constant source of comfort to me. In these past few weeks I have realized that indeed Michael was very well loved by very many people throughout his life. And I am so grateful to lovely Nancy Siegel for loving my son so well. He had much happiness in the few months before his death because of her.

The following Saturday, December 15, we had our own memorial service for Mike. I called it simply, "A Tribute to Michael" and we held it at Peninsula School, an old alternative school where Mike had spent 2 happy years in the seventh and eighth grades. I had prepared eight large posters with pictures of Michael through the years as well as pictures of Nancy Siegel, Yuri, Tanya, Natasha, my father, mother, grandmother, and two brothers, Philip and Sheldon, Michael's friends, and several scenes of Lagunitas, Marin County, where my grandmother's cabin is located and where we also plan to bury Michael's ashes. Again, it was a beautiful day and as the many people came, I had a chance to greet them on the porch of the school. I was pleased that

Michael's doctor, Dr. Barkin, was able to attend. We closed the tribute with a few moments of silence and then went into an adjoining room for Russian tea and breads of various kinds. It was a very moving and meaningful experience for me, one that left me feeling at peace with my acceptance of Michael's death. There was even a kind of joy present—again from the great sense of love that seemed to prevail.

The last thing we did for Michael was bury his ashes on our property at Lagunitas, Marin County (because the land is in an unincorporated area, this is permissible), and plant a small tree near Michael's grave. We have also established a memorial fund with the American Cancer Society where donations can be made in Michael's name and specified for leukemia research.

In closing, I can only say that it is the quality of our lives that matters, not the quantity. Michael seems to have given and received more love in his short 16 years than many of us have in our longer lives. I am very proud and happy to have had such a son.

SUPPORT OF MEDICAL STAFF

As a postscript to the story of my son's death, I want to say a few words about the role our physician, Dr. Alan Barkin, played throughout Michael's battle with leukemia. Both his attitude and that of other Kaiser Hospital staff members were important in helping us cope with Michael's illness and eventual death.

First of all, as soon as I knew of Michael's illness, I had an overwhelming need to trust the doctor, to feel free to ask any and all questions of him, and to expect honest, forthright answers. Being essentially a trusting person, I did just that. And indeed, he responded to my trust with honesty.

As Michael faced his first crisis in early July, with his life hanging in the balance, Dr. Barkin told me that his case did not warrant much optimism, that it would be "a matter of days" if his body did not respond to the Donnamycin, that his father should come from Toronto as soon as possible. These were all statements in response to my direct questions. As hard as it was for Dr. Barkin to say them and as hard as it was for me to hear them, communicating the truth was the best policy. I felt better knowing the truth. It told me just how hard we would have to fight. And, since Dr. Barkin had left the door open for the possibility of the Donnamycin halting the spread of the white cells, all of us put our energy and faith into making that possibility a reality. Again, it was important to us to know that Dr. Barkin appreciated and allowed our will and determination to fight the disease in spite of the very gloomy prognosis. I remember thinking when I first heard the news of Michael's illness, "No son of mine is going to die, not if I have anything to do with it."

As far as Michael was concerned, Dr. Barkin explained to me that it was his policy to answer only those questions that Michael himself might ask but not to offer information he did not ask for. Dr. Barkin also made this clear to Michael's girl friend, Nancy Siegel, who asked her own share of questions and who also received honest answers. Michael did seem to want to know the truth about himself and shared his innermost concerns with both Dr. Barkin and Nancy.

It was also of great importance to us that Dr. Barkin was compassionate, caring, and calm. He was always available and was very sensitive to Michael's personal welfare, and his need to enjoy life as much as possible. He saw to it that, whenever possible, Michael spent time at home rather than at the hospital. Dr. Barkin also came to welcome the constant presence of Nancy in Michael's hospital room. The devotion of these two 16-year-olds to one another was taken seriously and respected. I remember Dr. Barkin saying about Nancy that, "He'd never seen anyone like her." At another time he told me that it was good to see a family that was "so much together." In other words, Dr. Barkin's expressed sensitivity to the love that all of us felt for Michael increased our trust in him and helped us to cope.

Further, Dr. Barkin and the other staff members at Kaiser Hospital showed their empathy by occasionally stretching certain hospital rules. For instance, having fourteen visitors in Michael's hospital room the night of July 4 was overlooked (though later cautioned against!) as was our often staying a half-hour past visiting hours at night. For the two nights preceding Michael's death, Little Nancy was given permission to stay with him in his hospital room all night. Likewise, on the day that Michael died, the twelve of us who kept vigil all day, felt free to come and go to his hospital room and to use the adjoining lounge area. Never did the doctors or nurses make us feel that we were in the way. Thus, was Michael allowed to have a death of dignity and love. I remember being struck by the feeling that Michael's hospital room was charged with tremendous energy. It was as if intense love were being passed from person to person and between Michael and each one of us. It was truly awesome and I cannot imagine his death happening otherwise. It seemed so natural. We acted as if we had the right to be there, as many of us at a time as we wanted. Yet, it was only after Michael's passing that the doctor told me that Kaiser Hospital had changed its policy only a year and a half before, that previously relatives and friends of dying patients had not been accorded the freedom we had experienced. Again, for that freedom I am deeply grateful.

Lastly, I would like to offer a bit of humble advice to those members of the medical profession who must deal with dying patients and their families. Perhaps many doctors and nurses already know it but it came as a beautiful shock to me from Michael himself, and that is simply that death is not so bad and that we can and should have more trust in the patient's own ability to cope with terminal illness. I remember watching Michael the week before his death as his condition worsened each day. At first there were signs of depression and anger and a certain recklessness about him, almost as if he were courting death, wishing to get it over with. He spoke of "being tired of being sick" and of "wanting to go away someplace." After 5 months he was tired of fighting leukemia and seemed to be making the conscious choice to give in to the disease. When he told me he wanted to take Little Nancy out on a ride on his motorcycle and I expressed concern for his safety, he quickly assured me that everything would be all right and not to worry. It was only later, after he had died, that Little Nancy revealed to us that Michael had actually contemplated suicide on the ride, but, since this had upset her, he had dropped the idea. Still, as if knowing that death was imminent, he began planning with Little Nancy who should inherit his guitar, his coin collection, and his other prized possessions.

As his condition worsened, Michael entered the hospital for the last time 3 days before he died. I felt helpless as I watched Michael and Little Nancy coping with what now seemed inevitable. Yet, neither of them fell apart or became hysterical or morbid. Somehow I knew I could trust the two of them to face whatever would happen. Little Nancy did not lose her composure but continued to minister to Michael's needs.

Then, on the morning of the day he died, I sensed a change in Michael's attitude. Gone were the fear, anger, and depression. Instead, he was his usual sweet, unassuming, lovable self. When I first saw him that morning, I thought, *My God, my son knows he's going to die and look at him.* I did not say much to him at first, just smiled and held his hand. I felt like I was giving him a diploma for carrying off his own death so beautifully. And, indeed during the next 12 hours we all witnessed a beautiful death.

Now, 3½ years later, I find I am still positively affected by Michael's death. I sense his spirit in my daily life and take much comfort in just thinking about him. Whenever I am faced with an uptight situation I recall Michael and can almost hear him saying, "Be cool Mom, relax, you can do it." And I think to myself, *If Michael could face his death I guess I can face my life.* Furthermore, instead of totally losing Michael, I feel as if he belongs to us forever. In conclusion, death itself is not the worst thing that can happen to a person. A life without love is far worse. It is my hope that all of us including members of the medical profession will begin to see the wisdom of this truth.

Chapter 11

Dr. Strauss' Last Teaching Session

Walter Hollander, Jr.
T. Franklin Williams

In writing about the late Dr. Maurice B. Strauss, others have rightly stressed his extraordinary role as a teacher.[1, 2] It seems worthwhile to record the substance of what was probably his last "teaching session," which occurred with the two of us—both students of his throughout our medical careers—less than a week before he died.

As is generally known, the inoperable esophageal carcinoma that led to Dr. Strauss' death was only diagnosed when pain in the upper part of his chest and variable fever developed in February 1974. For several weeks thereafter, he was in such severe pain and was at times so mentally clouded as a result of the pain (and probably the high fever) that he avoided all direct contacts with anyone other than his wife and his immediate physicians. He remained at home, as was his strong desire, and spent what time he could arranging his affairs and writing friends about various matters, including frank discussions of his illness without pretense or sentimentality about its inevitable outcome. By the second week of April, however, he was feeling sufficiently better (for reasons described below) to agree to a visit from us when it was proposed. Accordingly, we arranged to spend as much of the afternoon of Saturday, April 13, with him as seemed appropriate.

Reprinted from *Archives of Internal Medicine,* **135**:1391–1392, October 1975.

Maurie talked with us for about two hours, sitting in the living room of his apartment overlooking the Boston Common. We had heard that he had lost weight, but it was hardly evident. He seemed in good spirits—no different, in fact, than as usual in prior times. Although hoarse, he spoke effectively most of the time and otherwise communicated in writing. Indeed, when he entered the room, he handed us a number of sheets of paper to read, mainly the detailed written records and charts he had kept of his hour-by-hour signs, symptoms, and treatment since soon after his illness had manifested itself. Characteristically, too, he expressed a lively enthusiasm and full commitment to what was a thoroughly lucid discussion of the topic under consideration. From the outset, and by his clear determination, that topic was his illness.

After we left, both of us were aware that the meeting had been a profound experience. Although we discovered later that our reactions had differed in certain limited respects, we agreed that, in addition to its emotional impact, the visit had also been one more valuable teaching session with Maurie. It had involved certain vivid lessons that we thought we would like to share with others, as we believe Maurie would be pleased to have us do. Ruth Strauss fully concurred when we discussed the possibility with her.

Rather than reviewing all the details of Maurie's perceptive analysis of his illness and its management, we would like simply to report several noteworthy highlights that are applicable to patients generally, not just to those who are, themselves, knowledgeable physicians.

The single most important item concerned a patient's right to participate as actively as possible—and with all pertinent information at his disposal—in decisions relating to the management of his terminal illness. Maurie told us briefly but with much forcefulness how, once his diagnosis was confirmed (followed by an apparently futile course of irradiation) and once the near certainty of his fairly imminent death was apparent, he insisted on a meeting of all his physicians, together with his wife and himself. At that meeting, he said he tried to make certain that his physicians understood his own views and agreed to be guided by them. One such view was his determination to avoid all heroic last-ditch stands, such as bypass surgery, intravenous alimentation, transfusions, and resuscitation efforts. Another was his very firm wish to avoid hospitalization so that he could live out his remaining days in the familiar and satisfying setting of his own apartment. He pointed out to us how many times he would inevitably have been disturbed—precisely because he would have had well-intentioned physicians and nurses—by uncomfortable and debilitating diagnostic procedures every time his fever spiked or some other of the many changes in his clinical course occurred had he been in any modern medical center hospital during the previous six weeks. Finally, he and his physicians determined that henceforth the single primary goal of therapy was to be his comfort. His family's acceptance of these decisions clearly was also an essential factor. Here Maurie, the patient, was (whether consciously or not) teaching us, his professional colleagues, about the patient's right to know his condition if he so wished, to discuss his future with any and all of his physicians in some organized and sensible fashion, and to make his own final decisions.

Second was our discussion of the control of pain. It seemed clear that Maurie wished, as do most people, to face death with dignity and self-respect, and there is no doubt that he did do so courageously. However, the extreme pain he had experienced during much of the preceding month or more, together with an awareness of his intermittently confused mental state, had apparently stripped him bare of these vital attributes that are so essential for any human being to face himself, much less others. Accordingly, it was of major importance to him that the pain be adequately controlled, and when we saw him, this had been accomplished. Earlier in his course, in the way many physicians prescribe and patients take potent analgesics, Maurie had delayed administration of opiates until pain became moderately severe. However, on that routine, each new dose took too long to work; within an hour or so afterwards, the pain would be even more severe, requiring a second injection that still did not provide adequate relief. Moreover, the second dose would often lead to several hours of somnolence, and thus a cycle of severe pain and mental depression was set up that was totally unsatisfactory. When we saw him, a change in his schedule had eliminated the problem: he was then receiving morphine routinely every four hours by the clock, which was preventing the pain without noticeably depressive side effects. When this more effective and satisfying approach was described by one of us to an eminent pharmacologist, he commented that he thought too few clinicians know how to use opiates successfully for their primary purpose, prevention and control of pain, particularly in terminally ill persons. Obviously, here was another lesson, this one regarding the proper management of pain. In addition, however, there was an even more important message: namely, that successful control of severe pain is of paramount importance in the management of patients with painful terminal illness and that, in frequently failing to provide it, we physicians deny our patients the opportunity to face death or even to face their family and close friends with self-respect and dignity.

Another matter almost surely relating to the control of pain, as well as to his periods of disorientation and incoherence, was the recognition that an active infectious mediastinitis, rather than side effects of irradiation or the cancer itself, was causing his high fever and contributing to his chest pain. He showed us his home-made temperature chart, which displayed increased fever during and following irradiation but, more importantly, a dramatic return to near normal soon after antibiotic therapy was initiated. Furthermore, the subsidence of fever was associated with mental clearing and a considerable decrease in chest pain.

An additional lesson related to the problem of adequate nutrition for the patient with dysphagia and whose esophagus was, as Maurie put it all too vividly, probably acting in part merely as a sieve into the mediastinum. For many weeks, Maurie had had great difficulty swallowing and could still only take liquids after the mediastinitis had subsided. As already noted, he had ruled firmly against gastrostomy or intravenous feeding; accordingly, recalling the high caloric value of ethanol, he devised his own oral liquid diet consisting of enough gin to provide 1,000 calories, mixed with enough orange juice to make a total daily intake of 1,200 calories. He sipped this very slowly without apparent discomfort or side effects while the three of us talked. To this he added one or two soft eggs each day to provide protein. On this regimen he had turned his previously downhill weight curve around during the preceding two to three weeks with a gain of 2 lb. In view of this, it was ironic and unfortunate that, since soon after his illness became apparent, and for no obvious reason, Maurie had totally lost his taste for any alcoholic beverage—and for his pipe—so that neither of these could any longer even provide diversionary value, nor could he swallow enough of the gin mixture at one time for its analgesic action to be useful.

Finally, there is a disruptive socioeconomic aspect of illness that Maurie also used his own case to illustrate, this involving one of the many absurd features of third-party payment for medical care. He pointed out that during the early part of his illness, there was a period of daily radiotherapy, which, since he insisted on living at home, required a round-trip taxi ride costing about $2. As he noted, it would have been easy to justify his admission to the medical center on several grounds, in which case the full cost of his care would have been paid by Medicare and other carriers. In fact, however, as he pointed out, there is no provision for paying the cost of transportation for a patient living at home and receiving hospital-based treatment, a factor that undoubtedly forces many patients to accept otherwise undesired and often undesirable hospitalization when their home is far enough from the medical center to make transportation financially burdensome.

Maurie lived six more days, then died (at home as he had wished). His own book, *Familiar Medical Quotations*,[3] has provided us with two apt quotations with which to end this commentary. One is from *Lectures on the Duties and Qualifications of a Physician*, by John Gregory (1725-1773): "It is as much the business of a physician to alleviate pain, and to smooth the avenues of death, when unavoidable, as to cure diseases."[3] (p.408) The other is anonymous and reads: "There is a dignity in dying that doctors should not dare to deny."[3] (p. 87)

REFERENCES

1   Papper S.: "Maurice B. Strauss, MD." *N Engl J Med* 291:47–48, 1974.
2   "Dr. M. B. Strauss, noted teacher, dies in Boston." *JAMA* 229:259, 1974.
3   Strauss M.B. (ed.): *Familiar Medical Quotations*. Boston, Little Brown & Co, 1968.

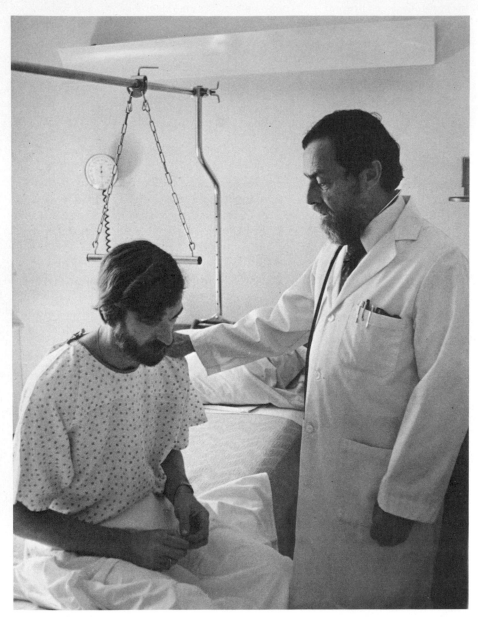

Courtesy of Katrin Achelis

Part Four

Doctor-Patient Relationships: Emotional Impact

Chapter 12

Treating the Dying—
the Doctor vs.
the Man Within the Doctor

Eric J. Cassell

In January of this year, I was asked to care for an 86-year-old man who had been admitted to the hospital on January 4th because of a stroke. He was aphasic and had severe right hemiparesis. These difficulties did not improve in the subsequent week. In the six months prior to admission, the family said, his health had been failing. Previously vigorous, his memory and mentation progressively declined so that before his stroke he was a failed old man. The neurologist, considering the progressive nature of his illness, raised the possibility of tumor and scheduled an angiogram for January 11th. The family indicated that no matter what the angiogram revealed, they would not consent to surgery.

Friday evening, the 7th, the patient developed a temperature of 103°F. and became comatose. I was not called, and on making rounds the next day read the events on the chart. The intern diagnosed pneumonia and ordered three blood cultures, nose, throat, and sputum cultures and a urine culture from the catheter. IV's were started and an appropriate dose of ampicillin added to the infusion.

I was distressed that antimicrobial therapy had been started that might delay the "acute, short, not often painful illness by which the old man escapes those 'cold degredations of decay.' " I started to write orders discontinuing his antibiotics and found

Reprinted from *Medical Dimensions*, 1:6–7, 11, 22, March 1972.

myself hesitating to do so—a hesitancy at odds with my belief that there is a time for everyone and that the time had come for this old man, giving me no right to interfere. I saw from the front of the chart that he was allergic to penicillin (these things happen) and with relief at the excuse, wrote the order stopping the ampicillin.

NO COMMON LANGUAGE

Two days later I asked the intern why she had treated the patient's pneumonia. In our discussion of the clinical problem we shared a common language and syntax and a common understanding of pathology and process. In the part of the discussion in which I suggested that it would have been better *not* to have started antibiotics—that it was one of her functions as a physician to allow a graceful death—our mutual comprehension ceased. We seemed to have no common language and no common understanding.

The case is not unusual and illustrates the dilemma that increasingly confronts us. The public cries increasingly that physicians seem more concerned with disease and science than with their patients. We ourselves have difficulty with what seem to be basic decisions.

Let us return to the case. Clinical experience is in conflict with the intern's actions. The overwhelming probability is that this 86-year-old man will soon die no matter what is done. There *are* miracles. Such patients do sometimes recover and live for months—institutionalized, with accumulating problems of incontinence and decubiti, infection and neglect. Further, there are few among us who would choose that slowly eroding death for ourselves or our parents. And yet the decision not to treat the pneumonia seems difficult for many physicians—particularly the younger ones (or even older ones in the glare of the hospital setting).

Let us dismiss the usual excuses promptly. *Malpractice:* I do not know of a single case in which the courts have decided against a physician who omitted further treatment in a terminal situation. *Playing God:* One no more plays God in withholding treatment than in giving treatment. By training and technological advance and with public consent, we have been given great power. With such power goes the need for professional judgment and responsibility. Abdicating in the name of God when such responsibility is most demanded is simple hypocrisy. *We've had no training in dealing with such problems:* That is not an excuse, that is fact. Guidance and experience are considered necessary in making difficult clinical decisions, but in these decisions—the most difficult of all—most of us have had little guidance and less training.

What are the problems that face us? When are we prolonging life and when are we merely prolonging death? Is there a difference between allowing death and killing? Is the quality of survival as important as the length of survival? And, finally, and perhaps most central, are we required to save life at any cost?

These are not new questions but have been given immediacy by our increasing technological power. For decades these basic questions have been avoided by resorting to the technological "fix"—another technical solution to solve the problem. If one has any question that those days of simply technical solutions are over, let him make rounds in a typical nursing home.

I cannot offer the answers to these questions, and, from my own hesitancy in discontinuing the antimicrobials, it must be clear that I myself remain in conflict. Nor do I know any source from which we can find immediate answers.

I would like to suggest, however, that there are ways of examining the problem and ways of talking together—as we do for so many other clinical problems—that can indeed help us.

It is important to remember that people come to us so that we can make them better; and, if we have come to a point where, in so doing, we are making a significant number worse—worse even in the face of the fact that the alternative is death—then there is good reason to take a hard look at the very basis for treatment.

However, if factors other than the patient's disease are going to enter thoughtful treatment choices, we should be able to understand the system from which these other factors come and how they are derived.

ILLNESS VS. DISEASE

When men become sick, they are sick in two distinctly different dimensions. In each sick person there is both an illness and a disease.

The illness is made up of the things patients feel and the meaning given to those feelings.

The disease occurs in that system of structural and biochemical alterations by which disease is diagnosed. As the illness is what the patient feels, the disease is what he has.

Sometimes the disease is considered the real part, the *illness only psychological and therefore less real. Such a distinction is not merely oversimplified but also is not true.* We tend to think and behave as though disease represents abstract truth; and while indeed it may, it is not the presence or absence of something that counts to us, but rather its meaning. The assignment of meaning—that is, giving precedence to the disease over illness—is a cultural decision, consonant with the growth and importance of science and technology throughout western culture.

As the culture gives meaning to things, it also assigns relative values. In its systems of care for the sick, our culture has assigned value to the presence of disease and has not assigned equivalent values to the presence of illness per se.

None the less, to most, the dimension of disease is largely theoretical (when did most of us last "see" a virus), while the dimension of illness is real. It is where men truly live.

Treatment decisions in the dimension of disease are generally based upon objective findings, and objectivity implies the absence of value judgments. It is important to note the implication that objective criteria are free of the disadvantages of humanness and human values.

Treatment choices based in the dimension of illness are generally subjective and, as such, are steeped in value judgments and human values and, because of that, are generally considered both unmeasurable and undesirable.

It is obvious that the two dimensions overlap—if they did not, disease would be a very poor explanation for illness—but they are not identical.

TREATMENT-RELATED ILLNESS

This is important to remember because in many diseases, especially in cancer, the determination of clinical status includes measurement of both improvement in the disease and the deterioration of the host due to treatment. There often comes to be two distinct illnesses: that secondary to the disease and that secondary to treatment. Both illnesses may feel the same to the patient, but they are given different value by the physician. Often the patient accepts the meaning given to the illness of treatment by the physician.

For example, the two illnesses are present with every surgical procedure. In ordinary or well-known operations the usual patient from our culture readily accepts the treatment illness as necessary to recovery. But we have become sufficiently sophisticated to be aware of the difficulties involved in trying to get patients from variant cultural backgrounds to accept the illness of treatment.

When we see a resentful sick patient unable to understand or accept his new treatment-related cluster of symptoms, we see why it is necessary to understand the process as a separate illness rather than to designate the symptoms as "side effects" or even "untoward side effects."

Furthermore, it is generally illness, not disease, that sends our patients to us in the first place. The patient brings us his symptoms, how he feels, we give him the disease. As an event in a complex life, illness is also surrounded by events in other lives, and so when sickness is profound, as in cancer or stroke, there may be, in addition to the patient's illness, an equally important illness of the family.

OBJECTIVE CRITERIA IN EVALUATING DISEASE

Our objective criteria for the evaluation of disease seem to offer the advantage of being separate from and free of human value. The advantage is more apparent than real. Ideally, objective criteria are free of human value only when we don't weigh one objective criterion more than another by adding human meaning to it. In fact, however, objective criteria are derived from human values. For example, in our society health is highly valued and human life even more highly valued, and the objective measures of life and health serve those values. *But it is a technological perversion of human values when the objective measurements meant to support them are dealt with as though the value is inherent in the measurement.* Thus, while a low serum sodium may threaten life, life is not merely a normal serum sodium, nor is it merely the presence of pulse, respiration, or even an intact electroencephalogram.

This confusion permeates and dangerously threatens medicine today. Objective criteria thus perverted are the entrance to a wondrous fairyland of medicine, free of the heavy responsibility of value judgment, a scientific playground, if you will. Unfortunately, that is not the real world nor the world of our patients. In the world in which we live, we are subject to the real doctor's dilemma—objectivity vs. empathy— and it is to that dilemma that we must address ourselves.

Knowing and crediting the concerns, fears and aspirations of patients and their families provide information as pertinent to therapeutic decisions as do the so-called objective criteria. But this knowledge requires understanding the subjective. Decades have been spent in avoiding the problem, in trying to find alternative objective measurements that when added together would somehow total the subjective.

There lie the two, thus far failed, promises of science—ultimate understanding of process and value-free decision. Just accepting the fact that neither promise is liable to be fulfilled is the first step out of our dilemma.

INFORMATION GATHERING

It should be clear by now that decisions based solely on information related to the patient's disease are being made on only part of the necessary information. But even allowing that all of this is true, how can we bring the important subjective information, unmeasurable as it is, into the decision-making process?

First, it is necessary to understand that because something is unmeasurable in usual scientific terms does not mean that it is unknowable or even that it cannot be given some order.

The characteristics of the subjective that give concern in illness can be systematized. There are, first, disordered feelings based in physiological distress: pain, hiccough, and dyspnea are examples. Second, there are disordered social feelings: the sense of being a threat to the group, of being foul in our impingement upon others by sight, smell, or sound, and the fear of being, as a consequence, cast out by the group. Feelings about illness or pain in our loved ones fall within this group. The behavior and feelings in tuberculous patients as described in Thomas Mann's *The Magic Mountain* are another example of disordered social feelings.

Finally, there are disorders of vanity: the self we compare with ourselves, noting the loss of our previous powers, previous looks, previous loves—to name a few. Although unable to evaluate the degree of distress, we all can recognize both the basis of the distress—that is, the system in which it occurs—and the theoretical validity of the distress—its right to be present.

There are only three sources of information from which to obtain a measure of the degree of distress the patient feels: the patient himself, ourselves the physicians, and the group around us.

The patient seems the obvious source from which to obtain a valuation of his distress. However, as physicians we know it is not that easy. If we wish to know *what* the patient feels, only he can tell us, but the question *how* do you feel *about* something is distinctly different; it is a question of relative values. The patient when he is well can assign relative values to hypothetical questions about himself when sick, but he cannot "imagine," in the physiological sense, the situation he will be in when sick. It doesn't take too much clinical experience to know the difficulty of doing for the sick person what he asked you to do when he was well. Furthermore, the sick person reasons in a manner qualitatively different than the well person and may be unable to assign relative value in a useful way. So, in absolute terms, the patient cannot always provide the value measurement and choice needed for his own treatment.

If the physician uses himself in assigning relative value, he can recognize the validity and basis for the distress and, were he to allow it, would find the resonance within himself that the patient's distress produces useful in assigning relative value to the different courses of treatment open to him. However, aside from the personal emotional cost, the battle of empathy and objectivity within the doctor makes his being the only assigner of values fraught with danger. (The unique place of physicians would be enhanced and the dangers lessened if doctors learn to work together to deal with these problems as they have with the objective aspects of disease.)

The use of the surrounding group to establish values has distinct advantages. It represents, properly selected, sufficient numbers to produce the objectivity of universality. It is also free from the physiological counter-demands of illness-pain. Group values change and thus represent the important outcome of the interplay between universal physiological demands and changing social mores. That lack of constancy is not as disadvantageous as it may seem, because such change is the characteristic of human values. The disadvantages of using the group values are basically those of all sample choices, but, as such, they are relatively well known and well worked out.

Any system that attempts to measure and assign human values in the evaluation of the subjective (illness as opposed to disease) must use all three factors—the patient, the physician, and the group—to test the correctness of the findings.

Part of the difficulty is that, for the discussion of values and the subjective elements of sickness, no boundaries have been established. Physicians have no language or syntax specific to the problem.

THE LIMITS OF PROFESSIONAL CONCERN

In discussing my patient with the intern, for example, we understood each other as long as our conversation was restricted to the patient's disease. We stumbled and failed when we tried to discuss those subjective elements that should have entered the treatment decision. We did have a common understanding of the family's desire that the patient undergo no undue distress. Also, we both had feelings about how we should like death to come to us and to ours. But this common understanding did not seem to be part of our shared professional interest, but rather only a private matter. But what we find out when we examine ourselves, our patients, and our group values is worthy of our *professional* effort.

When we start looking at illness afresh, we are not merely involved in fitting something else into our old biological frame. We are working in a different frame with a different language, and we must view this different language with equal professional seriousness.

An example pertinent to the case cited at the beginning of this article is how laymen and physicians differ in their definition of the dying patient.

Physicians tend to define the dying patient as one for whom they can do nothing. Given the example of an adult with acute leukemia, they may say he is dying whether he has symptoms or not and whether he knows it or not. Laymen react differently. Whether the man with leukemia is seen by them as dying depends on whether he knows what he has and how he reacts to the knowledge. Social and emotional factors enter into their determination as they recognize a state of being dying. For our patients and their families there is, in other words, an illness called dying. That illness is something the dying person has to offer the living, giving them the chance to accept what is coming. In the case presented, interfering with and prolonging the inevitable by treating the pneumonia prolonged both the death of the patient and the illness of dying in which the family participated.

But even allowing for all this, how can we make all the moral decisions that the world expects of us and for which we seem so poorly trained? Medicine is a pragmatic profession—we do not generally make global decisions. We treat each case as it comes along, realizing that knowledge is imperfect but trying, as it seems expected of us, to meet some larger set of standards. Here, too, knowledge is imperfect, and it is the larger set of standards of which we are most unsure.

We have come to realize the importance of these non disease elements in our work because of painful experience. We have, by virtue of that common experience, a shared community of insight to bring to bear on our problems. It is time to sit down together in what is essentially moral discourse, testing the particular case that troubles us against the general problem.

By sitting together I mean just that. Small groups of house staff and attending physicians—perhaps no more than 10 or so at a time. Stay rooted in specific cases, and, although the general problem seems too vague and unsolvable, the bases for decision will emerge. There are others to help, the clergy and philosophers—it won't hurt them either to see the pain of individual decisions in the real world.

Human survival is something larger than the survival of the individual—call it culture, or values, or what have you. We know that for ourselves, and we must extend it to our patients as part of our profession if we are ever to end the widening gap between the doctor and the man within the doctor.

Chapter 13

Help for the Young Physician with Death and Grieving

Morris D. Kerstein

The medical profession is so oriented as to circumvent, postpone, or meliorate death. Trapped by the direction of early medical education, the physician is often shocked by the inevitability of death and avoids a confrontation with its direct and indirect implications. Nevertheless, since the physician must deal with death, he develops patterns of response which enable him to function with a minimum of anxiety. Deviations reveal insufficient preparation for the reality of death. One must, therefore, question if there was a period of education for this responsibility. The doctor presides at countless deathbeds; yet, when does he get his orientation? Is it education under fire? Has he learned it from his basic family environment?

There is no formal period of education in today's society. Changes in the family structure have had a profound influence on the situation. Physicians, although encouraged to participate, appear increasingly unprepared to deal with death or to talk about it on a personal level. Several factors have contributed or reinforced this situation. Noteworthy has been the decrease in the number of families where three family generations live together. Newly married couples tend to settle in their own dwelling. Lateral mobility, the demands of executive competition, and obviously improved transportation find newlyweds often shifting cross-country from their families. The

Reprinted from *Surgery, Gynecology & Obstetrics*, **137**:479–480, September 1973.

deaths of older family members, once experienced by the group at large, are now total-ly segregated, physically and emotionally, from the younger family members. Public health accomplishments have obviously lowered the infant mortality rates and raised the age of term to the seventies. Children and families in general are, therefore, ex-posed less and less to death and the dying.

From the physician's point of view, learning the physiology of death and learning the interpersonal role of family co-ordinator following a death are two subjects not covered equally by the present medical school curriculum. The lay public relies on the physician for supportive aid and direction; he is accustomed to death as he deals with it all the time. This is an absolute fallacy. Physicians have not been trained to deal with the social and psychologic aspects of death. Exposure to an incident without the edu-cation or guidance to comprehend it produces little in the way of usable information. To be sure, the psychiatrist or psychologist and clergy could aid in this education, but it is the family physician, the internist, or the surgeon who deals with death and the dying in reality. It is he who must be educated to teach.

Rushing off to save those who are alive and need help does not mean rushing past the grieving family. It is interesting how much less attention is given to the dying patient's family when actually more is needed. Death must not be a failure for the physician and care does not terminate with the patient. It is, therefore, the responsi-bility of the attending physician to help with family transitions to roles of responsi-bility. The physician dealing with death is then the one who can and must share his experiences with interns, residents, and young practicing physicians. It is right that psychiatrists and clergy guide in medical school, but education is a co-operative effort. It is also interesting that psychiatrists seem to be the most involved, yet truly have the least experience. The clinician be he internist or surgeon sees death; it is he who must lead. He must be the teacher. Every patient who dies represents an example for study. More training programs must be designed to educate the physician to the sociologic and psychologic dimensions of death.

Once aware that the patient is not to be saved and euthanasia is not the alternative, the supportive role of comforter should be explored. There is a time when drugs are given ahead of the patient's request for pain medication. The physician caught in the usual dilemma of prolonging life must find that patient care is now on another level. The implications of the omnipotent physician being a failure in the role of healer must be irradicated, and the physician now assumes the role of comforter. The latter is a role which he can successfully carry out.

Since medical education is in a state of transition, let us use the opportunity to once again modify the curriculum. The physician is learning in depth of the physiology of death. He must be equally exposed and educated to the psychosocial aspects of the families who share the emotional intensity of death. The family must continue to function; someone must help them along the path. An awareness on the part of the physician of his role as first healer then mediator can only result in the improvement of care of the patient with a terminal disease.

Chapter 14

Elements of
Psychosocial Oncology:
Doctor-Patient Relationships
in Terminal Illness

Charles A. Garfield

INTRODUCTION

It is a sobering experience, indeed, to learn that between 1970 and 1974, 1,722,000 people died of cancer in the United States alone. Extrapolating that figure through 1975, cancer took the lives of approximately 2 million United States citizens, the equivalent of three times the population of San Francisco or fifty times the number of American citizens killed in the Vietnam war. If we assume that each terminally ill cancer patient was a member of a family of four, then in a 5-year period, an estimated 6 million grieving survivors (a group of individuals equal to one-half the population of New York City) were left to deal with the aftermath of a life-threatening illness. This army of the bereaved, often in intense emotional pain, appear to be extremely vulnerable to psychosomatic illness and the gamut of psychological distress. Despite the millions of dollars spent each year on biomedical research, the health care industry in this country is just beginning to sensitize itself to the need for developing effective psychosocial support systems for patients and families facing life-threatening illness. In the past several years, I have studied the psychological and social aspects of the dying process and attempted to develop a systematic psychosocial oncology. My colleagues and I have been in contact with many research and clinical efforts in this country

This paper is an expanded version of the author's keynote addresses presented at the First (1976) and Second (1977) National Training Conferences for Physicians on Psychosocial Care of the Dying Patient, sponsored by the Cancer Research Institute, University of California Medical Center, San Francisco.

and abroad. The primary purpose of this paper is to present some of the more salient observations we have made in our attempt to define the psychosocial issues basic to oncological practice.

I would like to begin by offering three observations central to my understanding of psychosocial oncology. (1) One learns far less about dying by interviewing several hundred patients for 30 minutes each than by spending many hours with fewer patients: In the past 3 years, I have spent 3 to 4 hours per week with each of 156 terminally ill cancer patients. Feelings about death and the process of dying, like feelings about human sexuality, are very intimate concerns that most people are unwilling to share with those constrained by the scientific rigors of a tightly designed research protocol. As one elderly man dying of lung cancer stated, "I'll be damned if I share my feelings about death and dying with anyone who makes 2-minute U-turns at the foot of my bed." (2) To date, no research or systematic clinical observation has verified any preprogrammed set of stages in the dying process; that is, researchers and practitioners have not yet empirically identified any set of linear, unidirectional, and invariant stages. Certainly many patients who are dying exhibit denial, anger, depression, and occasionally acceptance, but it is inaccurate to suppose that all individuals, regardless of belief system, age, race, culture, and historical period die in a uniform sequence. It is more likely that existing theoretical frameworks become self-fulfilling prophesies imposed by health care professionals who may coerce the dying person into conforming with a powerfully suggestive typology. I have heard nurses, in obvious distress, talk about "forcing a patient to move from stage three (bargaining) to stage four (depression)" because the patient's condition was deteriorating so fast that he or she might not have the time to reach stage five (acceptance). To needlessly add one more ponderous agenda to a patient's already heavily burdened psyche is an injustice to all concerned.* (3) There is a growing psychosocial literature, but most health care professionals pay little attention to this reservoir of information and expertise. At times, we hear statements like the following: "Why should I go to a seminar on death and dying when I work with dying people every day." This is an extremely regrettable attitude. As a psychologist, I work with individuals undergoing chemotherapy every day, but I would never assume mastery of the biochemical and pharmacological subtleties of chemotherapeutic treatment. The problems related to the psychosocial care of the terminally ill are every bit as profound and complex as those associated with medical and nursing practice. To perfunctorily dismiss psychosocial care as limited to merely chatting (or listening) for several minutes is to grossly underestimate the intricacies of human behavior and experience.

IDENTIFYING THE PROBLEM

It does seem symptomatic that few words if any are directed to medical students about how to help a patient die. House staff members may be criticized for failing

---

*Out of respect and appreciation for Elisabeth Kübler-Ross and her work I must note that she has made this point many times. With regard to all our theoretical models, I am reminded of Aristotle's observation: "Dear is Plato but dearer still is truth."

to carry out some relatively minor test or procedure, but seldom is there any evaluation of the care accorded to terminal patients' psyches during the last days. We all believe in treating the whole person and work hard at enhancing his physical and psychic comfort in small ways, which may have no influence on the final outcome of his illness, and yet it is not always noticed that a dying person very often seems to have less attention paid to him than to the patency of the multiplicity of tubes that are entering him from every direction and which will enable us to study his last, hopefully balanced, chemistries. Occasionally, it seems that more real effort is expended to get autopsy permission than to see to it that the patient does not die alone. It is as though, as doctors, we sometimes express our denial of death by focusing our attention upon the tubes, the chemistries, and the autopsy (Bulger, 1963).

In identifying the basic problems associated with the care of the terminally ill, it is necessary to examine at least two points of view: the professionals' and the patients'. Kastenbaum and Aisenberg (1972) consider the following sociomedical issues to be the major ones: (1) the imposition of emotional isolation upon the dying person; (2) the routinization of treatment; (3) the condescension of professionals who treat the patient as though he were an irresponsible child, unable to cope with his situation like an adult; (4) among those responsible for the patient's well-being, the inadequate and unreliable patterns of communication ranging from the choice of what is communicated to the patient and how it is stated, to all the little ways significant information is withheld or misinterpreted; and (5) the failure of all persons engaged in caring for the patient to recognize and fulfill their share of the total responsibility.

The major issues identified by patients are (1) that the dying person will become quietly isolated because of a decrease in communication resulting from the unwillingness of those responsible for his care to maintain the openness and emotional support essential for him to live out his life with some hope and participation in meaningful relationships; (2) that the patient will be subjected to painful, uncomfortable, and demanding procedures that might prolong existence without prolonging a desirable quality of life, and that the disease will force that patient to endure intense, chronic pain seemingly without end; and (3) that the terminally ill person will lose control of bodily, interpersonal, and cognitive functions, that will compel him or her to confront a terrifying and alien set of experiences, stripped of all decision-making powers.

The global problem encompassing both professional and patient identifications of the dilemma is epitomized by the question, "How do we know when we are treating a dying patient?" More specifically, "How do we decide when cure or prolonged life are still possibilities requiring aggressive treatment?" "When do we acknowledge that a patient is dying and that palliation and emotional support are the optimal strategies?" Having observed this dilemma many times, I am quite sure that a useful approach is to communicate the medical realities to the patient as skillfully, honestly, and clearly as possible and to allow the patient (with the help of his or her family or advocate) to decide upon the preferred treatment. To allow the patient to retain the basic right to choose comfort care and to accord him the opportunity to relate to his impending death in a meaningful way, health professionals must have the courage and willingness to acknowledge that the patient's wishes take priority over their own.

THE PHYSICIAN'S EXPERIENCE

What are the basic experiences of both physician and patient, the main participants, in the confrontation between life-threatening illness and medical expertise? It is clear that the physician and allied professionals are powerful figures for most patients facing life-threatening illness. We must, therefore, continually earn our positions of influence by earning respect and by showing we are worthy of this power. When the professional boxer commits violence against a person outside the ring, he is properly castigated, for his hands are registered lethal weapons; but at least he is conscious of his power. For the overworked and overburdened psychologist, nurse, or physician to commit emotional violence, even inadvertently, because he or she is unconscious of his or her personal power, is most unfortunate. The capriciousness of cancer is such that we can rarely outline a definitive time schedule or map out an accurate sequence of symptomatology for a given patient. Both physician and patient are often forced to confront considerable uncertainty. Prolonged and heightened ambiguity may result in the physicians' rejection of the largely untenable role as healer, psychological confidant, companion, and spiritual counselor. They may reluctantly, albeit correctly, conclude that they are unable to fulfill all the needs of the dying patient. Several medical colleagues have communicated observations similar to the following:

> When there's nothing more I can do medically my tools are gone. There's nothing I can do for the patient and that's upsetting for me. I would rather fulfill my promises and expectations or at least be able to make some headway. When I think of other people who have time for relationships, time to relate to my patient, to sit and talk, I sometimes become jealous. I don't have that time and it's annoying to think that I may lose the affection of my patient. This is something physicians don't talk about very often.

A more distressing attitude is revealed in the following:

> I've recently realized that for the past 25 years when a patient of mine has been terminally ill, I'd walk into the room talking constantly, approach the bed, and back out of the room talking. I do this because I have nothing to offer medically and I'm not willing to deal with the patient's emotional stress. That's not my training so it's probably better if I handle the situation that way. The psychologist or social worker or psychiatric nurse spends time with the patient and opens up a whole emotional can of worms and then who gets the brunt of it, I do, the physician. I don't have time to deal with these issues. It's better if physicians give brief general reassurance and don't dig too deeply.

Although the quality of the growing body of research on the psychosocial aspects of dying has improved markedly in recent years, relatively few studies have focused on the physician's reaction to the dying patient. Working for extended periods with dying patients is an emotionally charged experience, and physicians frequently sustain great stress when they must relate intimately to patients and families facing a protracted life-threatening illness. The psychological defenses and coping strategies elicited by this

stressful contact are legion. Physicians and allied professionals may view close relationships with patients as perplexing dilemmas to be avoided at all costs. Many regard the
patient's basic emotional needs as relatively insignificant compared to the primary task
of biomedical treatment. Other professionals consider long discussions about feelings
and emotional stress a waste of invaluable time.

When Freud observed that "the ego cannot comprehend its own dissolution," he
shared with a leukemic man named Ted Rosenthal (1971) an appreciation for that
emotionally incomprehensible question: "How could I not be among you?" (Garfield,
1977). Physicians who acknowledge the preeminence of the ultimate contest between
the possibilities of "ceasing to be" and survival become involved in supramedical issues
that affect physician and patient alike. Physicians and others may view this as a dangerous commitment and seek to protect their own personal and professional integrity
by indicating an unwillingness to entertain any questions that elicit feelings of vulnerability. As Artiss and Levine (1973) have noted, a physician's manner of coping with
the anxiety aroused by a patient's imminent death becomes the crucial element in
considering the relationship between patient and physician. However, physicians rarely
discuss their feelings about specific patients except in the company of other physicians
and then only seldom. It is a major drawback in medical practice that no professional
context exists in which physicians can share their feelings about their patients, the
demands of professional work, and especially the death of a patient with whom one
has worked for months or years. There are virtually no available emotional support
systems for physicians. Because a majority of practitioners manage to continue despite
the severe emotional stress inherent in those medical specialties requiring frequent
life-and-death decisions, the medical profession participates in society's perpetuation
of the "superhuman doctor" myth that has unnecessarily limited and isolated physicians.

At some point in a patient's terminal illness the physician must confront the even-
tuality that all efforts to prevent death will likely fail (Artiss and Levine, 1973). When
this point is reached, various aspects of the doctor-patient relationship become evident. If the concerned parties do not understand and adequately deal with all facets
of this interaction, the physician's effectiveness may be severely hampered. Just as it
is essential to understand the emotional realities of dying from the patient's perspective, it is equally important to comprehend its emotional impact on the physician and
other health personnel. Anger, denial, and depression/resignation are the three most
frequent physician reactions to the probable death of a patient. These are precisely
the three most common reactions of patients themselves. Physicians and patients alike
experience basic human reactions to loss. The prospect of losing one's own life or the
loss of a patient, the end of a relationship with a dying person or the sad conclusion
to a battle with an illness all may generate similar psychological repercussions.

Anger

Physicians may employ anger as a defense against anxiety, particularly if such anger
proves effective in establishing its possessor as the adversary of a shared "enemy"
(Artiss and Levine, 1973). This phenomenon, known as displacement, allows the

physician to trace the patient's death to external circumstances, overwhelming disease process, patient and family tardiness in seeking help, bureaucratic complications, etc. Given the superhuman qualities imputed to physicians and the high degree of physician-acceptance of these cultural projections, it may become necessary for physicians to explain death in a way that allows them to escape relating to it as a personal failure. For oncologists, for example, to relate to each death as a personal failure would result in an enormous blow to their self-esteem. Therefore, they may direct the anger mobilized after a patient's death toward a human, situational, or disease-related adversary that serves to "explain away the failure." The problem lies in equating death with the failure of the physician. This equation is most often erroneous and unfair to both physician and patient.

Denial

Physicians may deny that a patient's death appears imminent, claiming "heavy patient load or home and social obligations" to explain their reluctance to accept and confront the reality of impending death (Artiss and Levine, 1973). Physician denial sometimes reaches extreme proportions as in the case of one oncologist who told me that he had never had a patient who died. Surprised at the claim, I discussed it with him further and found that he took one of two precautions when a patient seemed near death; he either transferred the patient to another facility in order to avoid being the physician of record at the time of death, or he transferred the case to a younger colleague for similar reasons. Therefore, he was able to somewhat pathetically make the claim that he had never had a patient who died. A more common form of denial is the disavowal of a close relationship between physician and patient. No physician would deny the existence of the conventional, professional-client, doctor-patient relationship. However, when treatment toward maintenance, remission, or cure is no longer possible and emotional/physical comfort as well as the reduction of pain become the major issues, some physicians may deny that they have a responsibility to continue this relationship. This circumscribed definition of the doctor-patient relationship, as limited to the resolution of biomedical problems, is another way of avoiding or denying the emotional aspects of terminal illness.

Depression/Resignation

One of the most poorly understood physician reactions to prolonged contact with terminal patients is depression. Whereas denial and anger allow the physician to continue functioning, albeit sometimes at a fever pitch or in a somewhat disorganized fashion, depression can debilitate the physician and severely impair his or her efficiency. I have known physicians who, for years, via a sheer act of will, fought off incipient depression only to succumb finally to the cumulative emotional impact of patient deaths. Depression and its real or imagined emotional engulfment are extremely threatening to physicians whose heavy work schedule and personal expectations do not allow them the "luxury" of more modulated and frequent emotional expression. In the past several years, I have seen an increasing number of physicians in psychotherapy with presenting complaints related to a variety of emotional disorders. The majority have been highly productive in their careers but had not adequately attended to the emotional impact of their work. Most frequently, they suffered from one of a variety of psychosomatic disorders or depressions that had culminated in the impairment of work efficiency and severe emotional stress. For an individual, no matter how emotionally adaptive, to select as demanding a profession as clinical oncology without recognizing its emotional impact can only be detrimental to both physician and patient.

> Wheelis offers a vivid and literate picture of the professional man's final but necessary disillusionment. He writes of what happens when a man travels a long road to salvation and, until he is too far along to go back, doesn't realize that he is headed for the abyss. Nor could anyone have told him earlier. His hope then lies in finding that it would have been the same no matter which route he had chosen, and that he can help himself and others along the way. A mature resolution, but a poor one when compared with early dreams of ultimate conquest. For the man who cannot mature in his profession, every subsequent day of his life challenges his magic and with it, his identity. He has staked his life, like Faust, on learning the secret and he cannot turn back admitting failure. He knows well enough that he cannot win—that he will die, as will all his patients. He knows this not with equanimity but with the cynicism of the frustrated idealist. He less than other men is suited to face the dying; they are a personal affront, a symbol of his human helplessness, and an end to his life. He whose marriage is shaken because he cannot bear his wife's small complaints, whose children cry in their nights of illness for a father who has to be at an induced delivery—this man must often help a stranger die, and what can he do? He can be tough about it, maybe breezy, or maudlin—or maybe he can get an intern or nurse to drink the dregs of his heady wine while he is called to more positive and hopeful cases (Kasper, 1959).

THE PATIENT'S EXPERIENCE

The subjective experience of cancer is nearly unfathomable from the perspective of the observer. Whereas disease-related cellular and systemic metamorphoses have many identifiable and predictable characteristics, the phenomenology of the patient is in some ways harder to analyze. To help identify and meet the psychosocial needs of cancer patients, my optimal consultants are the patients themselves. It is only by communicating with these valuable sources of information that the possibilities for effective psychosocial support can emerge. It takes courage; but the courage necessary for us to minimize the differences between "Us" and "Them" is one prerequisite to really understanding the emotional impact on the patient of the words "and I, too, shall die."

The threat of ceasing to be, personality disintegration, or ego annihilation (i.e., the death of one's identity) has been identified as the core component of our fear of death (Choron, 1964). Despite the considerable magnitude of this fear for most of us, Annas (1974) cites seven studies from journals such as *Cancer, JAMA,* etc., that note that approximately 90 percent of all patients interviewed preferred to know their diagnosis, even if terminal, whereas 60 percent to 90 percent of their physicians opposed telling them. In my own research, over 85 percent of those terminal patients I have counseled strongly suspected they were dying before being formally told by house staff. It is very difficult to deny indefinitely as monumental a psychobiological phenomenon as a widely metastasized cancer. At times, we all use denial as a psychological defense to preserve our psychic integrity in the face of potentially traumatizing realities. What is not often recognized is that this process is both interpersonal (and selective) and most often time-bound (we all process information of a potentially traumatizing nature at differential rates). It is important to honor a patient's denial for as long as it is psychologically adaptive; that is, for as long as the individual chooses to admit into consciousness only those relatively nontraumatizing aspects of the illness— those with which he or she can cope more or less successfully. Through being emotionally accessible to the patient in the context of a caring, trusting relationship, a physician may provide the optimal occasion for a patient to choose to acknowledge the more traumatizing aspects of his illness—the possibility of death and his fear of dying.

Why then has so much been written about patient denial? I have consistently encountered as much denial by staff members as by patients. As health providers we experience ourselves as trained healers and view the death of a patient as an unacceptable conclusion to the health care process. As professionally skilled adversaries of illness and death, we may be less able to respond effectively to the dying patient. Our anxiety and sense of impotence may force us to keep our distance from a patient whose death appears inevitable, leaving the patient psychologically abandoned and emotionally and physically isolated. The vital question is not whether or not we have a "denier," but denial when and with whom and under what circumstances? I hope that we all subscribe to the notion that the dying patient has a right to know, but that this right is clearly contingent upon his or her right not to know. It is imperative that we honor a patient's denial until he chooses to admit into consciousness, frequently in symbolic form, a growing awareness of the life-threatening nature of his illness.

A 55-year-old truck driver with seriously advanced lymphosarcoma discussed his feelings about driving a large truck across country late at night. He spoke intensely of the dark, the shortage of gas, and how lonely and frightened he felt when it seemed as if it might not be possible to reach the next gas stop. He spoke of the loneliness of the open road, the trucker's lack of human contact and relationships, and his fear of the uncertainty of the situation. I honored his chosen metaphor and we spoke "truck language" for approximately one-half hour, after which time he made intense eye contact and said "I hope you realize that I'm not talking about trucks and the highway." I indicated that I understood what he was referring to and thanked him for sharing so intimate a set of feelings.

A 16-year-old girl dying of choriocarcinoma shared the following:

"I used to be a tremendous softball player. I could bat .900—I'd get nine hits each ten at-bats. Then my batting average began to fall. I started batting .500, then .400, and finally I couldn't hit the ball out of the infield and I had to bunt." I shared the observation that sometimes even the strongest hitter had to bunt. She smiled and said

"I realize now that I don't have to hit a home run each time. I just have to get on base and it doesn't matter how. The one thing I have to watch out for," she cautioned, "is hitting the ball to third base. If you hit it to third you're dead, third base is the coffin corner." This interchange opened up an extended discussion of the patient's fear of death, her feelings of isolation from her parents and the medical staff, and her sadness about being treated as a child when in reality she considered herself an adult.

A rule of thumb fundamental to the evolution of effective doctor-patient communications is that the physician answer all questions honestly, giving as much information as is asked for by the patient. For many people in extraordinarily high-stress situations, ambiguity produces far more emotional distress than even the most negative reality. I occasionally hear physician colleagues state that "the patient knows anyway." If this is true, then any reluctance to communicate honestly and openly merely compels the patient, his or her family, and the staff to collude in a lie that may severely increase the patient's anxiety. Situations similar to that faced by Tolstoy's Ivan Ilych are not rare.

> What tormented Ivan Ilych most was the deception, the lie, which for some reason they all accepted. That he was not dying but simply ill, and that he only need keep quiet and undergo a treatment and then something very good would result. He, however, knew that, do what they would, nothing would come of it only still more agonizing suffering and death. This deception tortured him—their not wishing to admit what they all knew and what he knew . . . . Those lies enacted over him on the eve of his death and destined to degrade this awful, solemn act to the level of their visiting, their curtains, their sturgeon for dinner—were terrible agony for Ivan Ilych.

Ambiguous or dishonest communication imposes needless emotional pain on patients and families facing life-threatening illness. The deleterious impact of the deliberate choice to withhold information without first accurately assessing the awareness of the patient is illustrated by the tragic case of an elderly couple from the Midwest. While the husband was dying of lung cancer, the physician and family firmly stood by their decision not to inform him that his illness was terminal. The wife, whom her husband described as his "bride of 50 years," tried valiantly not to leak the information to him. Given the fact that the latest research in nonverbal communication indicates that between 70 percent and 90 percent of what we communicate to one another is transmitted through nonverbal channels, how long could the wife maintain this facade without nonverbally leaking signs of her obvious distress? In minutes the tension resulting from her emotional stress was clearly perceived by her terminally ill husband who only hours before had confided to me that he had known he was dying for several weeks. He had long since noticed his wife's distress but had chosen not to tell her what he knew in an attempt to spare her the emotional pain of confronting his death. The inaccurate assessment of the patient's awareness of his prognosis resulted in a restricted system of communication that inflicted great stress on both husband and wife. Since both defined their relationship of 50 years as a "marriage made in heaven" what value existed in reducing their last set of interactions to a lie? The unfortunate and deceitful conclusion that such dishonesty prevents (rather than causes) pain results from a desire for mutual protection frequently observed among patients, families, and staff. A professional or volunteer who has been trained in communication skills, has more time, and is able to understand personal metaphor and symbolic communication is in a better position to assess the level of all concerned. Without such assistance, a conspiracy of silence (in which everyone knows and yet no one is willing to share the fact that he knows) can overwhelm and alienate the patient, his family, and the physician.

Anger

One of the most perplexing responses for hospital staff to cope with is patient anger. The patient may be furious at what he perceives as a capricious universe unjustly inflicting cruelty in the form of his cancer. The emotional stress may cause the patient to search incessantly for some psychological and/or spiritual explanation for the cruel fate that has befallen him. In counseling cancer patients, it is important to realize that no definitive research has indicated a clear etiological equation specifying the relation between causes and effect (malignancy); hence, to the lay public (as well as many health professionals) the selection of those who get cancer often appears random and chaotic. The possibility of a random and meaningless universe, or worse, a tyrannical and capricious god, operating without plan or with malevolent intent can be powerfully unsettling. Some people attempt to explain cancer as a form of severe retribution; such an "explanation" may evoke considerable fear and guilt in many cancer patients. It is not rare for terminally ill patients to direct their anger against the infuriating whimsy of their illness. The services instituted by many hospitals simply do not meet the psychosocial needs of patients, families, and staff under considerable emotional stress. Overburdened medical and nursing personnel and anxious family members may be too preoccupied with their own needs and demands to provide adequate support to the patient. At minimum, it is important for us to recognize the difference between anger directed against a seemingly random and whimsical "death-sentence" and anger directed against (1) a physician who may have been slow at making a diagnosis or who had inaccurately diagnosed the illness until it was too late to treat effectively; (2) nursing staff who seem too busy to attend to the emotional needs of the patient; and (3) family members who choose to withdraw in fear rather than engage in meaningful dialogue with the patient.

Anger is frequently a defense against terror and severe loss of control. An effective approach is to help the patient understand his response by actively listening as he vents his anger and then distinguishing with him the issues that are realistically subject to variation from those that are not. Anger can be a psychologically adaptive and important reaction to severe emotional stress. It is vital that we not assume that anger is an immature response directed at an inappropriate target. We have much to learn about the emotional realities of people facing life-threatening illness and must always guard against stereotyping their responses and rendering them invalid.

Depression

Another frequently observed patient response to life-threatening illness is depression, both reactive and preparatory. When a patient experiences the tremendous loss of self-esteem that often results from prolonged and painful hospitalization and treatment, emotional abandonment by family and friends, the real or imagined insensitivity of hospital personnel, and the depletion of finances due to expensive medical care, he may understandably become severely depressed. Those who take the time to listen will frequently find that this depression is traceable to concrete life circumstances. Furthermore, some of these circumstances may be subject to modification, and all available supports should be mobilized to this end. Facilitating communication with family members, helping to minimize financial burdens, diminishing the impact of severe body-image changes, and sensitizing staff to the emotional needs of patients are areas that can be explored in an effort to alleviate depression of a reactive nature.

Preparatory depression is primarily an anticipatory reaction to the threatened "loss of oneself," that is, a grief reaction to the impending cessation of embodiment. The patient is threatened "not only" with the loss of life, but also with the loss of self-esteem, physical potency, and personal relationships. Typical reactions include frightening dreams, irritability, extreme sadness, anorexia, and apathy. Intense and prolonged suffering can exacerbate preparatory depression to the point where it incorporates elements of suicidal preoccupation. It is not helpful to interrupt this preparatory response with false promises of cure or positive response to treatment. This is a classic mourning period that offers a true test of the professional's (or family members') ability to provide continuous emotional support to the patient. One can be extremely supportive by sitting with the patient, often in silence, in an attempt to convey a willingness to share this emotionally demanding period. The health professional or volunteer can help a patient cope successfully with reactive depression by assisting in the development of a sense of closure (i.e., a sense of completing life's "unfinished business"—personal, interpersonal, spiritual, and financial). To offer on-going support during the preparatory period we must become attuned to the emotional realities of each dying patient and the personal significance of his imminent death.

Acceptance

Recent research has focused on the fact that some terminal patients seem able to accept their impending death. I have found that 5 to 10 percent of those cancer patients who die in the hospital maintain a predominately consistent death-accepting attitude. However, 15 to 20 percent of those terminal patients who choose to die at home achieve a similar level of acceptance. In caring and supportive families capable of substantially meeting the needs of the terminally ill member, the acceptance of death may resemble not so much the resignation of a beleaguered soldier accepting defeat, but rather an emotionally and cognitively integrated sense of "alrightness" about the termination of one's life. The degree of this acceptance often fluctuates depending on shifts in mood due to pain, drug side effects, and assorted emotional conflicts. In some instances, a major difference between the hospital and home context may be the willingness to honor the patient's chosen attitude toward death. The influence of a powerful antideath institutional belief (the basic attitude toward life-threatening illness of medical and nursing staff) frequently precludes a patient's acceptance of death. Understanding the impact of a death-accepting or death-denying environment on the dying person is crucial. It is unreasonable to expect a terminal patient to accept death when he or she is embedded in a hospital social system that views disease as an evil adversary and death as unacceptable. It may be extremely difficult for a dying patient who is dependent upon a fiercely death-denying family or hospital staff to ever accept his own death. It is a rare individual (usually someone with a profound spiritual or philosophic commitment) who can counteract the pervasive death-denying institutional bias militating against death-acceptance. The heroic measures sometimes used to prolong the lives of patients who have peacefully and clearly indicated their preference for letting nature take its course bears witness to the institutional abhorrence of death under any conditions. Many patients are not physically capable of sufficient impact on the decision-making process to suspend these aggressive measures. The point is certainly not that death-acceptance is always the preferable response, but rather that patient input and the right of self-determination are fundamental. As health professionals, we must avoid those absurdly macabre scenarios wherein medical heroics are directed at the prolongation of the life of a patient who has clearly and nonhysterically expressed an aversion to such measures.

For many people, particularly the elderly, the completion of unfinished business—economic and work-related, psychological and related to self-esteem, interpersonal, religious—may enhance a sense of the appropriateness of their own death. The ability to derive a sense of purpose and meaning from life and perhaps death, to have, in Weisman's (1972a) terms, "an appropriate rather than an appropriated death," appears integral to any self-accepting experience of terminality. This is not to suggest that the acceptance of death is the equivalent of an emotionally or physically painless death, but rather that such acceptance may enhance a person's opportunity of relating to death in a more meaningful fashion. Few people realize that personal change and maturation often appear more possible on one's deathbed than perhaps at any other time in the life cycle. The fluidity of ego boundaries and the suspension of stereotypic modes of social interaction, of "the games people play," may allow for such maturation. The culturally dominant notion that death, the Grim Reaper, is nothing but tragic prevents us from realizing that even in the midst of painful chaos and parting, the possibility of positive change exists. However, such change can occur only with the patient's willing support and can often be facilitated by a person trained to develop these subtle but important possibilities.

As noted previously, the two main areas of serious concern to terminal patients are (1) extreme pain and (2) emotional and physical isolation and the threat of abandonment. The most cogent analysis of patient isolation and abandonment I have read is that of Erikson and Hyerstay (1974), who describe the psychosocial gestalt of a hospital death with considerable accuracy. The need for developing better palliation strategies has been discussed by LeShan (1964) and Marks and Sachar (1973). With the help of our colleagues at the hospices in Great Britain, we are beginning to learn that patients in the United States may, at times, endure much needless pain because of undereffective palliation strategies. Hospice physicians and patients claim that (1) effective pain management strategies exist for almost all patients facing life-threatening illness, (2) patients can remain lucid *and* pain-free throughout most of the dying process, and (3) addiction and habituation result from the ineffective administration of palliative drugs. There is no possible excuse for not thoroughly investigating these claims. My own clinical experience and observation has substantially borne out their validity (which does not derive from the fact that British pain-killers contain heroin as the active pharmacological ingredient since morphine is often the agent of preference). In studying the psychopharmacological aspects of pain, it is important to remember that making judgments about another person's pain is an extremely hazardous proposition. Physicians must use their patient's feedback as the most significant criterion. In evaluating the effectiveness of pain-management strategies, to say, as one professional did in reaction to a patient in extreme pain, "He's not in as much pain as he says he is," is most unfortunate. In general, physicians need to acknowledge as primary data the subjective reports of their patients and prescribe palliative strategies based on this acknowledgment.

Individualized Approaches to Psychosocial Care

I have found the following outline useful in determining and meeting the psychosocial needs of terminal patients.

1 With the assistance of the patient, define the major areas of emotional distress.

2 Respond to the patient's requests for information with an honest, complete, and accurate presentation of the major aspects of illness and treatment.

3 Inform the patient's family of the status of his health so that family members can assume their rightful status as members of the treatment team.

4 Make it possible for the patient to be aware of staff expectations concerning treatment, patient-staff relationships, etc., and conversely be aware of patient expectations.

5 Always compare your perceptions of the patient and his situation with those of your colleagues. It is hazardous to make unilateral judgments about another person's emotional reality.

6 Remember that psychosocial evaluation, like medical appraisal, is a continuous process. Two innovations that have proven successful in maintaining ongoing evaluation are (a) the institution of interdisciplinary psychosocial rounds the specific purpose of which is to evaluate staff success in meeting the emotional needs of all patients (the option of inviting patients to talk to staff about how to best care for them has been a successful aspect of these rounds), and (b) the use of a psychosocial log in which all health providers may record their feelings and thoughts on various aspects of working with seriously ill patients. This log can serve as a catalyst for discussion during psychosocial rounds.

Several premises are basic to the effective psychosocial care of patients and families facing life-threatening illness. First, it is important for those who work with the dying to monitor their own feelings. As Weisman (1972b) has pointed out, "We are not im-mune to denial, dissimilation, antipathy, and fears of personal annihilation." We must not be ashamed to recognize that caring for the dying is itself an "exposure to en-dangerment" that often necessitates enlisting the aid of key individuals and a variety of modes of support. Second, as Dobihal (1974) has noted, the dying patient and his or her family constitute the optimal unit of health care. It is extremely important for patients to live out and conclude family relationships in as emotionally satisfying a way as possible. It can be very distressing for critically ill persons and their families to be separated by the treatment milieu and forced to limit or terminate their relation-ships. Dobihal offers the following suggestons to health professionals:

1 Train family members to participate in treatment.
2 Encourage them to do such things as continue to cook special meals for the patient.
3 Allow unlimited visiting so that the total family, including children, can spend time with the patient.
4 Provide special hospital space for patient-family meetings, as well as space for family members to live when the patient's death is imminent.
5 Provide special social and educational programs for the family and patient, and continue these programs, adding home visits for the family, after the patient has died. Research in preventive health indicates that the bereaved are much more susceptible to mental and physical trauma (including early death) than people not suffering from the loss of a close friend or relation.

Third, as Schmale (1974) has observed, the capacity of the physician to accept and relate to the patient's awareness of dying is important. It is not easy to listen and respond to patients' statements about their readiness to die, but the opportunity to relate to patients approaching the end of their lives (when they often relinquish for-mer attitudes, behavioral patterns, and defensive strategies to become totally immersed in the present) may provide a unique learning experience for the health professional.

Fourth, staff members should make every attempt to relate to the patient as a col-league. This case of a woman labelled "difficult patient" for many months and who was the subject of endless discussions in rounds and case conferences offers a graphic example of the success of this orientation. Staff members were unable to develop an approach adequate to the situation. The woman appeared belligerent, demanding, and unresponsive to staff efforts. It was only when I suggested that she be allowed to attend management rounds as a colleague and speak to staff about how to best care for her that the situation changed. When presented with this alternative, she responded "Now, that's the first sensible thing I've heard since I got here." Following her care-fully outlined lecture, staff adopted many of her suggestions, negotiated others, and the situation changed substantially for the better.

Fifth, it is most useful for a patient-advocate or companion to be available for each patient, that is, someone who is able to listen and follow through on specific patient requests. Given the powerful conditioning inherent in our training as health profes-sionals, we may unconsciously adopt an ironclad distinction between professional and patient and further equate professional with *correct* and patient with *incorrect*. It is urgent for us to realize that as professionals we may require attitudinal reorientation as much as our patients. Having a patient-advocate or representative available to the patient in an unconditionally supportive manner may allow for more effective coping in the face of life-threatening illness.

Finally, we should recognize that the disease process and medical treatment may affect the patient's mental faculties, causing fluctuation between slightly altered levels of cognitive and perceptual functioning and states of consciousness distinctly discontinuous with the waking state (Pelletier and Garfield, 1976). In light of these alterations in psychological functioning, it is important to avoid pressuring the patient toward some staff ideal of how to successfully cope with his impending death. Each patient's "deathstyle" is as unique as his lifestyle, and it takes time and a willingness to understand the attitudes and behavior of a given patient before successful psychosocial support is possible.

CONCLUSION

Worchester (1935), in a fine book entitled *The Care of the Aged, the Dying and the Dead,* offers the following guidelines for care of the dying patient:

1 Disturb him not, let him pass peaceably. Even while only watchful waiting is needed, the physician must not underrate the help that his mere presence may afford in steadying and comforting both the dying patient and the family. They also serve who only stand and wait.

2 In the practice of our art it often matters little what medicine is given, but it matters much that we give ourselves with our pills. Until the doctor had had the sad experience of standing by to the very last those nearest and dearest to him, he can only imagine the heartache of his dying patient's family and their sore need of sympathy; nor until he himself has been nye onto death can he more than imagine the comfort that even the firm clasp of a friendly hand can give to one in such extremity.

Shortly after the First National Training Conference for Physicians on Psychosocial Care of the Dying Patient, I heard Walter Alvarez, one of the elder statesmen of America's medical community, comment that in 70 years of medical practice he had never seen a patient die. I was struck powerfully by the contrast between Dr. Alvarez's experience and my own. As mentioned earlier, in the past 3 years I have provided emotional support to 156 cancer patients who finally succumbed to their illnesses. On a number of occasions I have been present at the moment of death. I have experienced 156 times a few of the emotional realities of life-threatening illness but not nearly so intensely as those who have died. Their deaths and my enforced separation from them have been painful to varying degrees, but not nearly so painful as the loss experienced by their families and friends. I have wondered often what it will be like for me when I am compelled to face the deaths of those I love most and my own. The power of these reflections in reformulating the values that govern my life has been considerable. To say the least, we have much in common with many of our patients. Perhaps the best expression of this commonality in human experience was offered by a 38-year-old man dying of intestinal cancer.

> Several days before he died Roger asked me to read to him. As I proceeded slowly through the lines while he drifted in and out of waking-state consciousness, I wondered whether he even heard me at all. Suddenly, as though he had been stung by a needle, his eyes shot open and he looked at me and said, "Please read that line again." I read the entire paragraph again and he repeated his request. "The line near the end," he said, "please read the line near the end." I read the line three or four times and each time Roger nodded his head. Finally, with tears gently streaming down his face he said, "Please tell my doctor and the nurses that's why I'm so afraid." The line that Roger asked me to read was "The eternal silence of these infinite spaces frightens me."

As I reflect on Roger's words while writing during the hours before dawn, a time when my humility is apparently at its peak, I must confess with a sharp jolt of *ego-chill* (Erik Erikson's term) that "the eternal silence of these infinite spaces frightens me" also.

BIBLIOGRAPHY

Annas, G.: "Rights of the Terminally Ill Patient," *Journal of Nursing Administration,* 4:40–43, 1974.

Artiss, K. and A. Levine: "Doctor-Patient Relations in Severe Illness," *New England Journal of Medicine,* 288:1210–1214, 1973.

Bulger, R.: "Doctors and Dying," *Archives of Internal Medicine,* 70(3):327–332, 1963.

Choron, J.: *Death and Modern Man,* Collier, New York, 1964.

Dobihal, E.: "Talk or Terminal Care," *Connecticut Medicine,* 38:364–367, 1974.

Erikson, R. and B. Hyerstay: "The Dying Patient and the Double Bind Hypothesis," *Omega,* 5(4):287–298, 1974.

Garfield, C.: "The Impact of Death on the Healthcare Professional," in H. Feifel (ed.), *New Meanings of Death,* McGraw-Hill, New York, 1977.

Kasper, A.: "The Doctor and Death," in H. Feifel (ed.), *The Meaning of Death,* McGraw-Hill, New York, 1959.

Kastenbaum, R. and R. Aisenberg: *Psychology of Death,* Springer, New York, 1972.

LeShan, L.: "The World of the Patient in Severe Pain of Long Duration," *Journal of Chronic Diseases,* 17:119–126, 1964.

Marks, R. and E. Sachar: "Undertreatment of Medical Inpatients with Narcotic Analgesics," *Annals of Internal Medicine,* 78(2):173–181, 1973.

Pelletier, K. and C. Garfield: *Consciousness: East and West,* Harper and Row, New York, 1976.

Rosenthal, T.: *How Could I Not Be Among You?,* Braziller, New York, 1971.

Schmale, A.: "Principes of Psychosocial Oncology," in P. Rubin (ed.), *Clinical Oncology for Medical Students and Physicians,* American Cancer Society, Rochester, 1974.

Weisman, A.: *On Dying and Denying,* Behavioral Publications, New York, 1972a.

Weisman, A.: "Psychosocial Consideration in Terminal Care," in B. Schoenberg, A. Carr, D. Peretz, and A. Kutscher (eds.), *Psychosocial Aspects of Terminal Patient Care*, Columbia, New York, 1972b.

Worchester, A.: *The Care of the Aged, the Dying and the Dead*, Charles C. Thomas, Springfield, Illinois, 1935.

Chapter 15

The Changing Relationship Between Cancer Patient and Oncologist

Michael A. Friedman

The relationship between a patient with cancer and his or her physician is a complex and protean one. To provide a framework within which to understand this special oncologic interaction, I will analyze the generic aspects of the fundamental relationship between doctor and patient.

Throughout the past several decades Americans have increasingly sought to redefine the relationship between physician and patient. The need to explore patient-physician interaction as one aspect of the total health care system has been clearly articulated by such diverse groups as patients, insurance companies, social scientists, philosophers, and physicians. This important reexamination of medical care has resulted in much destructive criticism of current health care practices, which in turn has evoked needlessly strident responses in defense of the present system. A shouting match rather than a profitable dialogue has emerged, demonstrating that no single polar position can redress all the needs and requirements of the doctor, the patient, and other participants in the health care drama.

It is not my purpose to review, defend, or revile this redefinition process, nor do I wish to address the shortcomings of the health care system in the United States (there are many), or criticize the slowness and lack of flexibility this system has sometimes demonstrated, or discuss the reordering of national, local, and personal health care priorities (which I believe is mandatory now). Nor do I wish to defend the quality of medical care in the United States (which I believe in the main excellent but by no means perfect). Rather than critically examining the complexities of all the inter-relationships in the health care macrocosm, I would like to focus on the microcosm of the relationship between doctor and patient. Examining this relationship may be a step toward resolving some of the larger controversies over medical care in the United States, and can add to our understanding of the specific oncologic situation.

To determine what is to be criticized and redressed in the doctor-patient inter-action, it is necessary to recognize that when a person, ill or well, consults a physician, a formal relationship is established that has profound moral, legal, and social implica-tions. It is a contractual fiduciary agreement, and this dyadic arrangement may origi-nate within one of many valid and appropriate legal forms, including:

1 *Formal-written.* The patient may belong to a prepaid group health care plan in which, for a yearly premium, all medical services are supplied by a physician who is employed by the plan.

2 *Informal-unwritten.* The patient may be injured in an accident and roadside assistance may be given him by a passing physician.

3 *Partially mercantile.* The patient may be treated by an emergency room physi-cian whose salary is based on the number and type of patients treated.

4 *Primarily altruistic.* The patient may be indigent or socially disenfranchised and may be treated by a physician who receives no payment.

This list is not all-inclusive; rather it suggests some of the more common contexts and describes the skeletal form, but not necessarily the vital content, of the doctor-patient relationship.

Over the past two millennia attempts to flesh out these skeletal outlines have con-centrated on the philosophic, artistic, or religious aspects of medical practice. Some analyses, such as the Code of Hamurabi, the Hippocratic oath, and the writings of Maimonides, have been formalized and codified. Appropriately, these tests have achieved the stature of law. They have broadly outlined the standard of medical practice adequately, but they have never been completely successful in defining the qualitative aspects of clinical care. In the past 50 years there have been judicial deci-sions rendered in the United States to clarify some aspects of clinical practice. Moral and technical malpractice can be defined and therefore litigated. However, the extra-technical, psychological, and emotional aspects of medical care have escaped legal definition. Because there is no body of law that definitively characterizes the special aspects of the doctor-patient relationship, other methods of analysis become essential.

Any analytic attempt must address the obviously sensitive aspects of the doctor-patient relationship that make it uniquely difficult to define precisely. These sensitive aspects include bilateral attention to:

1 Life and death matters
2 Daily sense of health, well-being, and ability to enjoy life
3 The most intimate consideration of health and disease wherein no subject is taboo

Because this definition process is so difficult, the identification of an appropriate analogy may be of value.

The doctor-patient relationship is a cooperative venture comparable in some ways to contemporary Western marriage. The contract entered into by the doctor and patient bears some striking similarities to the spousal arrangement. Both relationships are:

1 Defined by formal, legally recognized, written contracts that are subject to judicial review

2 Defined by informal oral but legally binding contracts associated partially with romantic and vague illusions

3 Uniquely intimate relationships

4 Designed to last lifelong and to become more durable and rewarding with time

5 Destined to change with time to address the needs of each age and situation

6 Not bound by limits of time, financial situation, or state of being

7 Difficult to fulfill because the reality of the relationship is often discordant with its image

Both relationships are based on fidelity of emotional and physical support. Indeed, both should provide the participants with more than the simple sum of their abilities and strengths, and both relationships gain from this joint effort. To develop the potential of each of these relationships requires a considerable investment of trust and faith.

Because of the risks associated with marriage and/or doctor-patient interaction, it is difficult for the parties to these relationships to engage in unguaranteed trust. As a society we are increasingly suspicious of government, organized religion, and the law. As individuals we are even more wary about entrusting our love or our lives to another. Both marital and doctor-patient relationships are fragile. The oaths and ceremonies of ritualism lend weight and form and structure to them but do not insure success. Often these relationships do not thrive.

There are many ways to explain the increasing rate of failure, whether it takes the form of a divorce action or a malpractice suit. A frequent explanation is that there was a lack of communication in the relationship. Used in this sense, *communication* refers to a mutually active process of broadcasting and receiving messages dealing with issues ranging from the mundane and sterile to the most sensitive and emotionally charged. Often expectations are unmet and emotional needs unfulfilled because of an inability to communicate meaningfully.

Occasionally needs and expectations are unrealistic and remain unfulfilled because the parties involved are incapable of meeting them. More often, however, they are not satisfied because the parties lack communication skills; their failure to exchange messages could be corrected by more sensitive attention to each other's needs.

However, communication is not an end in itself, but rather a vehicle toward an end. Neither the marital nor the medical relationship exists in a social, economic, or psychological vacuum. The environment for each is a dynamic, changing one presenting new situations and problems that must be addressed by novel or ingenious solutions. The process of maintaining a viable relationship should include identification of any problems, mutual attention to them, and a cooperative solution for them.

The ability to deal flexibly with stresses characterizes the most satisfactory marriages and medical relationships. The sociobiologic concept that these relationships grow and mature is valid. For example, the doctor-patient interface is modified by specific pathophysiologic factors of illness, just as the marital interface is changed by specific socioeconomic ones. These associations are organic (growing, adapting, maturing) as opposed to static. They remain viable by constant attention and appropriate modification.

Like marriage partners, the participants in a doctor-patient relationship must dynamically balance adaptability and stability. The mutual commitment to the welfare of the cooperative partnership must be consistent. The frequently invoked marital pledge of an intimate bond unaffected by wealth or poverty, health or sickness, ease or travail, and dissolved only by death, rings curiously true for the physician and dying patient as well. This fidelity of purpose remains the ultimate goal, but to achieve it considerable adaptations may be necessary.

The interaction between spousal partners and medical partners can assume several forms, and Eric Berne's system of transactional analysis[1] provides a psychological model for analyzing this interaction. Simply stated, some interactions between two individuals can be characterized as occurring between the adult (active, controlling, authoritarian, directing) and the child (passive, dependent, and desiring direction). The four possible permutations of this model describe a variety of doctor-patient relationships. One of the most common situations, and perhaps the most criticized, is:

Adult → Child

Directing

Physician → Patient

This interaction is often appropriate for pediatric medical care and for some dependent adult patient-physician relationships. However, many adults object to oversimplified explanations, a paternalistic tone, direction instead of discussion. Patients who wish to participate actively in their own care desire:

Adult ⇆ Adult

Cooperation
Interaction

Physician ⇆ Patient

Doctors have a responsibility to fully educate and advise their patients, but the patients must then interact and assist the doctor in planning their therapy.

[1]Eric Berne, *Transactional Analysis in Psychotherapy*, Grove, New York, 1961.

There is no single model that is correct or incorrect in an absolute sense. Rather, there is an appropriate or inappropriate interaction. If a patient at a given time desires to play the role of a child and the physician is prepared to act as an adult then this is a proper arrangement. As more individuals demand an adult role (i.e., women, racial minority groups, and adolescents) the physician must be flexible enough to change his or her own posture.

One typical constraint on doctor-patient relationships is that often interactions occur during acute episodes of illness and not at times when bilateral interchange is possible. Serious illness does not allow time for intimate exploratory discussions but requires acute care in which the physician often acts as a director-father figure. Since many patients react to the acute stress of illness by assuming a more dependent posture, physicians may generalize from these episodes and treat patients in this fatherly way at all times. If both patient and doctor could identify and communicate their abilities and needs prior to these episodes, there might be a decrease in the number of dissatisfied patients and doctors.

Similarity between marriages and doctor-patient relationships as examples of unique and organic relationships is striking. Both are cooperative ventures predicated on mutual satisfaction. In a successful marriage both participants benefit. In a successful medical relationship the same is true. Although not always superficially apparent, the physician *often gains* as much from the therapeutic relationship as does the patient. The emotional and psychological benefits the physician enjoys from this interaction can be more meaningful than the associated intellectual or financial benefits.

Changing social expectations have influenced both types of relationships. The halcyon days of strict definition, if they ever existed, are gone forever. The success of marital or doctor-patient endeavors depends on adaptability not conformity, and on appreciation of common interests and objectives.

It is understandable that many doctors and patients, as well as husbands and wives, are dissatisfied with the status quo and anxious for change and improvement. This dissatisfaction is a sign of the times. It is not necessarily a reason for indicting institutions in general, but rather for constructively modifying them. Change in an institution is not only to be expected, it is necessary if the institution is to remain viable. However, modifications should not be dictated by one homogeneous group with clearly defined and identified goals. Many groups—including women, the elderly, the poor, the non-English speaking, and racial minorities—have voiced their growing dissatisfaction with their relations with doctors. Each group objects to certain aspects of the doctor-patient relationship and no one simple modification can alleviate all these dissatisfactions. However, doctors must attend to the specific needs of each individual patient—not each ethnic, racial, or financial subpopulation. The doctor-patient relationship can be durable, enriching, and the basis for emotional growth and health only if both partners give adequate attention to tending and maintaining it.

It is apparent that the model of physician-patient interaction that I have proposed can apply to any specialized medical field. The specific example of this generic relationship I would like to highlight is the interaction between the oncologist and the patient with cancer. The relationship has both special positive and special negative aspects.

Among the negative aspects is the fact that interactions between the participants may be severely limited by time. Unlike the general physician, the oncologist usually does not have the leisure to establish an intimate relationship. Too often an entire load of serious and critical messages must be broadcast and perceived by both parties in a short period of time. The dramatic stresses of disfiguring surgery or toxic anticancer therapy or imminent death place extra burdens on this interchange. In trying to establish the communication pathway, both doctor and patient must expend significant effort, and a frightened, ill patient may have difficulty dealing with a physician who is burdened with the concerns of caring for this patient. The financial costs of acute or subacute oncologic care and the patient's loss of job-generated income are further impediments to unencumbered doctor-patient interaction. A physician is charged with: giving every patient the most complete understanding of the biology of his or her disease as is possible; providing every patient the best advice about therapy; and implementing the informed wishes of the patient. How much harder this becomes under such adverse circumstances!

Paradoxically, the same intense problems that hamper this relationship can be its strengths as well. Because of the recognized time constraints, a more immediately intimate relationship is sometimes possible: the two parties need to establish agreements quickly that address the needs and concerns of each. The doctor's promises to discuss the patient's condition truthfully, to attend to simple bodily concerns (such as analgesia or relief of constipation), to provide unflagging care, and to remain accessible are among the most appreciated reassurances he or she can offer.

The oncologic patient desires above all fidelity in purpose and information. A patient frightened by a disease and the drastic treatment required for it needs to have an unfailingly stable, dependable, comfortable relationship with his or her physician. No matter what form this medical dyad takes, if it honestly addresses the needs of both parties it is proper, appropriate, morally correct, and most of all maximally satisfying.

Chapter 16

Self-willed Death or the Bone-pointing Syndrome

G. W. Milton

Doctors who treat dying patients or patients with malignant disease are often doubtful about the desirability of giving the patient details of his prognosis. As a general rule I believe that honesty is the best policy.[1] However, there is a small group of patients in whom the realization of impending death is a blow so terrible that they are quite unable to adjust to it, and they die rapidly before the malignancy seems to have developed enough to cause death. This problem of self-willed death is in some ways analogous to the death produced in primitive peoples by witchcraft ("pointing the bone").

The syndrome of a self-willed death nearly always affects a big man who is proud of his virility. The patient, when first confronted with the problem of his malignant disease, appears to disregard it and be extraordinarily cheerful; to the young doctor this spurious bonhomie is a matter for great admiration and wonder. Far from appearing to feel sorry for himself, the patient will laugh, joke, and be facetious with all who come near him. Overnight the patient's whole manner changes and he is physically and mentally transformed. He literally turns his face to the wall and lies inert in bed, covering his face with the bedclothes. He does not seem to be terrified but is vague, evasive, and shows blank indifference. If asked whether he has any pain, his eyes will avoid contact and he will answer, "No, no pain . . . ," "Are you alright, is anything worrying you?," "No, no complaints . . . everything is fine." Throughout questioning his

Reprinted from *The Lancet,* 1:1435–1436, June 23, 1973.

answers are minimal, and as soon as the questions stop he is silent. He rarely attempts to take the initiative in conversation with his wife, children, and medical attendants. He eats little but does not complain of lack of appetite. Although he will often be reported to be sleeping badly, he does not complain, in fact he has no complaints. If the patient is at home, his wife may nearly be driven to distraction by his lack of responsiveness. However, no amount of cajoling from well-meaning relatives will affect his attitude. He does not lament his fate nor does he look abjectly miserable, rather he gives the impression of being completely indifferent. He does not have the obvious signs of extreme anxiety or fear. Blood pressure, pulse, and respiration remain normal. He does not seem to be becoming either cachectic or dehydrated. He may eat and drink a little "to please his wife" but derives no pleasure from it. Within a month of the onset of this syndrome the patient will almost certainly be dead. If a necropsy is carried out, although the patient may have an extensive tumor, there will often appear to be no adequate explanation for the cause of death.

A similar syndrome is associated with the custom of "pointing the bone" in primitive societies. In bone pointing a spell is cast on the victim, who must be aware of the presence of a spell. The other form of willed death in primitive societies is one in which the patient himself wills his death without any external interference.

Pointing the bone is essentially a magic spell cast by a witch-doctor into the spirit of the victim. The Australian aborigines believe that all disease is the result of disharmony of the spirit.[2] If the spirit can be disturbed by such spells, illness should follow. It is believed that if the spirit is sufficiently manipulated any hope of escape becomes unthinkable and, provided the victim holds the necessary beliefs, death follows the witch-doctor's spell. Obviously, the method is ineffective against those who do not hold the necessary beliefs.

The similarity between the westernized man dying through fear of a disease from which there is no escape and the aborigine who dies from an all-powerful spell is illustrated by an account of the death of an aborigine tracker.[2] "Big Paddy" had worked as a tracker for the police in a small, isolated Western Australian town for 25 years, and he appeared to have become totally integrated into modern society. When out on patrol with two other Black trackers and a White police officer, the group surprised a tribe who were thought to have been responsible for a murder. The witch-doctor of the tribe was in a prominent situation when he cursed the invading party. Big Paddy and the other two aborigines knew that they had been cursed. Big Paddy seemed to be more affected than his companions and in less than 24 hours showed complete indifference to everything around him. He stayed in the saddle for the rest of the patrol but was indifferent to every remark or gesture made towards him. At first he would answer questions with a monosyllable, but soon he would not even respond in this way. He did not appear to be shaking with fear, but he seemed cut off from his surroundings. He would not look at his White companion, but with the greatest difficulty he could eat a little. Despite all efforts he became weaker and died within a few weeks.

Occasionally a patient who is discharged to a nursing home known to be used for terminal cases will demonstrate attitudes similar to those encountered in the bone-pointing syndrome. The reverse situation can be seen in young children or animals who have malignant disease but are unaware of it. In these cases the children and animals affected may behave normally until close to death from weakness.

Among Stone Age peoples[3,4] the patient may be saved from an evil spell by one of two mechanisms: if the original spell is found to be defective, a reprieve is possible; a more powerful witch-doctor may be able to overcome the curse of his rival. Both these mechanisms can operate in modern society. The patient who is told that an original diagnosis of malignant disease was incorrect may demonstrate remarkable responses, and the process of willed death can be reversed, provided he can be completely convinced that the original diagnosis was wrong. However, the doctor must be truthful, since further deception is unwarranted. A more dramatic reversal of willed dying is seen in some patients who are sent to special clinics. The Melanoma Clinic at Sydney Hospital often admits patients with incurable melanoma who are beginning to demonstrate all the features of self-willed death. As soon as the patient feels that something can be done to help him, even if all that can be achieved is to show an interest in him and relieve his symptoms, his mental attitude improves. This improvement may be so dramatic that there is a danger of the medical staff believing that various treatments offered by a special clinic have prolonged the patient's life by an organic effect. It is this psychological reversal that makes the investigative assessment of cancer therapy so difficult. Short-term remission of malignant disease in such circumstances, unless definitely substantiated by measurement of the tumor, is more likely to be the result of psychological changes than chemotherapy of the tumor. The quack clinic which purports to cure cancer trades on this psychological reversal of the bone-pointing effect.

In a charming book entitled *The Letters from an Indian Judge to an English Gentle-Woman* (London, 1934) the anonymous author wrote that it takes three generations for the Indian to shake off the powerful effect of his village upbringing, "The drums still beat for at least three generations." Patients who will their own death when confronted with a situation they believe to be hopeless demonstrate that the drums in fact continue to beat for longer than three generations.

REFERENCES

1   Milton, G. W. *Med. J. Aust.* 1972, ii, 177.
2   Elkins, A. P. The Australian Aborigines; p. 311. Sydney, 1968.
3   Idriess, I. L. Our Stone Age Mystery; p. 147. Sydney, 1964.
4   Idriess, I. L. Our Living Stone Age; p. 138. Sydney, 1963.

Chapter 17

The Art of Delivering Bad News

Howard P. Hogshead

Every physician derives satisfaction from delivering good news to a patient; and no physician that I know enjoys delivering bad news. Still, there are rare occasions when it becomes necessary for the physician to disclose a fatal or crippling diagnosis and prognosis to the patient. There is no greater test of the physician's skill and courage than this task of delivering medical bad news. Some physicians delay or avoid this unpleasant task for fear of provoking an emotional scene which they are ill prepared to handle, fear of producing a serious depression, or perhaps fear of losing the trust and confidence of the patient. All of these are valid possibilities which need to be considered.

There are as many ways of handling bad news conferences as there are physicians. There is probably no "right" way, and no "wrong" way to handle this. No thinking physician would use the same stock techniques with every patient. Patients are much too different and too sophisticated to be handled in such a fashion. The particular method of delivering bad news must be varied to meet the needs of the situation. The following are some general guidelines that I have found useful over the years. Most of these rules are not original with me, but I haven't found a single source that covers the subject.

Reprinted from *Journal of the Florida Medical Association,* **63**:807, October 1976.

1 *Keep it simple.* Perhaps as a result of apprehension or uneasiness, there is a tendency to go into too many details and technicalities.

2 Ask yourself, *"What does this diagnosis mean to this patient?"* Many patients are simply unable to comprehend the nature of the diagnosis, in which case methods must be found to gradually educate them.

3 *Meet on "cool ground" first.* It is very unpleasant to walk in to meet people whom you have never met before, knowing you have to give them a piece of really bad news. It is always easier to handle if you have some earlier relationship to the patient or his family, and have some notion of their background and possible reactions to the news.

4 *Don't deliver all the news at once.* It is a good idea to try not to provide too much information at the first sitting. People have a marvelous way of letting you know how much they are able to handle. Like the newspaper that printed "all the news that's fit to print," I feel that the patient has the right to all information that he is prepared to handle. This may mean that the full disclosure has to be spread out over two or three sessions.

5 *Wait for questions.* A long pause will allow the question that tells you where to go next.

6 *Do not argue with denial.* A characteristic response in many patients is outright denial of the reality of the situation. No matter how illogical the denial, it is serving a purpose, and there is nothing to gain by battering down the denial with logic. This usually leads to loss of rapport with the patient. In general, the patient will "hear" the message when he is ready to accept it. It is sufficient that he has been told at least once in some form that condition "x" has been discovered.

7 *Ask questions yourself.* Ask the patient to tell you what you have told him, or ask him what it means. Oftentimes you will be surprised at the answer. Or, ask the patient what the doctors at such-and-such a hospital have told him.

8 *Do not destroy all hope.* There are a hundred ways of handling this, and it requires real tact and experience to be able to acquire the necessary skill. "Most people with this kind of injury don't walk again" is a useful kind of treatment.

9 *Do not say anything that is not true.* This would be the most cruel blow of all.

Again, perhaps there is no right way, only varying degrees of wrong ways. The assistance of a minister, social worker, nurse, or friend may be invaluable. Common sense and human compassion are the prerequisites for the physician who must artfully deliver the bad news.

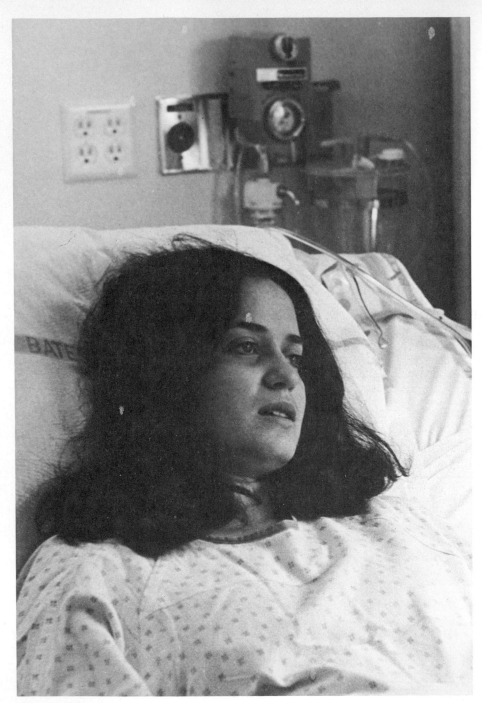

Courtesy of Katrin Achelis

Part Five

Psychological Needs: Recognition and Action

Chapter 18

The Living-Dying Process

E. Mansell Pattison

The purpose of my presentation is to describe the personal dimensions of the living-dying experience. This includes the subjective viewpoint of the dying person; and our objective observations of psychological and social coping mechanisms used by the dying person. We need both the subjective and objective views to comprehend the dying experience. And to begin, we must first look at our own attitudes toward death.

FACING OUR OWN DEATH

We are asked to understand and respond to the dying person. Yet to understand another person in his or her life requires that we understand the same conflicts, the same feelings, and the same situations located within ourselves—for all humans partake of universal feelings and reactions. To understand dying in others demands that we deal with dying within ourselves.

Freud[22] suggested that the unconscious does not recognize its own death, but regards itself as immortal: "It is indeed impossible to imagine our own death; and whenever we attempt to do so, we can perceive that we are, in fact, still present as spectators."

This Freudian view says we fear the unknownness of death. On the other hand, more recent observations suggest that death anxiety does not pertain to physical death, but to the primordial feelings of helplessness and abandonment. The fear of the un-known of death is the fear of the unknown of annihilation of self, of being, of iden-tity. Leveton[31] describes this sense of *ego chill* as: "a shudder which comes from the sudden awareness that our non-existence is entirely possible."

This unknown threat cannot easily be processed within the self. Robert Jay Lifton[34] has graphically described his personal reactions while interviewing the survivors of the Hiroshima atomic bomb. At first he was profoundly shocked and emotionally spent as he sensed his own frail, human mortality, but as the interviews went on he found him-self becoming detached and developing the objective attitude of the scientific observer. He did not become insensitive, but found himself inexorably developing a sense of "psychic closing-off"—the development of a distance between the experiencers of death and his own personal relationship to death—in order for him to function effec-tively as a physician and as a scientist.

This personal account by Lifton points to a critical observation: *we cannot for long look at our own nonbeing.* In fact, the central theme of Becker in his book *Denial of Death* is that life is an unordered chaos in which there is no predictability or sense. To survive, says Becker, the human organism *must repress* its sense of fraility, must sub-merge its awareness of mortality, and must construct a mythology of existence—which we call our mature sense of reality. Reality is *not* out there, to be rationally compre-hended. Reality is the construction we make in order to exist. To sense our own non-being is perhaps vital, but we cannot for long look directly at it. It is like the sun. We can only look directly at the sun for a few fleeting, blinding moments at one time. For the most part, we look at the sun in the same fashion as we look at our own non-being, that is, indirectly.

There are many ways that we face death and our own nonbeing. In general, our culture has been *death-denying.*[3] It is curious to note that although the care of the dying has been handed over to the medical profession and to hospitals, Feifel[21] reports that physicians deny death more than the general populace. Even psychiatrists, who are trained to be sensitive to human emotion, avoid death . . . they just use more abstruse mechanisms. Thus Wahl[57] notes:

It is interesting also to note that anxiety about death when it is noted in the psy-chiatric literature, is usually described solely as a derivative and secondary phenom-enon, often as a more easily endurable form of the "castration fear" . . . it is impor-tant to consider if these formulations also subserve a defensive need on the part of psychiatrists, themselves.

The denial of death is seen in hospitals in the apprehension and avoidance of the dying patient. Often hospital staff suggest that it is unwise to talk to dying patients about their dying because such patients will become nervous, upset, hurt, anxious, or injured. Kübler-Ross[30] reports that only 2 percent of dying patients rejected the opportunity to discuss their dying, but that many staff members became emotionally upset. Similarly, I have found that most dying patients are not only willing but also want to share their dying experience with others. It is rare that such discussions upset the dying person. But I have seen many nurses, physicians, and mental health personnel become nervous, anxious, upset, and distraught. At times they angrily denounce what they perceive as my inhumaneness for frankly discussing death with the dying. Is it possible that such fear and anger are not demonstrations of concern for the patient, but a projection of the anxieties that professional persons experience about their own feelings of death?

The *death-defying* attitude is rooted in the traditions of our Judeo-Christian heritage. We can all recall many instances of people who have fought for causes, ideologies, families, or countries in defiance of the fact that they might die in the process.

The *death-desiring* attitude is much more common in our culture than we admit, for it is not considered acceptable to desire death either for oneself or for others.

A death-desiring attitude is found in those who are severely debilitated, disabled, and the unhappy elderly, who seek release and escape from the misery of their lives. And there are those happy people who have reached fulfillment and look toward death as the satisfying and acceptable end of their lives.

We must also be aware that there are many circumstances where we may desire the death of others. We may have a humane desire to see the end of suffering and misery. We may desire relief from personal, emotional, and financial responsibilities and burdens. There may be people who are a source of anger, frustration, or resentment, whose death may be a welcome termination of the relationship. Death-desiring attitudes and emotions may be neither neurotic nor abnormal. Yet this probably still remains the most taboo attitude toward death.

Death-accepting attitudes place death in perspective as a part of life and one that is integral to existence. Death as the concluding episode of one's life plan is eloquently described by Bertrand Russell:[45]

> An individual's human existence should be like a river—small at first, narrowly contained within its banks, and rushing passionately past boulders and over waterfalls. Gradually, the river grows wider, the banks recede, the waters flow more quietly, and in the end, without any visible break, they become merged in the sea, and painlessly lose their individual being.

This might be termed *death as conclusion*. But this is a romantic view. For as Schneidman[47] points out, this view makes accidental death or early death a tragic and nonnatural event—the romantic progress of life has been interrupted!

A very different death-accepting attitude might be termed *death integrating*. Existential thought has placed death at the center stage of life. Death is not physiological termination; it is our frail mortality. It is not the threat of body stoppage; it is the threat of one's own nonbeing. If we do not face and come to terms with the existential fraility of our existence—the fact that we plan life trajectories that will lead us to old age when, in reality, our life may be snuffed out at any moment—if we deny this fragile life, we become vulnerable to all the neurotic processes of denial. Jacques Choron[13] notes: "postponement of death is not a solution to the problem of the fear of death . . . there still will remain the fear of dying prematurely." So it is not the integration of death, but the integration of a sense of being-meaning that is at issue. As Becker[6] says:

Fear of death is not the only motive of life; heroic transcendence, victory over evil for mankind as a whole, for unborn generations, consecration of one's existence to higher meanings—these motives are just as vital and they are what give the human animal his nobility even in the face of his animal fears.

Becker suggests what has been a traditional religious solution, and one that finds its expression in the Judeo-Christian heritage: "For whosoever will save his life shall lose it; and whosoever will lose his life for my sake shall find it" (Matthew 16:25). Death integration is perhaps then not just an individual psychological solution, but may only be integrated within a transcendent belief.

What is the practical import here? To talk to, work with, and understand the dying person evokes intense personal feelings. As Weisman[59] notes, the care of the dying arouses some of the most pervasive fears of all people—fears such as extinction, helplessness, abandonment, disfigurement, and loss of self-esteem. We could not long survive, much less serve our fellow man, if we had to struggle continuously on the raw edge of our own existence.

Too often we encourage the denial of death, but the remedy is not a defenseless wallowing in the blinding acuteness of our own mortality. Rather, there is that psychic distance to be achieved: *compassionate detachment. Appropriate repression* of our death anxieties is a necessary prelude to effective professional care. By this I mean the capacity to bring into one's consciousness the fundamental awareness of death anxiety, and the ability to feel acceptably comfortable about one's own finite mortality, and thus to allow the fundamental concerns to lie out of conscious sight most of the time. When necessary, or when evoked by life circumstance, one can then respond without major conflict to the stirrings of one's own concerns about death.

Helping Ourselves

Death is ultimately personal. To respond to the fears and human condition of the dying person will always involve responding to ourselves. We face a continuing tension within ourselves: to be in touch with the meanings of death for ourselves so as to be emphatically sensitive, and yet to be able to maintain our psychic composure and objectivity so that we can respond to the dying person as he or she is in life. As Pogo once said: "We have sought the enemy, and found him, and he is us."

So to help with dying, we must first face death for ourselves. Then, hopefully, we may avoid fearful rejection of the dying person, and also avoid the counterphobic mechanism of fusion and identification with the dying. We may then assume a posture of detached compassion.

Our own attitudes toward the dying are a panoply of positives and negatives, as they also are for the dying person, his family, relatives, and friends, and all professional staff. It is unrealistic to only expect positive attitudes in ourselves or in others. Sometimes we will be angered and frustrated by the dying. The situation of dying does not suddenly make people nice! Dying people are all types of human beings, some likeable, some not. Some people are easy to relate to, others not. Some dying persons we will feel like helping, others not. Some people who die will cause us sorrow, others who die will provide us with a sense of relief, or maybe even with vindictive feelings of satisfaction! It is our task to identify and assimilate all these feelings in ourselves and others; to establish a pattern of nondenial of all such feelings; to recognize that the range of emotions is part of the human experience; to integrate both positive and negative feelings; and, finally, not to act upon raw emotion, but to filter our feelings through our conscious self, and act in accord with responsible integrity to ourselves and the dying.

Another aspect of self-helping is to recognize the phenomenon of *death saturation*; that is, we can only work with dying persons for so long, and with so much personal investment, and with so much intensity, before we have reached the limits of our personal tolerance. Helping the dying is a personally demanding task. We each have limits to our intimate exposure to dying. We must be able to identify our personal limits of saturation. Then we need to back off, to gain distance, relief, and reconstitution of ourselves. We readily recognize that our bodies need sleep in order to be fit to face the next day. Yet we less readily acknowledge that our human spirits get exhausted too. It is unrealistic to demand of ourselves the ability to face dying all the time on an intense basis and expect to survive psychically. If we do not build into our work and life schedule appropriate spaces for reprieve and reconstitution, our psychic defenses will do it for us, but not in desirable ways, for then we see the emergence of denial, callousness, emotional withdrawal, disinterest, and so on that are the probable manifestations of psychic exhaustion.

Finally, we need to establish and maintain an ethical attitude that places our professional responsibility in perspective.[40] We cannot be perfect. We can and will make mistakes. But we do need to try to do a decent job to the best of our ability. Maurice Levine[32] sums up an ethical stance that I find most germane:

1 to avoid hostile reactions that harm the patient
2 to avoid self-aggrandizement that may lead to operations or treatments for which one is not prepared
3 to avoid sexually distorted attitudes that lead to possible sexually evoked rejection or seduction of the patient
4 To avoid revealing the confidences of patients for the sake of gossip, or to appear important in the eyes of one's spouse, friends, or colleagues
5 to avoid excessive therapeutic ambition that leads to unnecessary procedures
6 to avoid unnecessary stimulation of anxiety in the patient

Professional Distortions

A posture of compassionate detachment is difficult to attain and maintain. Over the past decade of professional interest in the problem of the dying, two major distortions of compassionate detachment have emerged.

The first is *exaggerated detachment*. Instead of denial of death in a gross and crass manner, emotional distance is achieved through professionalization. Dying is made an object of scientific inquiry. Death is made a disease, a thing. Death is no longer a threat because it can be therapized, so we can now turn to the right treatment of dying. Dying is no longer a subjective experience of persons, but an impersonal objective external problem. Such professionals often demand that specific regimens be set up for dying persons. People are now supposed to die in the right way. They look for logical and rigid patterns of the progression of dying, so that they can rigorously follow the scientific course of action. I have had such professional people seek my consultation because dying persons were no in the right stage, not reacting in the right way, or otherwise failing to respond to the professional and scientific treatment of the dying. In a word, dying is made acceptable through professional *objectification*.

The second distortion is *exaggerated compassion*. Here, instead of separation from the dying, there is psychological fusion with the dying. Such professionals not only identify with the dying person, but also may seek in their work to undo past guilts, relieve past shame, restore personal self-esteem, rework their own prior death experiences, and anticipate their own death anxieties. They live, die, and are reborn with each dying person. Such vicarious identification is also a defense. The dying person is me, but then the miraculous occurs, for when the dying is dead, I am still alive. I have beaten death after all. Such professionals often become personally and professionally overinvolved in the life of the dying person. I have seen these persons angrily denounce any distance or detachment they see in others who work with the dying. How can you have compassion if you are not totally involved? Here dying is made acceptable through professional *subjectification*.

Love and Hate: The Ambivalence Toward Dying

In the recent past we have hated and despised death—and now at least some would have us welcome, embrace, and even love death! I am reminded of those who hate or love the fact that they were born. But birth *is*; we had no say. Even so, death *is*; we have no say. Feelings of love or hate are irrelevant. Life *is*.

However, most people do have feelings of love and hate. All important relationships are a mixture of love and hate. No important person fails to disappoint and frustrate us, and, indeed, the deeper the love and degree of emotional involvement, the higher the probability of disappointment. For the most part we accept and tolerate the negative hateful emotions, and tend to experience in our consciousness only the positive emotions. But it is clear that all of us harbor feelings of love and hate together. Our capacity to accept, tolerate, and even utilize the ambivalence of our feelings is one major hallmark of emotional maturity.

The importance of universal ambivalence is central to our attitude toward the dying. The dying person who is important to us evokes not only feelings of tender, loving compassion, but also feelings of anger, despair, frustration, disappointment, and, yes, even hatred. If we expect that loving feelings are the only dimension of caring for the dying, we shall delude ourselves, and fail to appropriately cope with the arousal of hateful feelings.

The process of appropriate grief and mourning revolves around the successful recognition and integration of our feelings of love and hatred for the dead person we mourn. Similarly, our attitudes toward the dying are rooted in our attitudes toward ourselves and toward others: an integration of the likeable and the despicable. So it turns out that the process of dying is a part of our life that can be best understood as we understand the nature of human nature.

THE DYING EXPERIENCE

Death itself is not a problem of life, for death is not amenable to treatment or intervention. We may consider death only as an issue between man and God. But the process of dying is very much a part of a person's life. Advances in medical technology now make it possible to prolong the period of dying, so that the process dying may stretch out over days, weeks, months, and even many years. For perhaps the first time in history we have many people who experience a new phase of life, *the living-dying interval*.

The human dilemma of this living-dying process was first illuminated for me on a personal level by a letter from a lady unknown to me:

> Dear Dr. Pattison: Quite by accident I read your treatise on dying. Because I am so grateful for your guidance I am writing not only to thank you but to suggest that the article be made available to relatives who care for patients . . . . My husband has been treated for chronic glomeruli nephritis for 9 years. For the past 5 years, he has had biweekly dialysis that equates to a living-dying stage of long duration. In these times, when there is no doctor-patient relationship in this type of indirect care, the entire burden of sharing the responsibility of death falls to the member of the family . . . . Your listing of the fears was so apparent when I read your paper, yet when my husband experienced them I was unprepared to see them or even acknowledge them. When a patient is accepted on a kidney program, he knows he is dying. Would it not be a kindness to the person caring for him to know his fears and how to help?

As said so clearly by this wife, the period of living-dying is most important to the patient, family, friends, relatives, and professional staff.

The Living-Dying Interval

All of us live with the potential for death at any moment. All of us project ahead a *trajectory* of our life; that is, we anticipate a certain life span within which we arrange our activities and plan our lives. And then abruptly we may be confronted with a crisis—*the crisis of knowledge of death*. Whether by illness or accident our potential trajectory is suddenly changed. We find that we shall die in days, weeks, months, or several years. Our life has been foreshortened. Our activities must be rearranged. We cannot plan for the potential; we must deal with the actual. It is then the period between the *crisis knowledge of death* and the *point of death* that is the living-dying interval. This is shown in Figure 1.

Stages or Phases of Dying?

In her landmark book, *On Death and Dying*, Elizabeth Kübler-Ross[30] organized her observations on the dying process around a series of stages; that is, she felt that dying persons typically go through a specific series of psychological reactions in response to their dying. Her series began with initial shock and numbness, followed by denial and isolation, anger, bargaining, and finally depression. If the person successfully moved through these stages he or she would end up in a state of acceptance, and live in hope.

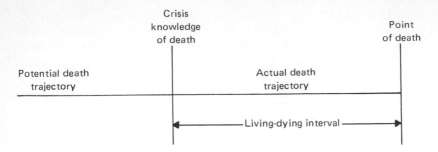

Figure 1 The living-dying interval.

Now it should be noted that Kübler-Ross did not present these stages of dying as an ineluctable process. A careful reading of her book will reveal that she gives many illustrations where these stages were not followed. Nevertheless, many people quickly concretized her clinical sequence into hard fact. And soon there were many references in the literature to the stages of dying, as if this sequence were really so for most dying persons.

Other consequences soon followed. Dying persons who did not follow these stages were labelled deviant, neurotic, or pathological diers. Clinical personnel became angry at patients who did not move from one stage to the next. I have often had professional people ask me what was wrong with one of their dying patients who was stuck in one stage, and who could not be moved on to the next stage. In the professionalization of dying, I began to observe professional personnel demand that the dying persons die in the right way! It was no longer acceptable to respond to the dying person in terms of his or her individual dying experience. Rather, the dying were being pushed and forced into a procrustean process of dying that had been scientifically established.

As this phenomenon of *staging dying* spread, there have been reactions by both lay people and professionals who find that the concept of stages is not only inaccurate, but also misleading to both the dying person and his helpers. For example, in her autobiography of her dying experience, Joanne Smith[53] reports that she became bewildered and began to doubt her own sanity, when her self-observations revealed that she did not follow the stages of dying. She finally concluded: "The stages of dying are not necessarily chronological. In my own experience I have moved back and forth through several of these a number of times."

In his book on the psychological autopsy, Weisman finds no clinical justification for the concept of stages. Rather, he suggests that there is a continual intermingling of emotional responses that go on throughout the dying process. Weisman[60] comments:

> Look how difficult it is to isolate a single characteristic, denial, depression, anger and so forth, and make pronouncements about the process . . . the idea of staging psychosocial episodes is very artificial . . . patients cope and fail to cope with various problems, and their emotional responses are simply indicators of personal conflict and crises . . . the concept of psychosocial staging appeals to me, because

patients are apt to have social and emotional problems anyway . . . it would be very orderly if psychosocial issues followed as neatly as anatomical and clinical staging seem to do . . . but there is no well-recognized succession of emotional responses that are typical of people facing incipient death.

There have also been careful reviews of the published scientific literature that examine the concept of stages. Here again no support is found for the concept. Shibles[51] concludes his recent evaluation of stages thus:

The stages are too procrustean, narrow and fixed, even though they overlap, to adequately account for thoughts, images, perceptual and motor abilities which a person has regarding dying.

In another review Schulz and Aderman[50] also conclude:

The findings again cast doubt on the validity of a stage theory. Patients were not observed to go through stages but rather to adopt a pattern of behavior which persisted until death occurred.

In reviewing the clinical evidence in my book, *The Experience of Dying*,[42] I find *no* evidence therein to support specific stages of dying. Rather, dying persons demonstrate a wide variety of emotions that ebb and flow throughout our entire life as we face conflicts and crises. It does seem misleading then to search for and determine stages of dying. Rather, I suggest that our task is to determine the stress and crisis at a specific time, to respond to the emotions generated by that issue, and in essence to *respond to where the patient is at* in his or her living-dying. We do not make the patient conform to our idealized concept of dying, but respond to the person's actual dying experience.

However, rather than *stages*, Weisman does suggest that there may be *phases* of dying. I concur with this latter way of looking at the living-dying interval. The period of living-dying can be conveniently divided into three clinical phases: (1) the acute crisis phase, (2) the chronic living-dying phase, and (3) the terminal phase. We can respond to the acute phase in terms of crisis intervention, so that it does not result in a chaotic disintegration of the person's life during the rest of the living-dying interval. Thus, our first task is to deal appropriately with the crisis of knowledge of death, so that the dying person can move into an appropriate trajectory that integrates his dying into his lifestyle and life circumstances. The second task is to respond to the adaptive issues of the chronic living-dying phase. Finally, the third task is to assist the patient to move ineluctably into the terminal phase when it becomes appropriate. These phases are illustrated in Figure 2.

Dying Trajectories

The phases of dying are related to several different types of trajectories or *death expectations* that are set up by the crisis of knowledge of death. Glaser and Straus[24, 25, 54]

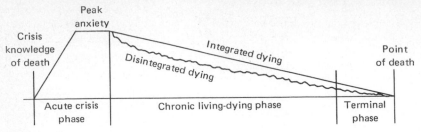

Figure 2   The dying trajectory.

suggest four different trajectories, the first of which is *certain death at a known time.* In this trajectory it is possible to move rapidly from the acute phase to the chronic phase, because the time frame for resolving dying issues is quite clear. In very rapid trajectories, such as in acute leukemias or accidents, the dying process may remain only within the acute phase. The second is *certain death at an unknown time.* This is the typical trajectory of chronic fatal illness. Here the problems tend to center on the maintenance of effective living in an ambiguous and uncertain time frame. The third trajectory is *uncertain death, but a known time when the question will be resolved.* One example of this is radical surgery, where a successful outcome may be known. Thus the patient and family must live through a continuing period of acute crisis. On the other hand, there are long-term problems, such as the possible arresting of cancer, where ambiguity may remain for years. Finally, there is *uncertain death, and an unknown time when the question will be resolved.* Examples are multiple sclerosis and genetic diseases that leave the person beset with a life of uncertainty.

Let us examine some effects of these dying trajectories. First, *certain* trajectories are easier to cope with than *uncertain* trajectories. Ambiguity is always difficult to manage in life. Anxiety is generated by ambiguity and uncertainty. On the other hand, although the certainty of death may not be good news, one can plan for the specific fact of death at a known time. Thus, trajectory 1 (certain; known time) provides the dying person and the people around him or her with a relatively specific time frame in which to order their responses. The time of most acute anxiety for the dying person is in the initial acute phase of dying when the uncertainty of events is highest, while as the person approaches the increased certainty of exact time of death, anxiety diminishes.[38]

Trajectory 3 (uncertain; known time) is somewhat similar. Here there may be prolonged anxiety in an acute phase of uncertainty—waiting for the pathology report after surgery, waiting to see if the organ transplant will work, waiting to see if the severely injured person will survive, waiting to see if the malformed infant will survive. In all of these instances, the dying trajectory is suspended in space, for no actions can be taken while the expectation is in doubt. Here the person and/or the family and staff may entertain high hopes and a positive expectation. It is understandable, then, that here there may be sudden disappointment, and frustration and anger when the hopeful expectation is suddenly dashed by the fact that the person does have a fatal diagnosis, or the illness does not respond to treatment, or the patient suddenly deteriorates and dies. Consequently, this trajectory is likely fraught with intense emotion for all involved.

Trajectory 2 (certain; unknown time) where there is an uncertain time of death is most characteristic of chronic fatal illness. Here there is certainty of death, but the living-dying interval may stretch out over several years. It is clear that here we have prolonged emotional stress for the dying person and for the family. They live with dying. To follow the principle of certainty, the lesson here seems to be the importance of *focusing on what is certain*. Since the exact time of death cannot be reasonably predicted, it is important here to shift the focus to predictable daily issues of life. Thus the dying person and the family can turn to specific issues and deal with life on a predictable day-by-day basis. Whereas in the acute trajectories one is faced with the imminent expectation of death, in this chronic trajectory it is important to shift the focus from death per se to the issues of living while dying.

Trajectory 4 (uncertain; unknown time) appears to be the most problematic for death itself is an uncertainty, and it is ambiguous as to when the issue will be resolved. On the one hand, this overall uncertainty seems to breed a high degree of anxiety that cannot be resolved, leading to dysfunctional defenses and hypochondriacal fixation on one's physical state. Examples are multiple sclerosis and hemodialysis.

On the other hand, where medical technology has produced means of management of uncertain illnesses, it would appear that at least younger patients are able to make a successful adaptation. In fact, they may perceive a reprieve from death in their chronic stable condition. This is illustrated in cases of hemophilia, and in those heart conditions that utilize cardiac pacemakers.

Overall, different trajectories require different coping mechanisms, they vary in their evocation of anxiety and stress, and they pose different clinical management problems.

Denial and Openness

Before we examine the phases of living-dying we must clarify our approach to the dying patient. Ten years ago a common question was: Should we tell the patient or keep it a secret? The question is false. For the care of the dying does not revolve around telling or not telling, but rather around the whole panorama of human interactions that surround the dying person.

There are many levels of communication between people, and many degrees of awareness. For example, the acutely ill patient who is barely conscious should not be subjected to long discussions about the severity of his illness. He knows he is ill and may well die. Care and comfort are foremost. On the other hand, a patient who is experiencing progressive physical deterioration and is told there is nothing to worry about may say nothing but wonder much.

It is difficult to keep secrets. The problem is when our actions say one thing and our words another. This is what is termed *closed awareness* of dying. You know and I know, but we both know we cannot let each other know. This blockage of communication does nothing but set up trouble for all involved.

The questions that a patient has are many. "Am I going to die?" is only the *first* of many questions that the patient may well need to pose and receive specific answers to, not only from the physician, but also from the many people around him. To avoid questions about death means that one must also avoid all other questions about his life that the patient has. Kalish[28] has listed a variety of information inputs that come to the patient:

1   direct statements from the physician
2   overheard comments of the physician to others
3   direct statements from other personnel, including aides, nurses, technologists
4   overheard comments by staff to each other
5   direct statements from family, friends, clergy, lawyer
6   changes in the behavior of others toward the patient
7   changes in the medical care routines, procedures, medications
8   changes in physical location
9   self-diagnosis, including reading of medical books, records, and charts
10 signals from the body and changes in physical status
11 altered responses by others toward the future

It is evident that the dying person is engaged in multiple communications with many people. If the messages are clear the dying person can make sense out of his experience. But if the messages are confused, ambiguous, or contradictory, the result is needless apprehension, anxiety, and the blockage of appropriate actions on the part of both the dying person and those around him.

Now on some fronts we have seen an attack on denial, as if it were a terrible pathology. As a result we sometimes see brutal, blunt, and tactless confrontations in the name of openness.

What do we mean by *denial*? I suggest four levels of denial. The first is *existential denial*. Here I mean our fundamental approach to mortality and the place of death in one's life. We all engage in degrees of existential denial as a necessary mechanism for existence. Second, there is *psychological denial*. This is an unconscious defense mechanism by which we repress that which is known. Both staff and patients use denial mechanisms rather frequently. It is doubtful we could eradicate denial mechanisms, and they often fulfill useful purposes. It is only when denial is pervasive, and the sole or predominant defense, that it becomes a major problem. The third is *nonaccepting denial*. Here we are aware of the facts, but we find it difficult to keep them in emotional awareness, so we tend to suppress our awareness. Fourth, there is *nonattention denial*. We engage our attention elsewhere, and for the moment we are unaware of the undesirable.

One of the persistent themes in the thanatology literature has been that denial of death is pathogenic, whereas acceptance of death is desirable. Unfortunately this is often posed as a black-or-white, either-or, phenomenon. Either we deny death or we accept it. As I see it, denial is a multilayered human process. When we say denial, we actually refer to *various* levels of human awareness of death. Likewise, acceptance may refer to our existential acceptance, or psychological acceptance, or our behavioral evidence of acceptance.

Dumont and Foss[18] have devoted a whole book to the issue of denial-acceptance, in which they examine the evidence at a cultural, social, and personal level. They find the evidence contradictory; there is both denial and acceptance present at the same time. At the center of this contradiction in evidence is the fact that *reason and emotion conflict.* They state: "On a conscious, intellectual level the individual accepts his death, while on a generally unconscious, emotional plane he denies it."

From this discussion I would draw the following conclusions. First, there are different degrees of denial and acceptance of death within each individual that vary over the living-dying interval. Second, there are always contradictions between the conscious-rational and unconscious-emotional aspects of both denial and acceptance. Third, our task as helpers is not to eliminate denial and attain absolute acceptance of death on the part of the dying. Rather, we face the more human task of responding to a flowing process of both denial and acceptance in both ourselves and the dying.

We should not expect at all times to be able to look at ourselves and others in the stark cold light of reality. There is an interplay between levels of denial and levels of awareness. Human communication is full of nuances. Thus, it seems absurd to me that we should expect that suddenly when it comes to discussions with the dying all of our patterns of human communication should change. If we are able to talk with people about their lives in many ways that are comfortable and acceptable to both them and us, then we should be able to talk about dying in many ways that are acceptable and comfortable. Thus I am not concerned with the issue of how much denial or openness there is. But I am concerned that there be *opportunity*, *availability* and *possibility* for open communication with the dying.

The Acute Phase

The crisis of knowledge of death can be seen as a crisis in the life of the person. During the period of acute crisis anxiety increases until it reaches a peak at the person's tolerance level. No one can continue to function long at peak anxiety, and therefore the patient will call upon whatever psychological mechanisms are available to reduce the anxiety. If ineffective mechanisms are used then a disintegrative dying style will follow.

The knowledge of death as a crisis event can be analyzed in terms of five aspects of crisis.[39]

1 This stressful event poses a problem that by definition is insolvable in the immediate future. In this sense dying is the most stressful crisis because it is a crisis to which we bow, not solve.

2 The problem taxes one's psychological resources since it is beyond one's traditional problem-solving methods. One is faced with a new experience with no prior experience to draw from, for although one has lived amidst death, that is far different from facing one's own death.

3 The situation is perceived as a threat or danger to the life goals of the person. Dying interrupts a person in the midst of life; and even in old age it abruptly confronts one with the goals one set in life.

4 The crisis period is characterized by a tension that mounts to a peak, then falls. As one faces the crisis of death knowledge, there is mobilization of either integrative or disintegrative mechanisms. The peak of anxiety usually occurs considerably before death.

5 The crisis situation awakens unresolved key problems from both the near and distant past. Problems of dependency, passivity, narcissism, identity, and more may be activated during the dying process. Hence one is faced not only with the immediate dying process but also with the unresolved feelings from one's own lifetime and its inevitable conflicts.

The first response to this state may be one of immobilization. It is as if life is standing still. One's life flashes before one. There may be no panic, no anxiety, no trace of despair, no pain, but rather an altered state of consciousness. Noyes and Kletti[38] term this a *depersonalization* phenomenon. "This is not really happening to me, I'm just watching."

Then may come an overwhelming, insuperable feeling of inadequacy—a potential dissolution of the self. There is bewilderment, confusion, indefinable anxiety, and unspecified fear.[38] There is seemingly no answer and the anxiety makes it difficult to look at what needs to be done.

We should not be surprised to see many pathological defenses in this acute stage, and we should perhaps not react too vigorously to them. For if we focus on the reduction of anxiety through a focusing on reality issues and appropriate emotional support, it is likely that the dying person will move toward appropriate emotional responses to his living-dying.

The Chronic Living-Dying Phase

During the chronic phase the dying patient faces a number of fears. During this time it is important to specify the precise issues that the dying person faces so that he or she can resolve each specific issue in an appropriate manner. One cannot deal with all issues of dying simultaneously. Rather, our task is to separate apart each issue and take one at a time as they occur. Then the dying person can resolve the issues of dying in a rewarding fashion that enhances his or her self-esteem, dignity, and integrity. The dying person can take pride then in having faced his crisis of dying with hope and courage and come away having dealt successfully with his or her dying. One might call this healthy dying!

Now let us consider the specific fears of the living-dying interval as these are listed in Figure 3.

```
1  Fear of the unknown
2  Fear of loneliness
3  Fear of sorrow
4  Fear of loss of body
5  Fear of loss of self-control
6  Fear of suffering and pain
7  Fear of loss of identity
8  Fear of regression
```

Figure 3   Fears of the dying.

Fear of the Unknown The initial phase of crisis may involve a bewildering array of concerns. However, as the dying person looks forward on his dying trajectory he may fear the fact that he does not know what lies ahead. It is important to separate apart those things that can be known from those for which there are no answers. Diggory and Rothman[17] suggest the following fears of the unknown:

1 What life experiences will I not be able to have?
2 What is my fate in the hereafter?
3 What will happen to my body after death?
4 What will happen to my survivors?
5 How will my family and friends respond to my dying?
6 What will happen to my life plans and projects?
7 What changes will occur in my body?
8 What will be my emotional reactions?

It is evident that some of the above questions can be answered immediately, some answers will be found in the process of time, and some will never be answered. The issue is summed up rather well in the ancient prayer of serenity:

Grant me the serenity to accept the things I cannot change, the courage to change the things I can, and the wisdom to know the difference.

Fear of Loneliness When one is sick there is a sense of isolation from oneself and from others. This is reinforced by the fact that others tend to naturally avoid a sick person and leave him alone.

This mutual process of withdrawal is even more evident when a person is dying. The isolation attendant to dying is not only a psychological phenomenon, but also a reflection of our social management of dying. No longer does our culture afford us the luxury of dying amidst our family, friends, and belongings, for over 60 percent of deaths now occur in impersonal, isolated hospital rooms. We have given medicine and hospitals the social responsibility of caring for the dying, yet the hospital is not geared up to care for the dying.

There have been many critiques of the depersonalized and mechanized care of the dying in general hospitals. Yet our criticism of hospitals and their staff may be misplaced. Most hospitals are socially constructed to provide acute remedial care. To then ask the same social institution to provide chronic supportive care is to place the hospital staff in a doublebind. Which priorities do they respond to? Hospital staff do not necessarily ignore dying patients, but they give priority to patients for whom they can provide life-saving measures. This is not unreasonable.[15]

The dilemma is that acute care hospitals are not well equipped to care for the dying. As a result, the dying are isolated, ignored, and left with little human contact, although perhaps given good technical care.[29] The solution, to my mind, does not lie in the depreciation of acute care hospital staff, but rather in the provision of chronic care facilities that are devoted to the appropriate care of the dying. An example is St. Christopher's Hospice, directed by Cicely Saunders in London, which is a hospital for the dying.

The acute care hospital is necessarily geared toward *curative* functions. Whereas, the dying require *caring* functions. Oliver Wendell Holmes stated the difference nicely: "Our task is to cure rarely, relieve sometimes, and comfort always."

The fear of loneliness is perhaps sensed by the dying from the beginning. The necessary withdrawal from work or recreational activities may begin to accentuate the loss of everyday contacts. It may become difficult to maintain social relations. The dying person may not know what to say to others, while others do not know what to say in return. This social awkwardness is revealed in the autobiography of a dying woman.[53] An insurance salesman came to the door. When asked if she was interested in life insurance, she replied: "Yes, I'm dying and need the insurance right away!"

Increasing physical debilitation and confinement to bed may further limit the patient's social contacts with family and friends, and hospitalization may do so even more. In the hospital the dying person may well be placed in a private room, yet this isolates the dying person even more. Where only supportive technical care is provided, the dying person may be left essentially alone most of the time.

The impact of this social isolation is a sense of human deprivation. As shown in many experiments of sensory deprivation, the human deprived of contact with other humans quickly disintegrates and loses a sense of ego integrity. For the human who is dying, human isolation and deprivation sets the stage for what may be termed *anaclitic depression*. This depression is not due to loss, but due to *separation*—the sense of being away from those we love and depend upon.

Without human interaction the dying person is vulnerable to that syndrome of human deprivation we term *loneliness*. It is one thing to choose to be alone at times— as we all desire—it is another to be left alone. It seems that the fear of loneliness is paramount when the person first faces the prospect of death and fears that he will be deserted in his dying.

Fear of Sorrow We do not like to face situations of grief and sorrow; if possible we prefer to avoid them. Yet the dying person is faced with many losses, which he may fear to face. "Can I stand thinking about what I am losing?" There is the fear that one cannot tolerate the painful experience of sorrow. There is the loss of job, of future plans, of strength and ability, of the ongoing pleasure of relationships and activities.

The task that faces the dying person may seem formidable. Yet not all these losses are likely to occur simultaneously; some joys and pleasures may be taken from some aspects of life during the living-dying interval. This requires that we help the dying person to avoid *premature* sorrow that cuts the person off from available satisfactions.[23]

On the other hand, it is also necessary to help the dying person engage in *anticipatory grief*; that is, to handle each episode of grief as it occurs, so that one can work through that grief and set it aside. Thus one is not beset by constant grief and sorrow, but may have interludes of satisfaction and accomplishment. One may grieve over what must be given up, but may then proceed to engage in what is present in life now.[12, 48, 49]

Fear of Loss of Family and Friends The process of dying confronts the person with the reality of losing one's family and friends through one's death, just as much as if they were dying. This is a real loss to be mourned and worked through.[1] Rather than denying this real separation and preventing the grief work, it is possible for both the person and his or her family to engage in anticipatory grief work. The completion of such grief work may allow the person and his family to work through the emotions of separation and part in peace.

The grief of separation before death is akin to the Eskimo custom of having a ritual feast of separation before the old person steps onto an ice floe, waves good-bye, and drifts off into the sea. Similarly, in the Auca tribe of South America, after a farewell ceremony, the old person leaves the village, and then climbs into a hammock to lie alone until death.

Failure to recognize this real loss ahead of time may block the normal and healthy process of grief. This makes it difficult for the dying person to distinguish between his own problem of death and the problem of grief and separation from those he is leaving. Thus the grief of separation should be accomplished *before* death.

Fear of Loss of Body Our bodies are not just appendages, but a vital part of our self-concept. When illness distorts our bodies there is not only physical loss, but also a loss of self-image and self-integrity. This narcissistic blow to the integrity of self may result in shame, feelings of disgrace and inadequacy, and loss of self-esteem. As before, we may help the dying person to grieve over these losses of body without incurring a loss of integrity or esteem.

Since we humans do not tolerate ambiguity well, it is difficult for us to tolerate ambiguous distortions of the body. External disfiguring disease may be more acceptable because one can see what is wrong, whereas an internal silent process, such as a failing heart or brain, may be more dismaying.

On the other hand, external disfigurement may provoke a sense of being ugly and unacceptable. The dying person may despise his distorted body image and may feel like rejecting his ugly body. Then the dying person may try to hide his unlovely self from his loved ones for fear that his family will likewise despise his ugly body, reject him, and leave him alone.

Fear of Loss of Self-Control As debilitating disease progresses one is less capable of self-control. There is less energy, less vitality, less strength, less responsiveness. These all are part of one organism. We think less quickly, less accurately, and we may fear this loss of body and mind.

This problem is particularly acute in our society, which has placed strong emphasis on self-control, self-determination, and rationality. As a result, most people in our culture become anxious and feel threatened by experiential states that pose loss of control or obtundation of consciousness. This is reflected in our cultural ambivalence over the use of psychedelic drugs and alcohol, which produce diminished states of self-control and altered states of consciousness. In contrast to Eastern mystical experiential states that many participate in, it is unusual in Western culture to experience any acceptable loss of self-control. Even alcoholic highs are viewed with ambivalence. Thus we come ill-prepared to those times of life when we must give up some degree of control over ourselves.

When we come to the experience of dying, the loss of control over body and mind with a diminished sense of consciousness may then create anxiety and fear about the integrity of ourselves. One is placed in a position of dependency and inadequacy so that in a sense the ego is no longer master of its fate, nor captain of the self.

Therefore, it is important to encourage and allow the dying person to retain whatever authority he can, to sustain him in retaining control of his daily tasks and decisions, and thus help him avert feelings of shame for failing to exert such control, and to help him find rewarding experience in the self-determination available to him.

Fear of Suffering and Pain   Our social and cultural experience precondition is in our response to pain. Some ethnic groups are pain-accentuators, while others are pain-minimizers. But more importantly, we learn what *meaning* to give to pain. Thus pain is not the issue per se, but our response to pain that makes it either *sufferable* or *suffering*.

A certain level of awareness of one's body and one's consciousness is necessary to engage in the experience of suffering. Suffering does not occur when we are unaware. This self-awareness may either diminish or exacerbate pain and transform it into suffering.[52]

We may deal with the problem of pain by using medical means of pain relief and thus diminish suffering. This is all to the good, and those who say that pain is not a problem have likely neither felt much pain nor had to live with it. But the mere diminuation of pain does not eradicate suffering, and oblivion is not the answer.

Another alternative is to diminish suffering through awareness and understanding. David Bakan[4] suggests that a humanistic approach to pain and suffering lies in our understanding of and awareness of pain. The patient who fears pain is more likely expressing a fear of suffering. And what is suffering? It is pain that has no meaning, no location, no explanation. Clinical studies of pain in the dying bear this out: pain relief is not closely related to the dosage of pain-killing drugs, but rather relief is closely tied to the person's attitude toward pain.

The fear is not just a physical fear, but a fear of the unknown and unmanageable. Senseless pain is perhaps intolerable. On the other hand, pain may be accepted and dealt with if that pain does not mean punishment, or being ignored, or not being cared for. People will not suffer long, but they will endure pain.

Fear of Loss of Identity   The loss of human contact, the loss of family and friends, the loss of body structure and function, the loss of self-control and total consciousness all threaten the sense of one's identity. Human contacts affirm who we are, family contacts affirm who we have been, and contact with our own body and mind affirm our own being-self.

We can see that the dying process faces the person with many threats to self-identity. How does one maintain identity and integrity in the face of these forces of dissolution? Bowers[7] concludes:

> When life cannot be restored, then one can accept the fact with a meaning that gives dignity to his life, and purpose even to the process that is encroaching on his own vitality.

Willie Loman, the salesman, says of his own death: "A man must not be allowed to fall into his grave as an old dog." It is not that we die, but how we die. The tasks are to retain self-esteem and respect for the self until death, to retain the dignity and integrity of the self throughout the process of living we call dying. There are three major mechanisms for this.

The first mechanism is most important. We maintain our identity through contact with those who have been and are part of our life. We do not become a number, a case, an object if others continue to see us, react to us, talk to us, relate to us, *as the unique people we are.* Here again is the familiar theme of dying: maintaining contact with the familiar that keeps on reaffirming to the dying person that he is the person he has always been.

A second mechanism is reinforcement of identity through the continuity of one's life in family and friends. One sees one's self in one's children, one's life work, and in the bequeathing of one's possessions to others. One cannot only leave a will, but also leave parts of one's body in bone banks and eye banks. This personal sense of continuity was illustrated by a middle-aged man who was dying of lung cancer. I had spent much time talking with him about his life as he lay dying on my ward. He was transferred to another ward where the surgeons wanted to perform a biopsy. He refused until he could talk to me. I explained to him that the biopsy would not change his disease, but it would help my understanding of the disease. Then he was pleased to comply, for he felt he was giving me something, his diseased tissue, that in a sense I would carry with me in my professional life. He had given me a part of himself to be with me after his death.

A third mechanism is maintenance of identity through a desire for reunion with loved ones who have died before or who will die and join one. These reunion fantasies include the sense of return to the primordial mother figure as well as reunion with specific loved ones.[8, 26] There will be reunion with one's parents and one's progeny. Hence one can place oneself at one point in the continuum of ongoing human relationships, of which one's death is merely one point in the more universal span of existence.

Fear of Regression   Finally, there is fear of those internal instincts that pull one into retreat from the outer world of reality into a primordial sense of being where there is no sense of time or space, no boundaries of self and others. We have all had this sense of pull toward regression into self when we awaken in the morning. As the alarm rings we drowsily douse the noise, turn over, feel the immense weight of our sleep pulling us back into slumber. We luxuriate in the indefinite sense of our boundaries, the relaxation of our awareness, the freedom from the demands and constrictions of the real world that await our awakening. With exquisite pleasure we allow ourselves to float back off into a timeless, spaceless, selfless state of nonbeing.[35, 46] Certain religious mystical experiences, psychedelic experiences, and body awareness exercises produce similar altered states of consciousness.

In most of life the ego fights against this instinctual regression into selflessness. In our culture we have difficulty regarding such states as acceptable. We fear such states.

For the dying person, especially as he approaches and enters the terminal phase of living-dying, the fear of regression begins to loom. With the diminution of physical capacity and the clouding of consciousness, the sense of regression may be frightening. The dying person may fight against the regression, trying to hold onto a concrete, hard, reality-bound consciousness of himself. This may produce the so-called death agonies—the struggle against regression of the self.

It is here that we must help the person shift away from reality and turn inward toward the self, that is, we must allow regression and withdrawal to occur. With such support the dying person may then accept the surrender to the internal self, allow himself to turn away from life, and seek reunion with the world out of which he or she has sprung. Then psychic death is acceptable, desirable, and at hand.

The Terminal Phase

The onset of the terminal phase of living-dying is not precise. However, we can roughly state that it begins when the dying person begins to withdraw into himself in response to internal body signals that tell him he must now conserve his energies unto himself.[44] Perhaps it is like the experience we have all had with a bad case of the flu. We feel terribly sick, lose interest in food, activities, and friends. All we want to do is curl up in a warm bed and be left alone in peace and quiet. The onset of such a withdrawal in the dying process is the onset of the terminal phase.

Lieberman[33] has found that the terminal phase is marked by both physical withdrawal and by the appearance of subtle signs of emotional disorganization. Hinton[27] observed that there is a decrease in anxiety and an increase in depressive involution. Davies et al.[16] found that this psychological withdrawal is a type of "apathetic giving-up" that accompanies a deterioration of the physical state of the person.

This turning from the outside world to the internal self is clearly described in this case report by Janice Norton:[38]

> She told me her only remaining fear was that dying was strange and unknown to her, that she had never done it before. Like birth, it was something that only happened once to any individual, and similarly one might not remember what it was really . . . . She no longer worried about what was to happen to her after death . . . she felt that she might be unnecessarily concerned with the actual process of death itself.

Changes of Hope   At the outset of the living-dying interval, the dying patient has an *expectational hope*; that is, a set of expectations that have some possibility for fulfillment. There may be remissions, arrests, sometimes possible cures. There may be weeks, months, years of some rewarding life yet to be fulfilled. And it may well be that the dying person will cling to this expectational hope in a useful sense throughout the living-dying interval.[41]

On the other hand, a person's entering the terminal phase may be signalled by a change in hope. Stotland[55] has clarified the point that expectational hope now changes to *desirable hope*; that is, the patient may still hope that he might not die and this is a desirable thought, but it is no longer expectable as a hope. This transformation from expectancy to desire may herald the psychological process of giving-up. It is for this reason, as Cappon[11] notes, that hope should not cease until shortly before psychic death. However, we should also attend to the fact that we may aid the dying person in making the necessary transition from expectancy hope to desirability hope as he or she enters the terminal phase.

Types of Death When we consider the terminal phase we must take into account the various definitions of death, of which there are four.

First, there is *sociological death*; that is, the withdrawal and separation from the patient by others. This may occur days or weeks before terminus if the patient is left alone to die. The person is treated as if he or she is already dead. Some families desert the aged in nursing homes, where they may live as if dead for several years. The second of these is *psychic death*. Here the person accepts his death and regresses into himself. Such psychic death may accompany the appropriate diminution of the physical body status. But anomalies can occur; psychic death can precede terminus as in voodoo death,[10] or in patients who predict their own death and refuse to continue living.[5, 58, 61] Third, there is *biological death*. Here the organism as a human entity no longer exists. There is neither consciousness nor awareness, such as in the case of irreversible coma. The heart and lungs may function with artificial support but the biological organism as a self-sustaining, mind-body is dead. The fourth is *physiological death*, where vital organs such as lungs, heart, and brain no longer function.

The importance of these four types of death is that they can occur out of phase with each other, and that becomes a major source of ethical and personal confusion. As shown in Figure 4, as the person enters the terminal phase, it is reasonable to suppose that he or she has begun to give up and withdraw. The process of sociological death would allow the dying person to withdraw, and lead directly to psychic death, which is usually shortly followed by biological and then physiological death.

However, there are distortions of this process which are also shown in Figure 4. Where there is social rejection of the patient, he or she may become socially dead long before the other aspects of death occur. On the other hand, where there is social and personal rejection of the dying process, we have the problem of precipitous death that has neither been anticipated nor dealt with. This can also occur when a patient suddenly deteriorates and dies contrary to expectation. This often precipitates a shocked reaction in all involved, because the anticipated trajectory has been upset. Another example is where the patient rejects life. This usually meets with social disapproval. For example, old people are not supposed to say they are ready to die, nor is the acutely ill person. We want people to want to live. In so doing, we may interfere with their own dying trajectory. And finally, there is the case of death of mind and body and the preservation of life by artificial means in which there is social denial

1 Ideal proximity (note termination of hope)

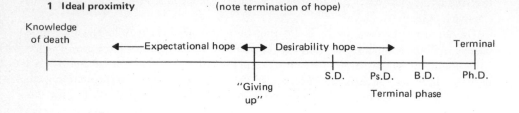

2 Social rejection of patient

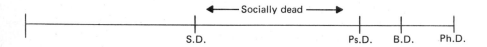

3 Social and patient rejection of death

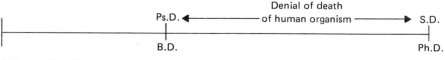

4 Patient rejection of life

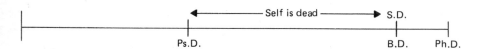

5 Social rejection of death with artificial maintenance

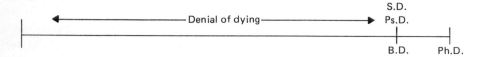

B.D. = Biological death
Ph.D. = Physiological death
Ps.D. = Psychic death
S.D. = Sociological death

Figure 4 Types of death sequences.

.of the fact that both psychic death and biological death have occurred. This is currently a source of much medical-ethical controversy in our culture.

In summary, our task is to synchronize each type of death dimension so that they will converge together in an optimal and appropriate fashion, rather than being disjointed and out of phase with each other.

COPING WITH DYING THROUGHOUT THE LIFE CYCLE

Thus far we have considered the dying process as if it were the same throughout the life cycle. However, the stage of life profoundly influences one's sense of identity, one's sense of self, and therefore one's sense of death.[2, 14, 19, 62]

In the young, preschool child, there is little sense of personal identity. The young child has no appreciation of the intellectual notions of death and dying. Rather, there are two aspects to identity: the bodily self, and the self as part of the parents.

Here the issues of death and dying are not intellectual but experiential. The young child does experience pain, discomfort, bodily dysfunction if he or she is ill. Therefore, the goal of coping with dying in the young child is to help him feel comfortable and to relieve bodily distress. The second aspect deals with presence and separation. Separation from mother and father is loss of the security and sense of self. To be with one's family is to be oneself. To be alone is to experience annihilation of oneself. Therefore, the care of the dying young child centers around maintaining the young child with his family if possible. If hospital care is necessary, then a stable and reliable parent substitute must meet the child's need for someone to love him and maintain his sense of being.

As the older preschool child (between the ages of 3 to 6) grows, he begins to develop a more unique sense of himself. The capacity to think, to reflect, and to inquire begins to emerge. He acquires a sense of self-control and self-direction. He feels a sense of action and result. This is the age of fantasy and daydream, of dreams and nightmares, of magic and mystery in the world. In the world of fairytales there are manifold possibilities.

The dawning intellectual appreciation of death appears. But death is still separation; death is not-being-here-anymore. So death is not pretend. It is real, but not permanent.

Again we have two motifs: magical fantasy, and real but impermanent death. The lively play of fantasy, not yet modified into tested reality, leaves this age child vulnerable to misinterpretation and misunderstanding of sickness and death. The child may view illness and disability as punishment for real or imagined actions. He may experience treatment procedures in magnified fantasies, and may see hospitalization as abandonment and rejection by his parents. He may interpret the grief, sorrow, and unhappiness of his parents as anger or disappointment in him. Thus, dealing with dying calls for the careful explanation of the causes of illness and the need for procedures and treatment. The child needs to understand the emotional reactions of his parents, so that he does not feel guilty, does not feel rejected, does not feel unwanted or unloved.

The grade school child is a doer. For him, life and being are synonymous with action. "Look ma, I can ride the bike—no hands." "I can run faster than you can." There is pride in achievement, affirmation of self in accomplishments, the definition of who I am by what I can do.

The school-age child now begins to see the distant horizon of a life to be lived. Fantasies now relate to a possible reality. There are heroes and idols and great deeds to be done. There is death in this world, but it is distant, it is not personal. It is the end of play, the interruption of the game. "Aw, do we have to quit now, we're just in the middle, I don't want to come home for supper." But if I must come home I will, and I will live with that frustration and disappointment, for life is here and now and I can dream about tomorrow.

As we turn to death and dying then, we can see that the child here must cope with bodily disability and dysfunction as an interference with his capacity to be a person. He needs to be able to do, to do what he can, to do what gives him satisfaction, to continue his involvement in his activities. Further, he needs his friends, the daily concourse of interchange that tells the child that he is O.K. He can appreciate the intellectual notion of his death, but his experience is still rooted in the life of today. He can and will dream of tomorrow, even if that tomorrow will not come, for at this age who knows what tomorrow there will be. Thus, the key to coping with dying is in the life of the present where life and identity are squarely placed, and let us dream of the possibility of a tomorrow.

One might think that the adolescent had a strong identity indeed. It is time for bringing up father, and putting mother in line. Parents are a reflection of exquisite self-consciousness. Who am I? is the central question. Adolescence is a time of intense intellectual and emotional preoccupation with oneself. It is the time to grasp oneself firmly, to shout "I am." The doing is subordinated to being. There is a subtle but critical transformation from what I do makes me important, to being what I am makes what I do important. The sense of respect for the integrity of my unique self is paramount.

Here the concept of death acquires an intellectual importance that meets the emotional experience of oneself. The adolescent now has a sense of being, a sense of person, a sense of *me*. Characteristically, the adolescent does *not* have a sense of longevity. The length of life is not at issue, but the quality is. Thus we see many romantic notions of death in the thoughts of adolescents. Who cares how long I live, so long as I live and die as the real me. So adolescents make brave soldiers, because they do not fear annihilation so much as whether they are brave and glorious. The image of oneself is important, the life of oneself much less so.

So, in coping with dying in the adolescent we are faced with the youth who may fear the loss of his or her newly gained sense of true-being. Am I strong, am I beautiful? Am I a decent human being? Am I really me? Or will I die before I know who I am? Will I die before I have a chance to show others who I am? The affirmation, confirmation, and clarification of the adolescent as a unique and real human being may be the most important task in coping with dying at this age.

The young adult is on the threshold. All has been preparation for life and now here it is. It is the beginning of a career, a home, a marriage, or a family. There are hopes and aspirations. Goals are now set to be tested by experience. How will it go? I can hardly wait. There is intensity, fervor, impatience, excitement, new ideas and places waiting.

The young adult's awareness of his own death causes much frustration and disappointment. The task for the dying is to reconcile what might have been with what is.

There may be a sense of being cheated, of unfairness, of not getting one's fair share of life. Why me? Perhaps the sense of frustration is greater here than in any other dying situation.

To cope with dying in the young adult is to deal with his disappointment, his rage and frustration, his anger at the world and at himself. Perhaps more than any other age group, young adults fight death and tenaciously hold onto their existence. I am here now, ready and able to live. A young woman of 25 with leukemia, another of 30 with carcinoma, both wanted to live with vitality, read, talk, and keep their houses as long as they could. They wanted to maintain the integrity of their adult mandate to live their lives. Perhaps this sustenance of the active, striving, coping, able adult is good. Dying with the harness on is what the young adult seems to prefer.

The middle years of adulthood are a neglected time. Certainly adulthood is not a plateau. Each decade of life brings new challenges and new perspectives. The impetuous drive of youth mellows to the steady pull of maturity. A growing sense of the surety and familiarity of oneself, one's marriage, one's spouse, leads toward a possible appreciation of the more subtle and muted rewards of life. It is interesting to interview couples at different decades of their lives. Each couple claims to like the decade they are living in the best. But they appreciate the value and perspective of each decade gone before. For the man, he will likely come to a more realistic appraisal of his goals and abilities. For the woman, there will be a greater freedom and opportunity for expanded selfhood. As one moves from one decade to another there is usually more security, more time for reflection, the opportunity to gather some fruits from the labors of life.

The issue of death in the middle years is more likely to take on an interpersonal tone. The middle years have usually seen the development of meaningful ongoing relations with spouse, children, relatives, friends, and neighbors. Hence death is a disruption of the involvement with others. It is not that you cannot leave the ones you love, it is that you do not want to. They fill your life. There are responsibilities and obligations. Who will fulfill them? Thus, coping with dying involves coping with the involvements you have with others. This may then become the focal issue in our response to dying at this age.

In old age more and more people now live longer. To be old does not mean that death is perceived as being just around the corner. A man of 70 told me recently: "Just because I am retired doesn't mean I don't enjoy life every bit as much as you do." Retirement and old age does not mean that one has come to peace with life and is now ready to accept death. In *Death of a Salesman*, Willy Loman says wryly: "A man can't go out just the way he came into it. He's got to amount to something." Old age brings one to reflect upon the whole of one's life. One's identity is still at issue. Was I a real person and am I a person still? Can I respect myself and love myself in the face of what my life has been? Robert Butler[9] has pointed out that many old people engage in a type of perseverative reminiscence of their lives. They go over and over their lives. Did it make sense? Was it worthwhile? Are they O.K.? In my conversations with old people, I find many who are not yet ready to die. They have not made peace with themselves. They still question and doubt their existence. Death will be an intrusion, unless and until they can affirm that their lives were unique and unlike that of anyone else. So again, coping with dying involves the affirmation of the real personhood of the aged person.

Ego Coping versus Defense Mechanisms

Before we turn to examine how people cope with dying throughout the life cycle, we must briefly examine the nature of coping mechanisms of the ego. The concept of *ego* is derived from the psychoanalytic observations of Freud, but the term has passed into common usage and lost its specificity. In psychodynamic terms, when we speak of ego, we do not refer to a thing in the mind, but rather to a set of mental operations that are conveniently summarized in the term ego. This *ego set* contains several functions: the sense of self, the center of personal identity, the experiencing self that receives input from different parts of the human organism, the seat of thinking and decision making. In brief, we may conceive of the ego as the control center of the self—interposited between the unconscious drives, images, fantasies, and impulses, and the external world of reality.

Freud observed that when the ego had problems resolving conflicts between the internal unconscious self and the external world of reality, a variety of *ego defenses* gave rise to neurotic symptoms. Hence it seemed that ego defenses were pathological.

However, not all ego defenses are equally pathological. Some defenses are used frequently by all of us, for example, rationalization and conscious suppression. On the other hand, some ego defenses are relatively unusual and represent gross distortions of reality, for example, delusions and hallucinations. Thus, we must consider a hierarchy of ego defenses in terms of their utility, the degree to which they distort reality, and the degree to which they comprise the total psychological function of the ego.

The development of ego defenses is part of psychological development. Thus, the young infant probably hallucinates. The toddler and preschool child use delusional thinking and projection. The older child begins to discard these gross mechanisms and adds passive-aggressive behavior, acting-out mechanisms, and fantasy, while the adolescent moves on to acquire the use of altruism, humor, suppression, and avoidance. Thus, we cannot look at the use of defense mechanisms without also taking into account the developmental stage of the life of the person.

Further, the concept of *defense* mechanisms has long had a negative connotation, as if it is bad to have or use defense mechanisms. In fact, we must be able to protect and defend ourselves psychologically. Thus, it is more appropriate to use the term *coping* mechanisms. Vaillant[56] has pointed out in a careful study of adaptive ego mechanisms that all people use a variety of coping mechanisms throughout their lives. Thus normal, psychologically healthy, and well-adapted people occasionally use immature ego-coping mechanisms. Under stress, all of us will most likely resort to some use of immature ego-coping mechanisms. Thus, the issue is *not* that we all use ego-coping mechanisms, but rather whether the coping mechanisms we use are adaptive to the context in which we find ourselves.

I have spent a bit of time here reviewing the meaning of ego-coping mechanisms, because these concepts have been much abused in the literature on dying. It is simple to observe classical *neurotic* defense mechanisms in dying patients. We can see denial, anger, depression, acting out, bargaining, ritualization, obsessiveness, hypochondriasis, rationalization, intellectualization, projection, fantasy, withdrawal, avoidance, and so on. The temptation is to say: "Aha, see how neurotic dying people are . . . look what pathological coping mechanisms they are using!" We go on to conclude: "Now we need to treat these psychologically neurotic dying people so that they will give up all these defenses, and proceed to die in a nonneurotic manner."

But the above attitude is an overinterpretation of psychopathology. As I have stated above, we all use ego-coping mechanisms that can be labelled immature or neurotic. Usually we do not use them all the time, nor in a fixed pattern. None of us is so perfectly developed psychologically that we can cope with the stress and conflict of life in a perfectly adaptive manner! In fact, I have no idea of what kind of person that would be. But I do understand that we are frail mortals who have various degrees of ability to cope with life in a reasonable fashion. Sometimes our ego-coping styles get out of hand, and then it is helpful to switch back to more adaptive ego-coping styles. Most of this therapeutic change in our ego-coping styles does not occur in psychotherapy, but rather occurs as the result of discipline, counsel, advice from our friends, confrontations with our loved ones, learning from experience, and other corrective experiences in life.

When we turn to the dying and observe their ego-coping styles why should we suddenly expect perfection in dying when there is no perfection in life? Nor should we need to label maladaptive coping styles as neurosis that need to be eradicated through treatment. I believe it would be preferable to respond to the dying as normal persons who may invoke a variety of ego-coping mechanisms. Hopefully, where necessary and possible we may guide the dying in paths of rewarding styles of coping with dying.

With this background let us examine the ego-coping mechanisms of the dying. First, I am struck by the fact that *all* people involved with dying experience high degrees of stress, from which none are immune. It is obvious that nurses, doctors, social workers, psychologists, and psychiatrists all sustain emotional assaults on their ego functioning as they work with dying patients. Nor do they respond with aplomb and equanimity. Well-seasoned mental health professionals experience anguish, pain, despair, anger, fear. These normal professionals use projection, denial, passive-aggressiveness, acting out, etc. So the pathologies, if such, are not the sole province of the dying; they are part of us all.

Second, I am impressed by the fact that during the acute crisis stage of dying, more primitive and immature coping mechanisms are commonly utilized. As I have stated earlier, acute crisis brings out the most primitive defenses in all of us. We cope the best we can with what we have. And we should neither be surprised nor dismayed to see such primitive coping styles fleetingly emerge during acute crisis. For the most part, as I see people, the dying person and their family quickly discard these primitive responses, and move on to more mature coping mechanisms. Our concern should be not for the moment, but whether the dying person is able to move on to more adaptive mechanisms after the acute crisis has passed.

Third, we must not forget that the living-dying interval is a time of repetitive stress. The dying person is also physically sick, and that drains one's psychic energy. While the healthy person may effectively use many coping mechanisms, the range becomes limited for the sick and dying person. For example, because of physical disability, the dying person may not be able to engage in physical activities such as recreation, or in involvement in work, or even in such simple coping mechanisms as conversation or reading. Hence, the dying experience limits the repertoire of coping mechanisms available to a person.

Fourth, I have asked these questions: What ego-coping mechanisms may we anticipate in each stage of the life cycle? Do all dying persons revert back to primitive, immature, or neurotic coping styles? Or is ego-coping style related to the life cycle in which the dying person lives?

I have indicated that the coping mechanism of denial is to some extent present in all of us all the time in regard to death. Further, there are degrees of denial at different levels of awareness that are constantly present in the dying person. Thus, it seems reasonable to conclude that denial is a relatively universal part of coping with dying, so I shall not include denial in my subsequent analysis.

In my book, *The Experience of Dying*[42] I have analyzed the types of ego-coping mechanisms used in each life stage. Figure 5 contains a list of the major ego-coping

Ego-coping mechanisms	Early childhood	School-age child	Adolescence	Young adult	Middle age	Aged
Level 1: primitive						
Delusions	+	+				
Perceptual hallucination	+	+				
Depersonalization	+	+				
Reality-distoring denial	+	+				
Level 2: immature						
Projection	++	+++	+		+	
Denial through fantasy	++	+	+			
Hypochrondriasis		++	++	++	++	+++
Passive-aggressiveness		+++	++	+++	++	++
Acting-out behavior		+++	++	+++	++	
Level 3: neurotic						
Intellectualization			+++	+	+++	+
Displacement			++	++	+	
Reaction formation			++	+++	+	
Emotional dissociation			+++	+	+	+
Level 4: mature						
Altruism			+		+	++
Humor			+	+	+	+
Suppression			++	+++	+++	+
Anticipatory thought			+++	+++	+++	+++
Sublimation			+	+	++	+++

+ = occasional use
++ = moderate use
+++ = considerable use

Figure 5 Typical ego-coping mechanisms of the dying throughout the life cycle.

mechanisms arranged in a hierarchical sequence: *primitive, immature, neurotic, mature.* Again, I wish to caution that at any given cross section of time we may observe most of the ego-coping mechanisms being used in a transient fashion. What we are trying to determine, however, are the more typical coping mechanisms that the dying person uses.

Several points may be drawn from my observations of this process. First, there is a general trend for the dying to use the ego-coping mechanisms along a developmental sequence; that is, the youngest children only have the most primitive coping mechanisms available. As one grows older, in each stage of life, the dying person will typically use more advanced ego-coping mechanisms, and tend to rely less on earlier types of coping, so that when we come to the aged they have moved to a general mode of rather mature coping mechanisms.

Second, there is an obvious overlap of most of the ego-coping mechanisms for most life stages; but it is also obvious that the dying do *not* just use primitive or immature coping mechanisms. In fact, it is striking that the dying exhibit the frequent use of many mature coping mechanisms.

Third, in early childhood we can observe the dying process evoke primitive coping mechanisms, including delusional thought, perceptual distortions, and gross denial of reality. This is not psychosis. Rather it is the transient use of primitive coping mechanisms. The use of primitive defenses appears to extend into the preschool years, but does *not* typically appear thereafter.

Fourth, in the school-age child we see the emerging use of immature coping mechanisms. In particular, the child deals with the stress of dying through externalization mechanisms. This is, of course, typical of how the school-age child deals with stress and anxiety anyway.

Fifth, in the adolescent we see the appearance of the use of intellectual coping styles as a dominant pattern, although immature mechanisms are not abandoned. Some mature mechanisms also come into play, especially those of an intellectual type.

Sixth, in the young adult there appears a wider variety of coping mechanisms. It would seem that more immature mechanisms crop up in young adulthood. Adolescents appear to gain strength and coping ability from their parents and other adult figures, whereas the young adult may be making the transition to independence, and thus dying comes at a particularly vulnerable time that calls forth more immature mechanisms.

Seventh, in the middle-aged we observe the emergence of many mature mechanisms, and less use of immature mechanisms as seen in the young adult.

Eighth, in the aged, although hypochondriasis is a feature, the presence of predominantly mature coping mechanisms is manifest.

Finally, I want to reiterate that I have summarized *typical* mechanisms during the living-dying interval. As noted before, the initial acute crisis phase is likely to be marked by transient maladaptive coping mechanisms. In the above analysis, I have been concerned with the chronic living-dying interval. Finally, when we come to the terminal phase of dying, we may expect the typical coping mechanisms to recede, and be replaced by isolating mechanisms, withdrawal, and increasing detachment. I have suggested that this withdrawal may be misinterpreted as depression. No doubt there is some depression present; however, our task may not be to draw the person back into involvement with life, but rather allow him or her to appropriately withdraw from life.

In summary, then, the dying do not employ just a few stock coping mechanisms. As they did in the rest of life, they use all the many coping mechanisms of the human ego. It seems that the dying use the coping mechanisms most typical of their stage of life. The more mature the life stage, the more likely the dying will use more mature ego-coping mechanisms. It does not appear that people deal with the process of dying much differently from the way they have previously dealt with life. As people have coped throughout their life, so they will continue to cope in the same way with their dying.

HELPING THE DYING

To put the helping process in perspective, I should like to set forth four precepts about help in the dying process. First, I do not view dying as a pathological problem that should be treated.[20] Thus I do not want to present a set of treatment plans for the dying. Rather, I view dying as a part of normal living, so it would be more accurate to consider how we should respond to, relate to, and interact with the dying. Let us examine how we may behave in our personal and professional encounters with the dying in a manner consonant with human dignity.

Second, I view the concept of helping as a normal everyday response of human relationship, not as something special. All of us maintain a relative stability in life because of the helping interaction with the people in our social matrix of life. The once popular song by the Beatles says it: "I get along with a little help from my friends." Helping, to my mind, is the corrective, supportive, inquisitive, challenging, accepting, give and take that comprises our valued relationships with others.

Third, helping is not so much doing as being. In our anxiety to accomplish something, to do something about dying, to feel we are valuable, or whatever, I find a zealousness to do things. But this may be for our own benefit, not that of the dying. To comfort is to share. To share is the willingness to be, without having to do.

Fourth, I see helping with dying as the opposite of most helping. Usually we help people to move toward fuller engagement of life. With dying, we help people to disengage from life.

In working with the dying person, I do not propose some ideal pattern for dying, yet there are some general principles. The first is to achieve an integration of dying into the person's lifestyle. Weisman[59] describes this as an "appropriate death." The concept of an appropriate death is a style of dying that is adaptive to the specific person. We seek to assist the dying person to view his own death and live out his dying in a manner consonant with his own pattern of coping mechanisms, his own definition of the meaning of death, and his own life context. Thus the criteria for an appropriate death will be fulfilled in different ways for different people. Each person's death is different, but is appropriate for him or her.

Following Weisman, I propose the following criteria of an appropriate death.

1   The person is able to face and resolve the initial crisis of acute anxiety without disintegration.

2   The person is able to reconcile the reality of his life as it is to his ego-ideal image of his life as he wanted it to be.

3   The person is able to preserve or restore the continuity of his important relationships during the living-dying interval and gradually achieve separation from his loved ones as death approaches.

4   The person is able to reasonably experience the emergence of basic instincts, wishes, and fantasies that lead without undue conflict to gradual withdrawal and the final acceptance of death.

A second principle involves the maintenance of *phase appropriate* responses. I have called attention to the different emotional issues and reality factors that face the dying person in each of the three phases of dying. Each phase calls for a different style of response from us. In the initial acute crisis phase we are faced with the issue of acute anxiety, and perhaps high ambiguity. In the chronic living-dying phase we are faced with reality issues and the necessity of coping with problems in daily living. In the terminal phase we are faced with providing support for achieving separation and withdrawal.

A third principle that involves the terminal phase is to achieve relative synchrony, so that the social, psychological, and physiological dimensions of death tend to merge together in a coherent fashion. This means that we must attempt to maintain social and psychological attitudes that are consistent with the physiological state of the dying person.

Now let us consider some specific ways to help the dying face and cope with the various types of fears, listed previously, that they face.

Fear of the Unknown

As suggested, this fear is most manifest in the initial acute crisis phase. It is important to establish a relationship of confidence and trust with the dying in which he or she can ask questions and receive reliable answers. It is important to provide specific answers when possible; to state when specific questions will be answered if that is possible; and to state what questions cannot be answered except through the process of time. Finally, it is helpful to distinguish between questions about the reality issues of life, for which real people can give real response, versus philosophical, religious, and speculative questions about which we may offer opinions but cannot give answers. This then helps the dying person to distinguish between the real and known aspects of dying, for which he or she can obtain some known answers, versus the unknownness of death that cannot be known.

Fear of Loneliness

The problem here differs with each phase of dying. In the initial acute phase the fear of rejection or of being deserted may be more fantasy than reality. In this phase it may be useful both to be present on a frequent basis and to carefully determine who will be with the dying person at what times. During the chronic phase, it is useful to not allow the dying process to become the sole focus of the person's life. Rather, the task is to engage the dying person's interest in everyday relations and everyday tasks. In the terminal phase, it is useful to assure the dying person of the continuing interest and availability of people to the extent that the dying person needs and desires such assurance and companionship. Thus the dying person need not fear loneliness, although he or she may at times be alone.

Fear of Sorrow

Here the task is to provide an atmosphere that conveys the message that grief is not out of place. But grief does have limits. If we can accept the experience of grief and sorrow in ourselves and share in sorrow with the dying, it then becomes possible to draw to a conclusion that grieving. We have shared the sorrow, expressed the grief, and completed that small task of mourning. This is the function of anticipatory grief. It allows us all to identify the source of sorrow and work through that emotion. Otherwise, the dying person and others are likely to accumulate a storehouse of small griefs that soon become an intolerable load. It is useful to help the dying person to identify the particular griefs of the dying process and deal with each one on its own terms, rather than attempting to cope with all the griefs at once. Finally, it is useful to distinguish between the sorrow over one's death versus the particular sorrows of specific events or persons.

Fear of Loss of Family and Friends

Often the process of dying reawakens the latent dimensions of interpersonal relations. Submerged feelings of both love and hate may be evoked in the dying person's network of social relations. Here the task may be to help the dying and their family and friends accept the variety of emotions that flow between them, and to help clarify ambiguous and conflicting emotions and achieve some acceptable resolution of the emotional tensions that arise. In this way it may be possible for the dying to reaffirm the basic meaning and values of his or her personal relationships. It is when this resolution occurs, when some peace has been achieved, that the dying may then begin to separate from their loved ones, work through that grieving experience, and no longer fear the loss of relationships even though there is now separation as death approaches.

Fear of Loss of Body

The first task is to keep the dying accurately informed as to their bodily processes. They need to know what is wrong and why it is wrong. This removes the mystery of ambiguous bodily processes. The dying need to be assured that loss of body functions or abilities is not shameful. We need to provide assistance with bodily functions only to the extent that the dying person cannot do so himself. Thus, we preserve both a respect for the body as it is, and preserve body control and body function to the extent that it is possible. It is important, again, to distinguish between body functions that are healthy versus those that are sickly. It is important to distinguish between real physical *ability* that is present in the dying versus their physical *disability*, that is, we must keep a good sense of body reality in the forefront. It is neither useful to ignore body dysfunction nor to overemphasize body dysfunction.

Fear of Loss of Self-Control

We might consider control here at several levels—control of one's life, control of one's self, and control of one's body. These dimensions can get interlocked, and then confusion abounds. Control over one's life may include fear of being unable to determine life or death. That is a general attitude that needs to be resolved in the beginning of the dying process. However, the dying can make specific decisions about their lives, such as those affecting wills, property, family concerns, funeral, burial, and other matters about how they shall live through their living-dying. Thus, this enables the dying to determine, to the extent possible, the direction of their living-dying lives. Similarly, the dying can be encouraged and supported to determine their own emotional and psychological style of living-dying. And finally, we can continue to provide the dying with the opportunity to exercise physical management of their bodies, to the extent that it is possible. So although the dying must ultimately relinquish self-control, it remains a gradual process.

Fear of Suffering and Pain

As noted earlier, suffering revolves around both loneliness and the unknown. Here as before, it is useful to assist the dying in the maintenance of life engagement. When the dying person has nothing to do except live in painful isolation, pain is likely to be suffering. Whereas the dying person who continues to be involved with life and persons can live with pain. Similarly, pain that is mysterious or that has no source or explanation is likely to be insufferable. Hence, the source of pain, the extent and duration of pain, need to be explained as reasonably as possible. It is not my purpose here to discuss the technical and/or medical aspects of pain management. I certainly do not suggest that stoical acceptance of all pain is either possible or desirable. I would strongly endorse the human value of using pain-relieving medications where appropriate. Only people who have never experienced severe physical pain would oppose the use of pain-reducing medications. But the opposite radical point of view that pills or shots will solve the problem of pain is also unrealistic. Suffering is a human problem that includes physical pain. Thus, our response must include both human interest and involvement, the provision of knowledge, and the personal participation of the dying person in his or her own pain management. Then it is possible to alleviate suffering and collaboratively work on the management of pain, which often cannot be eliminated but can be tolerated.

Fear of Regression

The fear of withdrawal is probably linked to past experience as well as to the reactions of others. If we insist on pulling people who are in the terminal phase toward active engagement we communicate the message that regression is indeed fearful and undesirable. On the other hand, we may accept and thereby communicate our own lack of fear of regression. This produces a setting where regression is not a shame, guilt, or fear-producing experience. Regression can then occur without undue conflict and relinquishment of self proceeds as a gradual process.

In the history of human culture we have rarely left people to fend for themselves when faced with death. Although I have focused on specific technical issues, I wish to reemphasize that to my mind the most important dimension of helping the dying is perhaps simply being with the dying.

Dying is that experience of life that simply reminds all of us that we are human and therefore mortal. Our goal—to achieve healthy dying—may seem paradoxical. But as we face our own mortality and the fact that death is part of our lives, we may begin to practice the high therapeutic art of helping people to die.

REFERENCES

1 Aldrich, C.K.: "The Dying Patient's Grief," *Journal of American Medical Association*, **184**:329–331, 1963.

2 Anthony, S.: *The Child's Discovery of Death*, Harcourt Brace, New York, 1940.

3 Aries, P.: *Western Attitudes Toward Death: From the Middle Ages to the Present*, Johns Hopkins, Baltimore, 1974.

4 Bakan, D.: *Disease, Pain, and Sacrifice: Toward a Psychology of Suffering*, University of Chicago, Chicago, 1968.

5 Barber, T.X.: "Death by Suggestion: A Critical Note," *Psychosomatic Medicine*, **23**:153–155, 1961.

6 Becker, E.: *The Denial of Death*, Macmillan, New York, 1973.

7 Bowers, M., (ed.): *Counseling the Dying*, Nelson, New York, 1964.

8 Brodsky, B.: "Liebestod Fantasies in a Patient Faced with a Fatal Illness," *International Journal of Psychoanalysis*, **40**:13–16, 1959.

9 Butler, R.N.: "The Life Review: An Interpretation of Reminiscence in the Aged," *Psychiatry*, **26**:65–76, 1963.

10 Cannon, W.: "Voodoo Death," *American Anthropologist*, **44**:169–181, 1942.

11 Cappon, D.: "The Dying," *Psychiatric Quarterly*, **33**:466–489, 1959.

12 Carr, A., D. Peretz, B. Schoenberg, and A. Kutscher (eds.): *Loss and Grief: Psychological Management in Medical Practice*, Columbia, New York, 1970.

13 Choron, J.: *Modern Man and Mortality*, Macmillan, New York, 1964.

14 Cook, S.S.: *Children and Dying: An Exploration and Selective Bibliographies*, Health Sciences Publishers, New York, 1974.

15 Crane, D.: "Decisions to Treat Critically Ill Patients. A Comparison of Social Versus Medical Considerations," *Health & Society*, **53**:1–34, 1975.

16 Davies, R.K., D.M. Quinland, F.P. McKegney, and C.P. Kimball: "Organic Factors and Psychological Adjustment in Advanced Cancer Patients," *Psychosomatic Medicine*, **35**:464–471, 1973.

17 Diggory, J.C. and D.Z. Rothman: "Values Destroyed by Death," *Journal of Abnormal and Social Psychology*, **63**:205–210, 1961.

18 Dumont, R.G. and D.C. Foss: *The American View of Death: Acceptance or Denial?*, Schenkman, Cambridge, Mass., 1972.

19 Easson, W.: *The Dying Child*, Thomas, Springfield, Ill., 1970.

20 Engel, G.: "Is Grief a Disease?," *Psychosomatic Medicine*, **23**:18–22, 1961.

21 Feifel, H.: "The Function of Attitudes Towards Death," in *Death and Dying: Attitudes of Patient and Doctor*, Group for the Advancement of Psychiatry, New York, 1965.

22 Freud, S.: "Thoughts for the Times on War and Death," *Collected Papers*, vol. 4, Hogarth, London, 1915.

23 Fulton, R. and J. Fulton: "A Psychosocial Aspect of Terminal Care: Anticipatory Grief," *Omega*, 2:91–100, 1971.

24 Glaser, B.G. and A.L. Strauss: *Awareness of Dying*, Aldine, Chicago, 1966.

25 ——and——: *Time for Dying*, Aldine, Chicago, 1966. Glaser, B.G. and A.L. Strauss.

26 Greenberg, I.M.: "An Exploratory Study of Reunion Fantasies," *Journal of Hillside Hospital*, 13:49–59, 1954.

27 Hinton, J.: "The Physiological and Mental Distress of Dying," *Quarterly Journal of Medicine*, 32:1–21, 1963.

28 Kalish, R.A.: "The Onset of the Dying Process," *Omega*, 1:57–69, 1970.

29 Krant, M.J.: *Dying and Dignity: The Meaning and Control of a Personal Death*, Thomas, Springfield, Ill., 1974.

30 Kübler-Ross, E.: *On Death and Dying*, Macmillan, New York, 1970.

31 Leveton, A.: "Time, Death, and the Ego-Chill," *Journal of Existentialism*, 6:69–80, 1965.

32 Levine, M.: "The Hippocratic Oath in Modern Dress," *Cincinnati Medical Journal*, 29:257–262, 1948.

33 Lieberman, M.A.: "Psychological Correlates of Impending Death," *Journal of Gerontology*, 20:181–190, 1965.

34 Lifton, R.J.: "On Death and Death Symbolism: The Hiroshima Disaster," *Psychiatry*, 27:191–210, 1964.

35 Montefiore, H.W., (ed.): *Death Anxiety*, MSS Info. Corp., New York, 1973.

36 Needleman, J.: "Imagining Absence, Non-existence, and Death: A Sketch," *Review of Existential Psychology and Psychiatry*, 6:230–236, 1966.

37 Norton, J.: "Treatment of a Dying Patient," *Psychoanalytic Study of the Child*, 18:541–560, 1963.

38 Noyes, R., Jr. and R. Kletti: "Depersonalization in the Face of Life-Threatening Danger: A Description," *Psychiatry*, 39:19–27, 1976.

39 Parad, H.J., (ed.): *Crisis Intervention: Selected Readings*, Family Service Association of America, New York, 1965.

40 Pattison, E.M.: "Psychosocial and Religious Aspects of Medical Ethics," in R.H. Williams (ed.), *To Live and to Die: When, Why, and How*, Springer-Verlag, New York, 1973.

41 —— : "Psychosocial Predictors of Death Prognosis," *Omega*, 5:145-160, 1974.

42 —— : *The Experience of Dying*, Prentice-Hall, Englewood Cliffs, N.J., 1976.

43 Petrie, A.: *Individuality in Pain and Suffering*, University of Chicago, Chicago, 1967.

44 Rioch, D.: "The Psychopathology of Death," in A. Simon (ed.), *The Physiology of Emotions*, Thomas, Springfield, Ill., 1961.

45 Russell, B.: *Portraits from Memory*, Simon & Schuster, New York, 1956.

46 Schneidman, E.S.: "Suicide, Sleep and Death: Some Possible Interrelations Among Cessation, Interruption and Continuous Phenomena," *Journal of Consulting Psychology*, 28:95-106, 1964.

47 —— : "On the Deromanticization of Death," *American Journal of Psychotherapy*, 25:4-17, 1971.

48 Schoenberg, B. et al. (eds.): *Loss and Grief: Psychological Management in Medical Practice*, Columbia, New York, 1970.

49 ——: *Anticipatory Grief*, Columbia, New York, 1974.

50 Schulz, R. and D. Aderman: "Clinical Research and the Stages of Dying," *Omega*, 5:137–143, 1974.

51 Shibles, W.: *Death: An Interdisciplinary Analysis*, Language Press, Whitewater, Wis., 1974.

52 Shontz, F.C. and S.L. Fink: "A Psychobiological Analysis of Discomfort, Pain, and Death," *Journal of General Psychology*, 60:275–287, 1959.

53 Smith, J.: *Free Fall*, Judson Press, Valley Forge, Pa., 1975.

54 Strauss, A.L. and B.G. Glaser: *Anguish: A Care History of a Dying Trajectory*, Sociology Press, Mill Valley, Calif., 1970.

55 Stotland, E.: *The Psychology of Hope*, Jossey-Bass, San Francisco, 1969.

56 Vaillant, G.E.: "Theoretical Hierarchy of Adaptive Ego Mechanisms," *Archives of General Psychiatry,* 24:107–118, 1971.

57 Wahl, C.W.: "The Fear of Death," *Bulletin Menninger Clinic*, 22:214–223, 1958.

58 Walters, M.J.: "Psychic Death: Report of a Possible Case," *Archives of Neurology and Psychiatry,* 52:84–85, 1944.

59 Weisman, A.D.: "Misgivings and Misconceptions in the Psychiatric Care of the Terminal Patient," *Psychiatry*, 33:67–81, 1970.

60 ——: *The Realization of Death*, Aronson, New York, 1974.

61 —— and T. Hackett: "Predilection for Death: Death and Dying as a Psychiatric Problem," *Psychosomatic Medicine*, 23:232–256, 1961.

62 Zeligs, R.: *Children's Experience with Death*, Thomas, Springfield, Ill., 1973.

Chapter 19

Oncology/Hematology and Psychosocial Support of the Cancer Patient

Ernest H. Rosenbaum

Good health is the greatest asset we have in life. When it is impaired because of an accident or an illness such as cancer, or kidney or heart disease, we are forced to make compromises. A 26-year-old woman with advanced melanoma who has made these compromises recently wrote me,

> I now see things in a much different light. Even though I probably will die young, I don't just sit around and wait for it. Actually, no one is given any more time than I am. We wake each morning to a new day, and that is all. No one is promised ahead of time that they will be here for the spring vacation, for the wedding in August, or even for the dentist appointment next Thursday. We are all equal in that we have one day to fill with anything we please. The quality of life lived each day is more important than how long we live. . . . I am not the only one in the boat but no one else can do my living or dying for me.

This woman is typical of a person who has a strong will to live, who continues to live even as she is dying. My goal as a doctor is to try to help each of my patients achieve a similar equilibrium. Sometimes I succeed, sometimes I fail; but the way I

With Isadora Rosenbaum and Tina Anderson.

handle each patient is based on a recognition of his or her special emotional needs as well as of the terror and anxiety that are common to anyone who has been diagnosed as having a potentially fatal disease.

When a patient is referred to me for a preliminary diagnosis or for reevaluation, it does not matter whether cancer is only suspected or whether it has been a reality for some time. The anxiety of each patient is extreme, the silent questions overwhelming. To begin to penetrate this terror, I explain at our first meeting by belief that the most beneficial relationship between us must be based on mutual trust and candor. To help him face his fears and anxieties, I explain the diagnostic procedures he will undergo. I discuss the reasons for doing each test, the range of possible results, positive and negative, and I assure him that if the results are positive, we have an arsenal of therapies with which to attack his problem. Finally, I continually ask each patient whether he has any questions and urge him to write them down as they occur to him so that he will not suppress these thoughts and add to his anxiety.

When testing is completed and the results indicate a malignancy, I arrange for the patient to come to my office at a time when I will be able to explain the situation to him or her without interruption. When possible, I prefer to have the closest family members present during the explanation. This eliminates the need for repetition and reduces the possibility of a misunderstanding. The presence of a close family member or friend also helps lessen a patient's fear of abandonment and reassures him that details about his condition are not being concealed from him.

Knowing that what I say in this interview is crucial and may affect the rest of a patient's life, I proceed slowly and carefully, ready to temper my approach as he reveals how much he wants to know at that moment. Although I encourage candor and full partnership between myself and each patient, it is still a patient's prerogative to choose how much he wants to hear at any given time. I give detailed explanations of his disease, repeating much of the basic information I gave him during the diagnostic procedures. Most important, I describe the treatments that are available to combat his disease and reassure him that although we will begin with one mode of therapy, there are others that may be equally good or will provide a backup if the first one is not effective.

For the past 2 years, for the benefit of both patient and family, I have tape recorded these 30-to-40-minute initial meetings of my explanation and of their questions and reactions and given them the recording to take home. I use this form of reinforcement for two reasons. The person who has just learned he or she has a serious disease is stunned and may hear little of what I say. He is busy thinking, "Why me?" or "How much will I suffer?" or "What will happen to my family?" The cassette recording, listened to at home in a more rational moment, will provide the same vital information and give reassurance to him and his family that there are concrete medical steps that can be taken to help him. Reviewing the information in this way also helps create openness between the patient and his family about the disease and the problems they will face as well as providing a springboard for future discussions between us. Many patients have told me that this procedure has added a new dimension to their understanding of their disease and their planned program of treatment.

Occasionally a situation will arise in which a patient or a member of his family will request that I keep information from the other one. In such cases I try to convince them of the desirability of openness with each other, but if I am ever forced to take a stand, I will side with the patient (except in an extreme case where a patient suffers from severe mental or emotional problems), for it is with him that I have made my covenant for honesty. It is his battle for life with which I am concerned, his feelings, his well-being. He, not his family, has come to me for service.

One of the obvious advantages of a well-informed patient who understands all of his options is his willingness to undergo therapy. Moreover, it is absurd to think of giving complicated treatments, with their possible side effects, to someone who is uninformed.

At no time during the course of treatment, even in the earliest stages of disease and medical therapy, should the subject of pain, suffering, or death be avoided. A patient always knows whether he can broach these terrifying subjects with his doctor. He will know intuitively whether his doctor is afraid and defensive. As one of my patients said,

It is in the earliest meetings, even before the diagnosis, that the tone of the relationship is set. In these encounters, the physician reveals his attitudes toward the disease and the patient. He establishes the foundation of confidence and support on which the patient will later rely. If he shows respect for the patient and his own courage in the face of cancer, he will immediately begin to win the patient's trust. It is important to achieve this before the diagnosis because the physician's manner in presenting the diagnosis and the patient's reaction to it have an enormous effect on the course of the disease.

Having had cancer for more than 2 years, I know what a doctor can mean in liberating one to live actively during the remaining time of one's life. Thus, a doctor should recognize that by his own courage and respect for the patient, he can relieve terror. If he shows confidence that he can remain in control of the disease and the pain, it removes an enormous burden from the patient's life.

When the doctor is afraid, the patient is afraid and communicates this fear to his family and friends, the very people who should be enlisted to support him in his ordeal.

The successful long-term treatment of any patient will depend to a great degree on a patient's attitude. If he can strive for and maintain a positive attitude, which means he is willing to fight for his life and believes he can live longer by doing so, he very often will respond better to treatment. I remember several instances where two patients who were similar in age, diagnosis, and degree of illness, and who were undergoing the same type of treatment, had different therapeutic results. The only discernible difference between them was the pessimism of those who did less well and the optimism and determination of the others to live as fully as possible despite their debilities.

I do not believe that I can *create* a positive attitude where none has existed before, but to the extent that I must know each patient intimately in order to prescribe and regulate therapy and to give him or her emotional support, I can also encourage a positive attitude in many ways. One way is to alleviate his or her fears concerning chemotherapy. Many people have heard frightening stories from uninformed relatives and friends about the side effects of treatment, both conventional and experimental. These stories make them more afraid of therapy than they are of cancer. I assure these patients that if side effects occur, I will try to alter the therapy or the method or the time of application, not only to reduce the side effects but also to enable them to coordinate treatment with their other commitments. For example, working people can often be put on a program that does not interfere with their work schedules by receiving therapy just before the week end. The side effects will have worn off by Monday.

Another source of anxiety and depression for a patient is his feeling of a loss of autonomy, of a new dependence on others—the medical team. From the day he seeks help for his symptoms, a person is questioned, poked, prodded, tested, and given treatment. I try to mitigate these unwelcome feelings of dependence by prescribing, when feasible, a program that includes oral chemotherapy that can be taken at home, and, in the later stages of disease, by encouraging home care and self-administered pain shots.

Fear of the unknown—of changes in therapy or of periodic test results—is always a source of acute anxiety for a cancer patient. For this reason I always describe the risks, side effects, and anticipated results of all the therapies appropriate to each person's disease in order to prevent unnecessary shocks in the present or the future. I also explain that it is not uncommon to change from one mode of therapy to another, to alter the dosage or content of a therapy, or even to cease therapy altogether for a time. I tell patients that such moves should not be misconstrued as a failure of therapy or a progression of disease. For those who worry whether their current therapy is effective, I can also reassure them that we will try something else if that one fails.

These are the kinds of anxieties that can be alleviated during regular office visits. Therefore, I encourage patients to always keep a list of questions that occur to them between visits. Many people are so fearful of receiving bad news during an office visit that they forget the worries that plagued them during the previous week or two.

Since any anxiety or worry can break down a patient's determination to fight, I also try to discern when there may be nonmedical problems that contribute to a patient's depression. The fear of losing a job, or a misunderstanding with a relative or a friend, should not be added to the ordeal of coping with cancer. I obviously cannot solve these dilemmas for my patients but I can, by listening to them, give emotional support.

Since it is not always possible to tell solely from talks during office visits what extra burdens a patient must endure in addition to cancer, I try, if requested, to make a house call early in a relationship. A very well-dressed patient may actually live in minimal circumstances or suffer from tension caused by another family member. One of my patients, a middle-aged man with colon cancer, became desperately ill one evening and finally telephoned me. I found him in a rooming house in a deteriorating part of town. He lived in one small room and shared a bathroom at the end of the hall with several other people, making colostomy care difficult when he had diarrhea. When he suffered side effects from chemotherapy, he had to depend on the manager of the rooming house to bring him his meals. He had been too proud to ask for help, but having discovered his true situation, I was able to mobilize nursing care and other assistance.

The causes of fear and anxiety and other types of problems I have mentioned all prevent a cancer patient from maintaining an attitude that will allow him to function maximally for his type and stage of disease. When these emotional problems are brought out in the open and possible remedies are discussed by doctor and patient, the patient gains a little more freedom to spend on the ordinary things of life—work, recreation, the pursuit of knowledge, the enjoyment of family and friends. It is this actuality of being able to participate in and enjoy the things one has always enjoyed that is the definition of having a positive attitude. One of my patients, a psychiatrist, is an excellent example of a person who has achieved this. He says,

> This is a very, very rich period in every single dimension of my life, whether that's family, sports, music, or my work. At least at this time I have no physical limitations and can maintain my former level of life. Cancer has not robbed or significantly diluted the capacity I have always had to enjoy life. I think most people are not transformed psychologically by having cancer, even though they may live their lives somewhat differently. Their victory is in the full continuation of their lives without being paralyzed by regressive fears and needs. Their victory is that of actively living while enduring cancer. This is made possible, in part, when doctor and patient are honest and open with each other. Then, although fears and fantasies don't disappear, they are put into a manageable perspective, and the individual is freed to do more than engage in solitary battle with his own phantoms.

Another person who approaches the problems of living with cancer in a positive manner is this woman of 35, who is married and the mother of a 7-year-old girl:

> Cancer is devastating. At first you can't even think about it. You're smacked hard and all the wind goes out of you. You don't begin to think until you reach a plateau where you know you're doing well. Then you begin to think about yourself and your family and your reasons for living.
>   I've seen people destroy themselves with their attitude in all kinds of situations, and although I don't believe your attitude can cure your disease, I do believe it can help you. Therefore, I reject my negative thought. It sounds insane, but it keeps me healthy. Negative thinking breaks down my energy level. Although my drive and my will and my pace are basically the same as they were before, I have changed in one way. I no longer fly off the handle over unimportant matters. My priorities are being alive and loving my family. I've always loved life, and the biggest pain is that I didn't have enough of it when this thing happened. So I said, "Screw you, world. I just ain't leaving."

The positive attitudes of these two patients represent what I call the *will to live*, and give a fifth dimension to the four traditional therapies—surgery, radiotherapy, chemotherapy, and experimental immunotherapy. I have said that patients with positive attitudes tend to respond better to therapy and are better able to cope with their disease-related problems. Some doctors and psychologists go further than this. They believe that the proper attitude may even have an effect upon cell function and consequently may be utilized to arrest, if not cure, cancer. In an effort to support their views, they are conducting studies to determine to what extent the mind and emotions are involved either as a contributing factor in the onset of cancer or as a means of altering its course.

Some researchers are exploring the possibility that people with certain personality traits may be more susceptible to developing cancer. Others are experimenting with methods of actively enlisting the mind in the body's combat with cancer, and to this end techniques such as meditation, biofeedback, and visualization are being employed. (Visualization involves the creation in a patient's mind of positive images about what is occurring in the body.) At present doctors and patients are divided on this issue of the degree of influence of mind over body. Personally, I do not think that any of the studies that have so far been conducted are scientifically valid. There is as yet no proof that a person can control his cancer with his mind. One of my patients, cured of leukemia, vigorously disagrees, however, and will not to this day even acknowledge that chemotherapy was the agent that pulled him through. He says,

> Chemotherapy was a crutch and I was willing to go along with all the crutches. I was willing to use any means available until I was able to do it myself. I don't respect it [cancer] at all because the moment I do, I'll be afraid of it, and fear is the greatest enemy in this thing. . . .
>
> Every disease, though real, is psychosomatically induced. There are no exceptions. The emotional and mental state of the individual triggers the germs and viruses in the body that cause disease. . . . I also subscribe to the notion that anything can be done if you believe in it strongly enough, and that includes the eradication of disease.

A second patient believes, as I do, that although a person cannot use his mind to effect a cure, a good attitude is still very important.

> Having acute leukemia in 1975 is somewhat akin to having the Black Plague in 1340 in Europe—namely, that one has no idea what the causality of it is. This can encourage magical thinking that somehow one has done something to provoke the forces of nature and that one only need do something else to regain control over them. This is the most fearsome thing to me—one's complete helplessness before the forces of nature. It would naturally be comforting to believe you brought about your cancer by your own emotions, actions, or state of mind. Scientifically, there may be some basis for believing that the emotional state has something to do with a person's response to cancer, but if the emotions do play a role, I don't think it's an obvious or a major one. On the other hand, I am certain that trying to maintain a state of psychological well-being won't hurt.
>
> When I speak of the will to live, I don't mean some kind of simple, blind faith or optimism. To me it has more to do with the kind of stance or posture that one adopts toward the disease, namely an aggressive, fighting posture. Having an attitude of doing battle with the disease and having some knowledge of the drugs, the program, and so on, makes it easier to cope with the discomfort because one then understands what is going on.

It will be many years before we know whether it is possible for the mind to control the immune defense system. In the meantime, the experiments of biofeedback and visualization are helpful to patients in that they encourage positive thinking and provide relaxation. However, these methods can also be damaging when a patient puts all his or her faith in them or ignores conventional therapy. For instance, in one of the current philosophies, Carl Simonton, M.D.[1], tells patients that they have unconsciously brought on their disease and that they have the power within them to decide whether they will live or die by changing their beliefs and improving their self-image. Through visualization the patient is taught to relax and mentally picture his disease, with the white blood cells attacking and overcoming the cancer cells. While such a procedure can lift a depressed patient who needs hope or a way to help himself, it can also prove psychologically devastating if he totally accepts the thesis that he has brought on all his discomfort and pain through his own personality and stressful way of life. The extreme guilt, disappointment—and often bitterness—when the disease progresses would not be necessary if realistic, rather than false, hope were given before participation in the program. Visualization is still in the theoretical stages. Perhaps it will turn out to be true that we cause our own cancer, but to create guilt and remorse before proof exists is a mistake, however well-intentioned and devoted the advocates of the theory.

My criticism is limited, however, for I do appreciate that these methods can increase the will to live and I recommend them to my patients. I also suggest to patients that they can, if they feel the need, avail themselves of one of the psychiatric support programs of private counseling or group therapy that are offered by a variety of institutions: hospitals; major cancer treatment centers; social welfare departments; and the American Cancer Society. Sharing frustrations with others in similar circumstances often relieves the sense of isolation that cancer patients experience. I think that none of us, even if we have been dangerously ill, can have any concept of the depths of despair and terror that are experienced by a person who has a terminal disease.

Thus, it is understandable why people grasp at straws. As cancer advances, the emotional and mental assaults increase, seriously compromising a person's self-image. After all, a sense of worth is directly related to what we do and how we interact with others. For instance, when a cancer patient is unable to work as hard as he did before his illness, or has less energy for family activities than he used to, he has feelings of shame and guilt. If his disease is terminal, his sense of being defective and even somehow to blame for his condition may be intensified. Unfortunately, these feelings of impotence and isolation are corroborated and reinforced by others in the worst way, for cancer does, unfortunately, make many people uncomfortable. Some even think it is infectious. The cancer patient of today has been equated with the leper of yesterday, so often does he encounter fear and avoidance in family and friends, nurses and doctors.

These attitudes contribute to psychological deterioration, which is intensified by the patient's awareness of his bodily deterioration. The paradox is that the more

[1] Grace Halsell, "Mind over Cancer," *Prevention*, January 1976, pp. 118–127.

physically dependent on others he becomes, the more psychologically and emotionally cut off he is. To better understand these devastating aspects of living with cancer, I sometimes tape record conversations with selected individuals who want to contribute their thoughts and feelings to help others. One such person is Dr. Arnon Fortgang,[2] a surgeon in San Francisco who describes what happened following his own diagnosis of cancer.

> Cancer, while a dreaded illness, does not necessarily totally immobilize the patient, nor render him an invalid. A decrease in productivity, however, can occur for various reasons. There is some physical weakness and increased fatigue, as well as some reduced drive and initiative. In addition, there are fewer opportunities open to the cancer patient—and very often he is not given an opportunity to return to his previous job or profession. Our society, which professes the need for rehabilitation and reconstitution of the injured or ill, tends, in reality, to shut the cancer patient out of the mainstream of his usual employment, severely curbing his productivity. This takes the form of inaccessibility to the previous job. In the case of professionals, such as self-employed physicians, medical practice becomes impractical because of the current exorbitant malpractice insurance fees, hospital rules, and disability schedules that do not allow for partial disability ratings. Thus, the medical cancer patient is often prevented from returning to work and similar experiences are common among cancer patients in other professions.
>
> There are also changes in the relationship between the cancer patient and his peers. Either there is a taboo around him, or his more enlightened friends may show empathy and sympathy, which usually stem from the attitude that "if it happened to him it could happen to me." Nevertheless, while there is a considerable amount of personal empathy and sympathy, there is as yet no organized structure geared to the rehabilitation and return to normalcy for the cancer patient. This situation creates, for the patient, a feeling of partial death. He is not wanted on the job, on committees, or on boards. His office starts looking like a morgue—full of old records and x-rays, but no new activity. What soon dawns on the patient is that he has been compromised over and over again. Initially, there is an illness that tends to render him less effective, on top of which there are limitations on his working opportunities. This often results in being offered a lesser job than he had before. Thus, while the illness itself forces him to compromise once, the other factors force him to compromise over and over again.
>
> As a cancer patient you try your darndest, every waking minute, to stay on top of your tragedy. Then you encounter these powerful negating roadblocks that counteract all your efforts. What is so painful about all of this is that although you cannot do much about being ill, you can sustain yourself by deciding to go back to work and be productive in the field in which you are trained. And yet, there are these external barriers that deprive you of what is most important to you and that become the most disabling feature of your illness. You get a feeling of running into a solid brick wall—total frustration.
>
> In recent years a considerable body of evidence has accumulated that the mind has the capacity to have a positive effect in illness on body healing, body resistance

---

[2] Arnon A. Fortgang, M.D., a surgeon in San Francisco, who planned to participate in the First National Training Conference for Physicians on "Psychosocial Care of the Dying Patient" by speaking of the patient's perspective on life-threatening illness, died on February 27, 1976.

to tumor, and body ability to develop immunity to tumors. By not being able to do one's work and to use one's mind positively, however, a double evil emerges. Because of the illness a person is limited generally, and on top of it he is rendered ineffective by forced compromises in work. Thus the mind, which could have a beneficial effect, is not allowed to fulfill its positive function in the struggle with the illness. Enforced idleness promotes depression that in turn reduces the will to live.

What can be done about all of this? Rehabilitation concepts similar to ones used in other disabilities have to be applied to the cancer patient. There are certainly no simple solutions. If the patient has a long-range, guaranteed remission, the possibilities of retraining can be considered even though this might need subsidizing from outside sources. If the remission is short or uncertain then the only acceptable solution would be that of being absorbed into the old job or profession. This might need special consideration initially in regard to financial help. There should be provisions for part-time work and allowances for partial disability to encourage the return to work. Unfortunately, a more practical solution is to accept a lesser job that requires less training than a person has had, and even a lesser income. This is a poor solution. It is a forced compromise on an already compromised patient. Such a setback would be difficult for a healthy person to accept and tolerate; it is even more difficult for a person who is ill.

As Dr. Fortgang says, there are no simple solutions. Fortunately, many patients are able to return to their jobs after the initial discovery and treatment of their disease. In the process of adjusting to living with cancer and returning to active living, they may receive help from doctors, nurses, social workers, or clergy; or from people associated with special organizations such as the American Cancer Society (including its Reach to Recovery Program), the United Ostomy Association, or the International Association of Laryngectomies.

If a person's disease becomes progressively worse, however, he or she will eventually experience all the depressing situations described by Dr. Fortgang. He will be forced to change his work or to work fewer hours; he will find that many people are uncomfortable in his presence. He will feel his sense of inner dignity and self-respect have been irretrievably compromised. And, in addition to these emotional struggles, he will not only feel physically weak from his disease but may also experience unpleasant side effects from radiotherapy or chemotherapy. Side effects unquestionably make some days worse than others for some people. If we knew in advance who was going to benefit from treatment, and who was not, we could spare the latter group the ordeal of unpleasant side effects but doctors are not prophets, and the percentages in favor of another remission indicate in most cases that further treatment is desirable.

One patient, however, who had a particularly bad time with chemotherapy, described it as follows:

It's an indescribably awful experience. It's like going every morning and having an injection of stomach flu. You do it every morning, and you do it yourself. It isn't like, "If I'd only worn boots, I wouldn't have caught stomach flu." You're going out to be whipped every day. You think people get depressed or are cowards because they're not willing to take it. But, goddammit, it takes away from you. When I think of the things I've gone through, I'm appalled. I don't know where I found the resources. I've got to be satisfied that I can still live with quality. I think treatment risks doing a great disservice to people who want not to be bothered anymore. But that isn't the same as folding up with no hope and going into a catatonic state, waiting to die. That's obviously one kind of reaction. But there are a whole bunch of people who just don't want to futz around anymore. They want to do their thing and then they want to drop dead. But treatment does terrible things. I could talk about the injections and get sick—actually throw up thinking about them—even though I haven't had them lately. A cerebral person like me doesn't want to be tied to a bodily function that affects his mind. The point is that you really change, Ernie.

The results of this man's treatment were only fair, since chemotherapy merely slowed down the growth of his tumor. But his side effects were out of proportion to the strength of the drug, a reaction I attribute to anxiety. The anticipation of bad results from a previous negative experience can actually increase toxicity. This case is a good example of why I feel I must be flexible and treat each person individually, and, at the same time, be ready to discern when a therapeutic change may have a good psychological effect. When a person is discouraged and depressed from the side effects of chemotherapy or from the routine of treatment, I sometimes suggest stopping therapy for a short time. This will at least give him a rest, and, because he feels better, it may also give him the impetus to travel, to work on an important project, or to participate more fully in family activities.

When a person is in an advanced state of decline, however, a change or cessation of therapy may provide only small respite. During this stage of an illness, the pressures on both patient and family are manifold. For this reason I urge them to continue their policy of candor with each other and with me concerning their feelings, fears, and questions. I remind them of the emotional relief that comes from frank talk, that they will be freed from the strain of hiding their own feelings while trying to guess what every other person is thinking and feeling. Fears and frustrations can then be dealt with as they arise and not left to fester until they become•too overwhelming to mention, or until the habit of withholding evolves into irretrievable isolation.

The candor I advocate between a patient and his or her family and friends includes a recognition of each other's needs as well as fears. Family members have a need to give, to feel they are doing something practical to contribute to the recovery or comfort of their loved one, whether he be at home or in the hospital. The separation caused by the hospitalization of the cancer patient is particularly traumatic. The wife or husband, child or parent, leaves the hospital each evening and worries whether his or her loved one will ever again lead a normal life or even leave the hospital. Feeling impotent, these family members need to give of themselves. Fortunately, there are many practical services they can perform for the patient while he or she is in the hospital—services such as feeding, walking, turning, and massaging. I encourage this kind of active participation because these acts, along with the offer of special foods or a favorite pillow, give solace to family and patient alike.

When a patient is at home, there are also many opportunities for the members of the family to give emotional support through practical means. For example, a patient may be anxious about his next visit to the doctor, wondering whether a new problem will be discovered or a new treatment recommended. He may not have transportation to and from the doctor's office or he may dread the side effects from the day's treatment. A spouse, parent, or friend can offer him a ride or accompany him on the bus; if they are working and unable to help in this way, they can still be present to give comfort and support in the evening when the patient may have to endure the side effects of therapy.

To be realistic, however, not every family is able to be open, loving, or intelligently supportive in the manner I have described, before or after a crisis. Even those people who have always assumed their family relationships were stable may find their traditional harmony is severely threatened by the pressures of a long-term illness. Under the strain of worry and fear, latent problems may emerge among those caring for the patient. Formerly controlled anger or guilt may surface in a sudden verbal attack upon him, or in indifferent or oversolicitous behavior toward him. The exhaustion and frustration of constant worry can break the most loyal supporter. I have also seen the most courageous of patients break under these pressures. When a person has fought long and hard against cancer, lost and regained hope many times, and then realizes the battle is not to be won, he often experiences a rage and depression that seek as their target the nearest available person—spouse, child, parent, or the nurse on duty. The anger is usually manifested as irritation over a trivial matter that in normal times would not even concern the patient. When these situations arise, I try to make the person under attack—patient or family member or friend—understand that this is not a rejection of him or her but a cry of anguish.

A cancer patient must also endure the endless boredom of being ill, as well as the fear of being a burden—the latter at a time when he or she wants and needs special attention. Unfortunately, the people from whom he needs this attention are also suffering from the tedium of the day-to-day routine of illness or, as I have mentioned, from feelings of inadequacy and guilt at not being able to relieve the patient's suffering. Unable to face the reality in which the patient is imprisoned, their attention diminishes, and the patient experiences added bitterness and increasing feelings of loneliness.

Even when these dire situations do not arise, when family and friends are candid, loving, and supportive, the cancer patient is alone in much of his physical and mental suffering, in his knowledge that death is not far off. Although the devastating experience of gaining and losing hope is shared by family and friends, it is actually lived by the patient in a way none of us can know until we experience it ourselves. The same 45-year-old man who described his reactions to chemotherapy, also described to me, upon his return from a business trip to Alaska, this experience of uncertainty and repeated loss of hope:

> I've seen any number of pictures of the tundra and the arctic wastes, but until I was up there I had not visualized how frightening, how truly frightening it is to

be up there. The size is beyond conception. It isn't like the photographs, with borders. It's without borders. It's without words. I chartered a small plane and flew across the north slope for hundreds of miles. There is nothing—no life, no polar bears, just snow. You can walk for eighteen hundred miles over the pole and down into Siberia. There is just nothing out there. I thought of the foolishness—or the incredible bravery—of the men in 1903 who started out across the ice cover, risking death. I've been close to death, but it's one thing to be there all of a sudden and not to whimper, and it's another to march across a plain resolutely, knowing that when you get there, you drop off. And it's another yet to know that you are marching across the plain to the edge, but kind of blindfolded so that you get to see only occasionally. Treatment is that experience. It's marching across a plain resolutely, sometimes blindfolded, which is when you are receiving treatment or are in a remission or whatever, but sometimes just seeing that you are getting closer. Suddenly the blindfold comes off and you are really close and it comes as a surprise. That is why people become freaked by their experience with treatment. And that's how people break. It's the uncertainty. There are lots of people who could march out there with certainty and with dignity. But there will be a breakthrough on the horizon, which is now so close, and it will suddenly be extended—perhaps to infinity. How many times can people take that? I don't think I can take it, and I consider myself a very strong person.

Thus, in the case of terminal illness, a patient suffers far more than physical deterioration. We have heard from the patients themselves what it is like to be forced into semiretirement, to lose their self-respect, to experience the discomfort of others in their presence, to gain and lose hope for recovery. As the 26-year-old girl said, "I am not the only one in the boat, but no one else can do my living or dying for me." The only thing a doctor or nurse, a husband, wife, child, or friend can do, is to *be* there, to communicate freely, and to show compassion.

None of us should add to the loneliness of a dying person by refusing to acknowledge what is happening to him or her. I emphasize this because the question so often arises as to whether a doctor should tell a patient when he is dying. The results of a recent study cited by John Hunt, M.D.,[3] at a conference in England in March 1975, illustrates the inappropriateness of such a question. The study revealed that 70 percent of doctors did not want to tell the truth while 80 percent of the patients expressed a desire to know what was happening to them. My own policy at such a time is the same as it was in the days of the diagnosis. I encourage discussion and candor. I let a patient know I am willing to answer all his questions, but I also try to be sensitive to his feelings and his ability to deal with bad news on any given day. The truth must not be allowed to extinguish realistic hope, even though that hope may extend no further than the next month or next week. Candor and the will to live must coexist in a delicate balance. When that balance is tipped and a patient is deprived of hope, the results are no different than if he had been the victim of a voodoo curse. In most cases his subsequent decline is inexplicably rapid. Thus, the will to live, the fifth dimension of

[3] John Hunt, "Life Before Death," *Proceedings of the Royal Society of Medicine,* **69**:124, February 1976.

cancer therapy, is as important to a patient's emotional and physical well-being at this time as it is in the months and years when he is actively living with his disease.

I almost always discuss with a patient every aspect of his or her condition during this period. We talk about when to stop anticancer therapy and how to control pain. I tell him my rule is to administer therapy as long as a patient responds well and has potential for a reasonably good quality of life, but that when all feasible therapies have been administered and a patient shows signs of rapid deterioration, I believe the continuation of therapy can cause more discomfort than cancer. I tell him I will then recommend surgery, radiotherapy, or chemotherapy only as a means of relieving pain. However, I assure him that if his condition should once again stabilize after the withdrawal of active therapy and if it should appear that he could still gain some good time, I will immediately reinstitute active therapy. I also assure each patient that there is an effective therapy to combat any degree of discomfort or pain and that I find the most effective procedure is simply to correlate the medication with the complaint. If he is nauseated, I will give him antinausea medicine. If he is unable to sleep, I will prescribe sedatives—barbiturate or nonbarbiturate, depending on his tolerance. And if he has pain, I will use an appropriate analgesic or narcotic, as often as needed. (These drugs can be administered in pill form, as a suppository, or by injection. A few patients even learn to administer their own shots, as a diabetic does, under medical supervision. Addiction is not a concern when a person has advanced cancer. Moreover, most patients report a tendency to use fewer drugs when they know drugs are readily available if needed.)

A patient has the right to give me instructions as to how he wants his last days handled. He can tell me where he wants to be and what he wishes in terms of medical support systems. He may sign a "Directive to my Physician" form that will prohibit me or any other physician from giving him cardiac resuscitation or from using heroic measures to prolong his life.

(The question often arises as to whether a cancer patient who is acutely ill should be treated with cardiac resuscitation and/or intensive care. I believe a patient merits these procedures automatically if he or she has not yet undergone an adequate trial of anticancer therapy. Every effort should be made with each patient to strive for remission. However, I do not recommend a code blue and/or intensive care when a patient's disease has proved refractory to anticancer therapy and he is failing from advanced disease. The only exception I make to this policy is when a patient specifically requests that such procedures be implemented and when there is a remote possibility of success with additional therapy.)

Although the decision as to where he or she will die is the prerogative of each patient, this may be determined in part by practical considerations. Although most people would prefer to be at home, not every household can easily accommodate a patient who needs round-the-clock care. Other family members may be working, or they may be physically unable to carry out some of the more strenuous nursing duties such as turning the patient or helping him to the bathroom. The result of these and other factors is that today more people die in nursing homes and hospitals than at home. Dying in this manner, separated from familiar sights and sounds, can be a doubly lonely ordeal, increasing a person's natural feelings of isolation and abandonment. However, if I had to choose between these latter alternatives, I would recommend a hospital. Most nursing homes need to be upgraded before they can provide the medical facilities or the proper warmth and dignity for anyone, especially for the dying.

An ideal of care exists at St. Christopher's Hospice, in London. Founded by Dr. Cicely Saunders in 1967, St. Christopher's is a research, treatment, and teaching facility devoted to meeting the needs of the dying and the long-term sick. Its aims are both control of physical pain and understanding of the emotional and spiritual problems of such patients and their families. Dr. Saunders wants her patients to live until they die. The atmosphere is informal, the building designed for maximum openness, space, and light. Families are encouraged to visit at any hour of the day; and the staff becomes as friendly with them as with the patients. Children are welcome visitors. In such an atmosphere, a patient and his or her family can say a loving good-bye. It is a time of sadness but not of depression and emptiness. Similar hospices are now being founded in the United States.

Clearly, there are better and worse circumstances in which to die, and what I would call a *bad* death is one that occurs in the sterile atmosphere of a hospital or in the loneliness of a nursing home. A bad death is one where there is little communication between the dying person and his family or friends or the medical personnel, where there is no acknowledgment of the significance and sorrow to the patient of what is happening to him.

One of the best examples of a *good* death is that of Charles A. Lindbergh who died in August 1974. Diagnosed as having a lymphoma in 1972, he continued to live actively while undergoing radiotherapy and chemotherapy. He traveled extensively on conservation missions, which included promoting the preservation of a rare species of eagle and encouraging the study of the Stone Age Tasaday tribe in the Phillippines. One of his doctors, Milton M. Howell, M.D.,[4] writes,

> Chemotherapy was instituted and continued to the limit of its effectiveness.
>
>   From time to time, he returned to his beloved Kipahulu Valley, on the island of Maui, in Hawaii, a living museum of tropical foliage and wildlife. His contributions of time and effort had been considerable in preserving the area as a national park. Near this valley of a thousand waterfalls, he had personally helped clear the neglected graveyard beside the picturesque church built by Yankee missionaries. In time, he made appropriate legal arrangements for his burial there and selected the site of his grave. Systematically, he arranged his personal affairs, and yet he maintained a sense of the past and an interest in the present. He planned for the next major event of his life but it did not become an obsession.
>
>   As time passed, the inexorable progress of the disease forced his hospitalization in a major university center for several months. The best of medical efforts were made in his behalf; the finest of medical skills were applied. All this was insufficient to the task, for the neoplasm was the navigator of this flight.

[4]Milton M. Howell, "The Lone Eagle's Last Flight," *Journal of the American Medical Association*, **232**(7):715–716, May 19, 1975.

Finally, in August 1974, a telephone call came to the village of Hana, Hawaii, from a hospital room in New York. "This is Charles Lindbergh. I have had a conference with my doctors, and they advise me that I have only a short time to live. Please find me a cottage or a cabin near the village. I am coming home to Maui." He did so. He was flown 5,000 miles on a litter.

He had made his decision, and he took full responsibility for it.

A cottage was found, overlooking the sea he loved. There, with two excellent nurses and his family, we participated along with him in the last eight days of his life.

He was elated for the first few days. His appetite improved. His fluid intake was adequate. There were regular morning conferences with the ranch superintendent to give instructions and receive reports on the progress of the construction of his grave and the building of his simple coffin. He planned his funeral service along with his family and requested that people attend in their work clothes. His days were full. There was time for reminiscing, time for discussion, and time for laughter. As his lungs filled, he required oxygen from time to time, and codeine, 15 mg as necessary. Finally, he lapsed into a coma and died 12 hours later. He wanted no respirator, defibrillator, or other complicated paraphernalia. None was available. He received excellent, prompt, responsive nursing care, oxygen when needed, a minimum of analgesia, and a great deal of love and consideration from his family and the medical staff.

He stated that he wished his death to be a constructive act in itself. His example of simplicity, his careful planning, his unfailing politeness and consideration for those around him, his public refusal of medical heroics, and his humble funeral are evidence of that wish. Death was another event in his life, as natural as his birth had been in Minnesota more than 72 years before.

Following the above article, Dr. Howell prints an excerpt from a letter written to him by Anne Morrow Lindbergh. It says, in part:

In the hospital in New York—excellent, thorough and tireless as the care was—there was always a veil between Charles and me, partly an inevitable physical veil because of the setup of a big hospital and routine . . . perhaps the veil was accidentally given by the doctors' and nurses' cheerful evasiveness . . . or perhaps due to my hesitancy in speaking first before Charles was ready to . . . and perhaps because Charles was trying to spare me from what I already knew . . . or perhaps he was not yet ready or able to broach such an emotional subject. Only in the last days there were we able to break through the veil, when Charles knew he was getting no better and he determined to go "home to Maui."

But it was the peace and beauty of Maui that we all could face together without fearing some of the fringes of its meaning. I am grateful for this opportunity to look at the mystery which everyone must meet in the end. For the boys it may have long-reaching effects down through their children and their children.

The death of Charles Lindbergh is an eloquent argument against the prolonged, futile use of advanced medical technology that sometimes results from a doctor's false optimism or unrealistic assessment of a patient's condition. In a manner similar to his,

I am often asked by a patient to make funeral arrangements as well as assure that he or she not be given heroic measures when the end is near. The only thing a patient cannot dictate to me is when he will die, for there are no yardsticks to measure that delicate, highly individual time. Often I have seen a patient and thought that this was his time, only to find him so improved in the next few days that he returned home a week later. Therefore, I no longer feel that I or anyone else has the ability to predict when another person will die. I prefer to withhold judgment, visit a patient frequently, and continually reassess his condition.

When a patient goes into a final state of coma, however, I keep him comfortable by providing a moderate amount of hydration, frequent turning, and skin care. In certain cases I may continue to administer narcotics or sedatives at regular intervals if there appears to be restlessness or pain. This reassures his family that any pain or discomfort is being alleviated.

When death comes, it is not easy for a patient's family to accept, even when it means that the patient's suffering is over. At this time family members need special attention, which I try to provide along with other family members and friends, nurses, clergy, social workers, and hospital volunteers. I always hope that a family will find solace in the knowledge that its loved one has received good medical care and sensitive emotional support, that he lived as long and as well as possible under adverse conditions, and that all possible comfort was provided to ease his dying.

About 10 days to 2 weeks after the death of a patient, the first flurry of attention from relatives and friends subsides, and the bereaved are alone with their despair. I try to help them by writing a letter in which I review the medical history of the patient, summarize his or her final days, and include any pertinent information obtained from the autopsy. I also discuss the important role played by the wife or husband or other family member in supporting the patient. Finally, I mention the normality of grieving and remind them that there will be a time when life will be less painful. I also invite them to visit me at any time if they feel I can help them with their problems of readjustment.

My goal, then, from the day I meet a patient until his cure, remission, or death, is to do everything I can to relieve the real and terrifying ordeal of living with cancer. Because I have witnessed it so often, I try to convince each patient that other people do live actively with disease; and I reassure him that if his disease is terminal, I can relieve his pain and suffering.

There is an understanding among people who work with cancer patients and the patients themselves—something we all know and few of us ever learn—that it is not the length of a person's life that is important, but the quality of his days.

Chapter 20

Misgivings and Misconceptions in the Psychiatric Care of Terminal Patients

Avery D. Weisman

Although medicine has always attempted to postpone or circumvent death by controlling the forces that cause it, until recently there has been very little study of psychiatric interventions in the care of the dying. Most medical schools do not offer courses in the care of terminal patients, nor do they provide for consideration of social problems related to death. For the most part, the student or young physician learns only incidentally about death during his assignments to medical and surgical wards, where demands on his time and limited skills do not encourage intimate study of any individual patient. The moribund patient is treated vigorously in some instances, or simply left alone to die as a result of incurable illness. He is seldom regarded as a challenging psychiatric problem. Consequently, whatever knowledge or understanding that many physicians acquire about death and dying is highly informal; foundations for future practice are put together as a patchwork of clinical impressions and earlier prejudices.

The situation is scarcely different for the incipient psychiatrist. Most psychiatrists rarely talk with gravely ill patients, except for brief periods in general hospital training,

Reprinted from *Psychiatry*, **33**(1):67–81, February 1970.

This investigation was supported in its early phase by the Foundations Fund for Research in Psychiatry (62–247) and later by PHS Grant No. MH 15903–01. "Psychological Autopsy Study of Preterminal Illness and Suicide."

and few psychiatrists have ever followed a patient until death. In the aggregate, most physicians, including psychiatrists, know far more about the causes of death than they care to know about the psychosocial context, environmental influences, and emotional factors that may contribute to death.

Misgivings about death and misconceptions about the dying patient may mutually reinforce each other and lead to drastic changes in management of dying patients. The more qualms a physician has about death, the more apt he is to shun interaction with terminal patients. If forced to participate in caring for incurable patients, the doctor may respond according to ill-founded beliefs, not upon dispassionate observations. As a result, such patients may suffer from their doctor's uncertainties and prejudices, and may not be permitted to find a dignified and acceptable atmosphere in which to die.

Understanding the psychological problems of the terminal patient is particularly important for the psychiatrist, because dying patients often respond favorably to effective interventions that heed the psychosocial factors and forces. Misgivings can be ameliorated; misconceptions can be rectified. With proper training and experience, health professionals—physicians, nurses, psychologists, social workers, and so forth— can learn how to approach a terminal patient with fewer apprehensions and greater appreciation of their contribution to the patient's management.

ATTITUDES TOWARD DEATH

It is well known that some patients are aware of impending death, and yet report little or no fear. No less a personage than John Hunter, who described the sense of calamity and dread in angina pectoris, is said to have acquired a tranquility and sense of pleasurable expectation in the waning hours of his own life (Lewin, chap. 18). Patients who have undergone severe anxiety attacks or deep, recurrent depressions volunteer that actual impending death is far less terrifying than were the fears and stormy conflicts of their healthier past.

Despite these observations, the belief still prevails that death is always and every- where an unmitigated evil to be avoided, opposed, and disguised just as long as pos- sible. Moreover, because the topic of death is taboo, and taboo subjects carry an aura of magic and mystery, we also consent to an implicit belief that if we do not talk about it, death can be discouraged, denied, and even banished.

Several years ago, Weisman and Hackett reported a small group of patients who were "predilected" to death, and anticipated its advent with comparative equanimity (1961). "Comparative" means that death was preferred to the prospect of continued life. None of these patients was deeply depressed, agitated, or suicidal. Most were resigned and, above all, not apprehensive about dying. Indeed, several even deplored efforts to keep them alive.

Contrary to common belief, these are not unusual observations. Many people in the final phase of life look to death as a release from a bleak and fruitless existence. In fact, even when they do not suffer from a fatal or high-risk malady, a significant number of patients will forecast their own death correctly. There are also patients who elect to die, despite the efforts of their doctors. Such patients compel us to recognize several facts about death: (1) Death need not always be construed as a bitter blow of fate, but instead can arrive in a seemingly appropriate and timely manner. (2) Misgivings and apprehensions about death may originate in doctors, and not always in the patients who risk dying. (3) Death may be a reasonable end-stage in the longitudinal process of living, and is not thereby an evil, tragic occasion. (4) Death with dignity and open awareness is more harmonious than death accompanied by a conspiracy of silence, deception, denial, and censorship.

SOCIAL ISOLATION AND EMOTIONAL QUARANTINE

The necessity and obligation to die is an inescapable fact of nature. Why then do we resist the reality of death? Mankind trembles at the thought of death largely because it implies untold mental and physical suffering. More specifically, we suffer in anticipating death because of an abiding belief that it always occurs prematurely, that it could be prevented, and that it deprives the world of those who can be spared the least, will be missed the most, and are unprepared to die (Parsons and Lidz). Moreover, we also maintain that death imposes an unjustifiable degree of pain, utter incapacity, and an atmosphere of defeat, hopelessness, and total extinction.

Beyond the personal agonies of the patient who dies, death is a source of suffering to survivors, for they, too, suffer from the belief that death is unnecessary, painful, and evil. Survivors sometimes suffer from a sense of guilt induced by a mistaken belief that death might have been prevented, or at least made easier.

Guilt, misgivings, apprehensions, grief, and misconceptions about death may cause bystanders at the deathbed to remove themselves prematurely, lest they feel more helpless and culpable. Even though the survivors may continue to stand by, it is with emotional isolation and even unreality feelings. They may shelter themselves behind a facade of formalities and socially acceptable but tedious platitudes. Habitual responses may change, speech becomes artificial, conciliatory, patronizing, and contrived. Ordinary interchange yields to circumspect rituals and routines. As a result, the terminal patient may find himself alone, unable to speak candidly or to respond effectively with familiar people. Even his physician may refrain from frankness. Instead, he may substitute brisk, unconvincing reassurances, couched in professional cant which hardly anyone could believe.

To be sure, we recognize that dying patients are suffering from fatal illnesses. Aside from the primary disease, however, some portion of secondary suffering may come from the social isolation and emotional quarantine imposed upon terminal patients by well-meaning, devoted people who stand to lose most by the death. Because death is an interpersonal crisis as well as a medical fact, it is sometimes possible to recognize a disorder called "Bereavement of the Dying." This is a condition of depression, loneliness, and regression found among terminal patients who have been emotionally isolated and abandoned during the final period of life. The syndrome may be traced to an enforced grieving for their own survivors! A hopeless diagnosis often amounts to a "condemnation" which creates a psychosocial void, and aggravates the threat of death. It is here that trained and compassionate intervention may be most helpful.

PSYCHIATRIC PARTICIPATION IN TERMINAL CARE

Why have psychiatrists tended to avoid dying patients? Suicide, depression, separation, broken object relationships, and severe invalidism belong within the psychiatric province. Moreover, general hospital psychiatry is a highly developed subspecialty. If it is suggested that psychiatrists as a group dread the hopelessness of terminal patients, we need only remind ourselves that schizophrenic patients can be far more alarming and less encouraging to treat than are most patients in the final phases of medical illness. We can also assume that psychiatrists are not more fearful of death than are other specialists, even though the dying patient seldom becomes a part of their daily practice.

I believe that one reason why psychiatrists do not treat the dying is found in the viewpoint of psychiatric training itself. Although we speak readily about "psychiatric illness" and "mental disease," our actual orientation assumes that psychiatric patients are physically healthy. Whatever theory we are inclined toward about the "cause" of mental and emotional disorders, the cause is not likely to be the same as that which produces organic diseases from which people die. Consequently, psychiatrists are diffident about treating patients who are "really sick," unless they also happen to have a readily identified psychiatric diagnosis. Despite brave words about the "patient as a whole," psychiatrists who forego treating the terminal patient do not understand that their contribution might be extremely significant in determining whether or not the final hours and days are reasonably harmonious.

Most psychiatrists are trained primarily for the office practice of psychotherapy and the hospital management of patients who are institutionalized for mental disorders. Although in their earlier days there were opportunities to consult about terminal patients, most senior psychiatrists are strikingly unsophisticated about the mental and emotional problems met with on medical and surgical wards. When asked to share his skill in understanding delicate human relationships and his knowledge of psychodynamics, the senior psychiatrist continues to shun the terminal patient. As a result, both psychiatrist and patient are deprived of an exceedingly important source of mutual enlightenment.

For entirely different reasons, as Duff and Hollingshead have demonstrated, other medical specialists also tend to turn away from psychological problems related to death. Prolongation of life, relief of pain, and resuscitation are their principal objectives. Emphasis on these aims alone sometimes leads to incongruous efforts to sustain life, long after the outcome has been decided and the patient is all but dead. Highly ingenious technical instruments and almost incomprehensible physiological measurements are brought into the heroic struggle to save patients who have in a sense already died, but, ironically, little is done to formulate and carry out intelligent management of concomitant social and emotional problems in the patient and his survivors. As a rule, psychosocial management is left to the informal, arbitrary improvisations of the nursing staff, even to the nonprofessional members of the attending personnel (Glaser and Strauss). Nurses may be highly skilled in ministering to nonmedical needs of terminal patients, but in the rush of simply doing their daily work, few nurses have the time, inclination, or training in which to carry out psychological treatment of patients for whom little else can be done. In the scale of professional priorities and values, talking well with patients and families has far lower status than more technical skills.

Until the very recent past, the plight of the terminal patient has lacked scientific respectability, particularly as contrasted with the high degree of interest in the causes of death and in autopsies. Eissler's *The Psychiatrist and the Dying Patient*, scholarly and humane, failed to stimulate a significant number of psychiatrists to devote more time to terminal patients. However, within the past decade or two, psychologists and other behavioral scientists have contributed so much to the field of thanatology that more psychiatrists are now affiliating themselves with scientific projects in which the actuality of death is prominent. Kalish is presently preparing a comprehensive bibliography of death literature. To mention only a few projects, psychiatric contributions to the study of kidney transplants, open heart surgery, serious myocardial infarctions, and self-inimical injuries and accidents point to the way in which skilled psychiatrists can effectively participate in the treatment of patients who may die. Less conspicuously, more physicians tend to be alert to how different lifestyles produce a predisposing psychosocial context in which organic causes then produce disease.

While the indications for a better understanding of death and dying seem brighter than ever, we should be more aware of how often skilled physicians bypass the psychosocial dimensions of their patient's mortality. Consequently, patients may suffer from an influx of prejudices, snap judgments, simple formulas, slogans, and, generally, misconceptions. One of the rewarding results of the recent growth of disciplined observations about dying patients has been the discovery of how readily such patients can be helped, when misgivings and misconceptions are confronted and controlled.

MISGIVINGS ABOUT DEATH

Intervention and treatment in psychiatry, as well as in medical practice, are frequently based upon folk-wisdom, custom, and expedience, instead of upon firm scientific principles. Although practice usually runs ahead of theory, and theory often leaves proof far behind, there are problems in which practice is unencumbered by explicit theory. Since no one is exempt from uncertainty about death, the way any physician intervenes in management of terminal patients may be decided arbitrarily by a cluster of prejudices, avoidances, superstitions, and misgivings. To preserve his professional equanimity, a physician may rely upon formulas, clichés, or moralisms, or he may simply abdicate all responsibility on one pretext or another.

Death and dying are untaught and taboo topics. Consequently, professionals— psychiatrists included—may maintain all the cultural avoidances, dreads, and cumulative fallacies that untrained people express about death. Medicine itself has a core of science surrounded by empiricism, rituals, and a rich magical tradition. Conversely, the medical practitioner has a core of presuppositions, mythology, and bias surrounded, if not encapsulated, by a scientific education. His own qualms about death may keep him from wondering what patients actually undergo during the process of dying. By consensus, investigation ceases, only to be replaced by the reassurance of common misconceptions.

To have qualms about death is a fact of living, not a symptom of emotional conflict. Guilt and anxiety may be properties of the human plight, not a sign of inner discordance. Yet, few clinicians readily acknowledge the depth or extent of their misgivings and apprehensions about death. As a rule, they prefer to conceal their reservations behind intellectualisms and other varieties of emotional isolation. It is, therefore, difficult to discover directly which reservation or what type of misgiving is hidden behind the clinical strategy. Because few psychiatrists can or do discuss this important issue with their colleagues, it is more practical to clarify the most common professional misconceptions first, and then draw inferences about the implicit personal misgivings of physicians. It would be clear throughout, however, that what may be true of doctors is also true of any professional who contends with patients in whom death is a threat.

TEN COMMON MISCONCEPTIONS

Let us admit misgivings about death, and concede that it has an unavoidable impact even upon the experienced professional who must be present at the deathbed. Let us also recognize that professional antipathy toward death may spill over upon the dying patient who confronts us with many of our own most fundamental fears. Furthermore, let us now realize that there are erroneous generalizations resulting from misgivings and antipathies about death, and that these unexamined beliefs may curtail effective understanding and management of terminal patients.

A misconception is an incorrect belief. There are people who act correctly despite erroneous beliefs, and others who act incorrectly because of inappropriate application of correct beliefs. While there are circumstances in which any so-called misconception might be true, these occur far less often than expected and never "as a rule." The following list of ten common misconceptions has been compiled from conversations with practitioners in various specialties, some of whom have frequent experience with terminal patients or patients in whom recovery is uncertain.

1   Even when death is inevitable, no one is willing to die. Unless he is suicidal or psychotic, no one really wants to die.

2   Reconciliation with the necessity of death is impossible, preparation for death is also impossible, and no one can therefore help anyone else to accept death.

3   Fear of death and dying is the most natural and fundamental fear. The closer one comes to death, the more intense this fear becomes.

4   Talking about death with a terminal patient will take away hope, and even may hasten his demise. This rule is particularly true for patients in whom recovery is still possible.

5   We must say as little as possible about death to dying patients. If questioned directly, a physician should turn queries aside, and use any means to deny, dissimulate, rationalize, and avoid open confrontations.

6   Dying people do not really want to know about their prognosis. Otherwise, they would ask about it. Unwelcome disclosure may involve the risk of suicide, psychosis, severe regression, and profound depression.

7   It is advisable that the physician, in consultation with the family, make decisions pertaining to treatment and giving information. When improvement or recovery

is impossible, the patient should be left alone, except when his pain must be relieved. In this way, he will gradually withdraw from the world and die in peace, without disturbance or anguish.

   8 Intensive scientific training, clinical experience, and knowledge of pathology automatically enable a physician to deal wisely with all phases of patient care, including the emotional and psychosocial dimensions of death.

   9 When the family does not want a patient to be told about his diagnosis and outlook for recovery, the physician should abide by that decision. The doctor's principal concern, after it has been established that recovery is not possible, is to relieve pain and to prolong survival. Psychological problems can be effectively managed with simple reassurance, adequate sedation, and, when death is imminent, referral to the clergy.

   10 Dying patients are doomed. It is therefore reckless, and perhaps heartless, to inflict unnecessary suffering. Nothing anyone can say or do will make a substantial difference. Survivors should accept this fact stoically and unequivocally. Unless a patient has a definite psychiatric disorder, such as a psychosis, psychiatric consultation is unlikely to help. After the patient dies, the family is no longer the responsibility of the hospital or the physician.

   Full documentation of why these are misconceptions or at least unwarranted generalizations is available in other publications (Weisman and Hackett, 1962). However, even such a brief list discloses many apparent inconsistencies and paradoxes, and much begging of questions. For example, a commonly cited expression, used to justify or omit certain interventions, is "to avoid unnecessary suffering." Exactly what kinds of suffering are there, and which kinds are necessary? Frequently, the decision that one intervention will relieve and another will inflict unnecessary suffering is based largely upon the uneasiness, misgivings, and sufferings of the family and physician, not upon the feelings of the patient, who is rarely consulted.

   What is there about a potentially fatal diagnosis that causes a family and physician to conspire, albeit with benevolent intentions, to deprive a patient of his "right" to know what is wrong with him, what can be done about it, and what future course he can expect? Only in pediatrics and in terminal care is it common practice to tell a patient as little as possible, and to ask responsible family members to decide for the patient. Were we to act consistently with what we already know about psychology and human responsibility, we would follow a policy of *first* telling an adult patient about the diagnosis and plans for treatment. Only then would the patient, in consultation with the doctor, decide what to tell, and to whom (Weisman, 1967; Oken).

   A physician has major responsibility for decisions about management and treatment. But do his special knowledge and clinical skills equip him to act judiciously about psychosocial problems? Patients usually know more about their illness than doctors suspect they do, and much more than they have been told. It is not unusual, for example, to hear a staff member say, "No, he hasn't been told what the trouble is, but I think he knows anyway." Few patients are so obtuse that they do not sense the quiet alarm of family and friends. In fact, many patients will restrain themselves, because they are aware of the distress and anguish felt by their family and friends. Random remarks and nonverbal behavior are often much more eloquent than formal statements. Although diagnosis, treatment, and prognosis belong within the physician's province, it does not follow that whatever a patient knows or senses about being sick comes from his doctor.

In deciding about the proper program of care for a high-risk patient, it does not violate medical responsibility to enlist the opinions of other specialists or to use the observations of others. The wishes of the family do, of course, need to be considered, but doctors are not obliged to yield when family members initially oppose candid discussion with the patient. Families suffer from shock, alarm, incipient bereavement, and repercussions of long-standing ambivalence. Is it therefore reasonable to expect unanimity, consistency, and judicious assessment? With the passage of time, family members may change their minds and come to appreciate someone who can help them restore communication. Furthermore, to share information about a limited prognosis and serious diagnosis does not mean that it is necessarily transmitted in a heavy-handed way, like the stroke of an executioner's axe. Nor does it mean that the dire information must be incessantly repeated, as if it were a dirge or melancholy litany. The principal value of sharing information is that it facilitates open, easier, and more honest communication.

Misconceptions about the role of the clergy in care of the dying are profound. Physicians often refer terminal patients to chaplains when psychosocial problems seem too immense, as if the clergy were an extension of social service. However, clergymen vary as much in ability to deal with problems of death and bereavement as do physicians and psychiatrists. Terminal patients, moreover, have different requirements, aside from religious formalities and spiritual consolation. It is wholly possible to share responsibility for a patient's welfare with a competent chaplain, who in many areas can contribute enormously (Ross). The hazard is that some physicians may be tempted to relinquish the patient in anticipation of death as if the patient were in fact ready for funeral services.

Survivors of terminal patients need additional help. Responsibility for the patient and his family need not end with signing the death certificate and autopsy permission. Parkes has demonstrated how often psychosomatic complications accompany prolonged bereavement.

All of this emphasizes that management of terminal patients does not begin and end with the simple questions of whether to tell, what to tell, how to tell, and how much to tell. These questions are scarcely even the beginning; what to do with the truth is more exacting than whether or not to tell the truth. It is as dogmatic and inexcusable to demand that full disclosure be made early in the course of fatal illness as it is to insist that no one should ever be told directly about his disease and outlook. Hard-cased recommendations, fixed policies, and formal techniques do not allow for either the patient's or the physician's individual idiosyncrasies and requirements.

HOPE AND DESPAIR AMONG DOCTORS

Underlying most misconceptions, and underlying the attitudes of even those who have deeper understanding about terminal patients, there are profound apprehensions about death that therapeutic and humanistic challenges are not likely to alleviate.

Nevertheless, physicians, and psychiatrists in particular, should be able to ask themselves questions and demand candid answers: How can I talk about death openly with someone who may die in the immediate future? What are the risks of such an open confrontation? Is the concern I feel produced by personal anxiety, my sense of failure in not being more effective, or my own awareness of mortality? Is it possible to preserve hope without deception and still realize that death is inevitable? Can I actually help this person to die, when I shall be spared? If I do want to encourage denial, how long can I keep it up?

Beyond these initial questions are philosophical but no less practical questions. Is hope or despair determined only by whether we shall live or die? We already know that despair is completely compatible with survival; why then is hope not consistent with the reality of death? What is the source of our misgivings about death? How can we come to terms with death so that, as physicians should, we can offer more to those who have less?

Never is it more evident that the personality of the physician is an essential ingredient of his profession than when he is involved with the psychological management of death. There is much which can be taught and learned about the terminal patient. Even after the element of the "forbidden" or "illicit" has been removed, a large and decisive proportion of a physician's technical interventions still arises from his status as a person. His specific contribution to the improvisations of the moment carries a spontaneity and authenticity not found in explicit strategies (Hackett and Weisman, 1960).

Professional defenses often take the form of emotional isolation, standoffishness, and intellectualized professionalism. Needless to say, physicians cannot regularly mourn for patients, nor regularly share their joys. Doctors perforce become accustomed to the clinical fact of death and to the frequency with which it occurs. But few physicians are wholly impervious to the individuality of the person who dies. A true professional in any area cultivates a sense of equanimity as well as challenge; he abrogates emotional extremes and stresses competence, not omnipotence or its accomplice, guilt. Except among doctors who never see patients, defeats and failure are part of a physician's life—but the doctor is not expected to feel like a defeated failure. More specifically, despite the inevitable death of another, he must not deprecate his own contributions, apologize for shortcomings, overcompensate by blaming another, or atone for someone else's misfortunes.

In brief, a physician is trained to outwit death whenever possible, and this is still an essential element in psychological management of patients. The doctor is not a magic healer, but a protagonist of health who believes that disease and death are his enemies. These are poignant issues for the doctor who looks after the dying. Patients facing death are often less apprehensive than their physicians, mainly because the patients have, in a sense, less to lose! Professional impersonality which denies vulnerability is a defense that itself is highly vulnerable. Consequently, in response to self-expectations and sense of failure, the physician may be subject to vacillations between hope and despair. Although death is a solitary crisis, to be a responsive as well as responsible physician is, in the long run, also a solitary and impossible occupation.

Hope may be defined as animal confidence in the desirability of survival and in our competence to control events. Consequently, hope depends more upon our self-esteem and inner confidence than it does upon whether or not we are able to survive. Despair is the antithesis of hope, and draws much of its anguish from our anxiety about being alive in the first place. The conflicts and dreaded calamities that induce despair are not equivalent to perception of imminent death. Many psychiatric patients are far more desperate than are patients with fatal illnesses or those in whom survival depends upon, say, the mechanical efficiency of a respirator. In other words, terminal patients may withstand conflict far more readily than do psychiatric patients who regard calamity and insoluble conflict as inevitable. For example, it is not uncommon for patients with a long history of depression to undergo brief remissions after serious, even life-threatening surgery. Their mood returns to normal during convalescence, with little or no evidence of paranoia, somatic elaboration, or perceptual disorder. Then, after recovery from the operation, these patients again relapse into depression and despair.

Physicians are prone to a kind of professional as well as personal despair. Death is always their enemy, but death cannot be defeated. The doctor may win a skirmish, even a battle, but sooner or later the struggle is over and his capitulation is ensured. In some instances, the incentive to care for a terminal patient may wane as cure becomes more remote. Yet, the solitude of dying and the dilemma of a conscientious physician can be relieved somewhat by paying closer attention to the agonies within the social field in which death occurs. It cannot be claimed that attention to psychosocial factors will extend life, even for an hour. There is evidence, however, that physicians, including psychiatrists, can help to prevent lonely and anguished deaths (LeShan and LeShan). To do so, the doctor must be accessible as a person, not only available as a physician. He can then maintain respect for the patient, because his primary antipathy will be directed only toward the cause of suffering, not toward the person who suffers, whether that person is the patient or the doctor himself.

Management based upon unexamined misgivings and dogmatic misconceptions tends to encourage denial, deception, and dissimulation. Such stratagems are not only harmful, but implausible and impractical. We may be grossly shocked by crude realities of death, but when we shun human confrontation we cast ourselves into the position of cultivating a phobia for an event which cannot be avoided. The physician then finds himself face-to-face with unyielding despair.

CASE REPORT

The following case has been chosen in order to illustrate how even a brief and therapeutically modest intervention may have a beneficial effect upon the final period of life.

A 61-year-old man had been treated for several months because of a rare blood disease. His condition deteriorated and, as a secondary complication, he was then found to have an acute leukemia that brought him to the brink of imminent death. For four weeks, his physician, a man of consummate skill and compassion, had urged the family to allow him to discuss the diagnosis and outcome with the patient. The patient's wife and physician brother-in-law were adamantly opposed to any disclosure, lest more anxiety and depression develop. Theirs was not an arbitrary decision based upon selfish considerations. For many years, the patient had been afflicted with recurring depressions. Sometimes these attacks came on without warning, but at other times he became morose and dejected after specific events. His only son was mentally retarded and in an institution. His elder daughter had been in a mental hospital for about five years, suffering from paranoid schizophrenia. The remaining daughter lived in a distant city and communicated only occasionally with her family. In brief, the patient was distinctly vulnerable to additional losses, had a low threshold of despair, and seemed to lack viable resources to combat fear of death.

During his recent deterioration, the patient had become more depressed. He slept poorly, complained of terrifying dreams, could not eat, vomited a soft diet, and had to be sustained with intravenous fluids and blood transfusions. Narcotics and sedatives only partially relieved his pain. Whenever pain seemed to abate, however, the patient became restless to the point of agitation. It was at this juncture that his physician suggested that a psychiatrist might recommend a more effective tranquilizer for the depression and anxiety. Finally the family consented to a referral to me, but stipulated that the patient must not, in any way, be informed about his serious condition.

When I first learned about the patient, it seemed likely that he had more than an inkling of information about his critical state. Therefore, I could agree to the restriction, and promised that only the topic of depression would be considered.

Later that day I visited the patient. Although he managed to sit up in bed, it was with great effort, and he was very sick indeed. After a few general remarks about his surroundings, and without any prompting from me, he spontaneously started to talk about his illness, its downward course, his thoughts about the probable outcome, and death. His speech was slow, interrupted often by trying another fresh position, seeking and never finding comfort. His mental state was clear, his words well chosen, as he described the threats which had afflicted him throughout his life. Largely these were internal problems. He spoke briefly about his children, as if this were a problem beyond his control. For more years than he could tally, he had, however, been prone to recurrent depressions and bouts of pessimism. He was convinced that any project he started was bound to fail. Despite full confidence in his preparation, he was sure that his knowledge would be inadequate and that the result would be disaster. Fortunately, his secure financial position depended upon inherited funds, so he had never worked for a living. But financial security did not insure him against deeper uncertainties. Nevertheless, until recently he had been sure that he would live to a ripe old age. When he had first become ill several months earlier, he had been certain that it was temporary. For the past few weeks, after his physical condition had deteriorated, he had become less confident about recovery. Fevers could not be controlled, mysterious bleeding under the skin appeared, and he was incessantly agonized by pains that mounted and did not relent. He told me that only the previous day his temperature had returned to normal, and he had believed that recovery might be feasible. However, the fever had returned, along with a fresh outbreak of pain in the distribution of the left sciatic nerve. Once again he was desperate, afraid to sleep, convinced that inability to retain food and fluids meant exhaustion, depletion, and death.

It was not necessary to introduce the topic of depression during the interview. The patient was explicit enough about his sickness and feared prognosis. I did not have to violate the conditions of the session because the patient himself brought up the topics I had been cautioned to avoid! As we talked, he rubbed his left leg intermittently because of pain, and then he began to bleed slightly from his nose. I started to interrupt the interview, not wanting to tire him further, but also realizing that it was because I did not wish to witness a fatal hemorrhage! The patient gestured for me to stay. After a long pause, he continued, "I want to survive very much; I'd come back regularly for transfusions." How often did he see himself coming back? "Once a month, maybe," he responded, his eyes filling with tears. "More often than that probably wouldn't be worthwhile."

At this point, I diverted the conversation from death toward the things he had enjoyed most during his life. Briefly, only two things had been a constant source of pleasure—his music and his marriage. He was an amateur organist, and although I had no way of judging his competence, I told him how much respect I had for anyone who could play the organ. He brightened unexpectedly and gestured toward a black leather case at the far end of the room. It was a silent keyboard that he had brought to the hospital so he could practice and keep his hands supple. Shortly before admission, he had bought a new organ, fully expecting to enjoy it after discharge. Now, of course, he wasn't sure about any recovery.

The interview ended shortly afterward, but I asked permission to return. His answer was similar to what he had said about blood transfusions—it might make him feel better for a time, but was it worthwhile? My response was that I only wanted to see him again; besides, I planned to order new medicine for his depression, as his doctor had promised, and I wanted to check on this. He then agreed that I might come back on the day after next. As I left, his wife entered. She was crisp, but cordial. Although she addressed her husband in a semi-bantering manner, she was clearly very concerned about him. We had only a few moments to chat alone, and she was in no mood to offer further details about his history. However, once she ascertained that I had not brought up the dire prognosis with her husband, she relaxed somewhat, and told me how eager she was that he be relieved of pain and depression—"But isn't it a little late for psychotherapy?"

During the next 48 hours, he became substantially worse. When I next saw him, he was decidedly terminal. Conversation was difficult because of a large, fresh hemorrhage beneath his tongue. His words were almost unintelligible, as they slowly emerged. Nevertheless, he was mentally clear. I took hold of his hand and said nothing for several minutes. I was not sure if he was dozing or simply too tired to speak, until he opened his eyes and, with a trace of a wry smile, asked what advice I had for him. My answer, based upon our previous conversation, was that he should only think about his organ music and his good wife—things that had meant most to him. He seemed curiously satisfied with my response, as if this was what he had prepared me to say.

Twenty-four hours later he was almost comatose, rousing himself briefly to sip water, then dropping off to sleep again. He recognized me as I opened the door, but his wife announced my arrival anyway. She was sitting by the bedside, busily sorting a large collection of get-well cards. She explained, in response to no one's question, that she was way behind in correspondence. The patient seemed ready to die at any moment, but his wife took me aside and asked if it would be all right for the barber to shave him!

Under the bleak circumstances, her question might have been considered incongruous, even downright frivolous. But she did not intend it as a casual question. Therefore, I spoke seriously about her request. I explained that, in her husband's condition, even a slight nick might cause bleeding that would be difficult to control. Then I helped her to find an electric shaver, so that in preparation for the very last he would be clean-shaven.

I never saw the patient again. That night he awakened from an undisturbed sleep, after a day in which he had been relatively pain-free. He was unusually alert and refreshed, asked for food, and even finished a soft diet. Soon afterward he lapsed into sleep once more and never awakened.

When I later spoke with his wife about the terminal events, there was not much to add. Had he said anything about his impending death during the past few days? No, he had never spoken about it, even earlier, and no one had ventured to ask him. Once more, she explained that because he had been so prone to depression, the family had thought that the less said, the better. But she was glad that after I gave him the new medicine his "terrible nightmares" had ceased. Then, almost as an afterthought, she added, "You know, Doctor, in the past couple of days, he was much, much less depressed, and for some reason, at the very end, he didn't seem at all afraid of death."

COMMENT

Although from a psychiatric viewpoint the patient seemed to improve, the entire contact was much too brief to assess adequately. However, we are justified in drawing several inferences, based upon his previous personality and his response during the final hours. In the first place, even though he was highly vulnerable to depression, he was also clearly aware of his incipient death. Consequently, to talk about what he already knew could not have made him more dejected, apprehensive, or discouraged. Rather, as a result of his having an opportunity to voice misgivings and concern, much of his anxiety seemed to be relieved. It was not necessary to introduce the topic of death. The patient spontaneously brought it up, did not seek confirmation or reassurance, but continued to elaborate his ideas as if they had been stored up, waiting for an appropriate outlet. In the second place, the patient disclosed how uncertain he had been about interpreting his symptoms and steady deterioration. Slight improvement and remission had been seized upon as optimistic signs, but after his relapse there was little tendency to further denial. He was now almost wholly certain about his foreshortened future.

The state of uncertain certainty has been called "middle knowledge" (Weisman and Hackett, 1962). It frequently appears when a patient becomes worse and develops new symptoms or recurrences. Most often, middle knowledge is marked by heightened denial, as if the patient were desperately trying to nullify his own perceptions. Such a finding is apt to be confusing for the physician and family. If, for example, a patient

has already spoken about death, he will seem to have forgotten all that had been discussed. As a result, observers are inclined to say, "Isn't it good that he doesn't know
how sick he is!" On the other hand, if the patient has never been interviewed before,
and seems not to recognize how serious his condition is, unfamiliar observers, including professional staff, may conclude that the patient is using full-scale denial and,
therefore, they will leave well enough alone. This conclusion is a fallacy and the procedure is ill-advised because the patient's denial is deceptive; he is *not* well, *not* unaware of his plight, and should *not* be left alone.

Middle knowledge is usually very transient. A patient may tend to disavow familiar symptoms and to ignore fresh symptoms. However, he is thoroughly capable of
sharing his limited awareness with an observer who is not shocked into silence by his
impending demise. The postulated "mechanism of denial" is not a mechanism which
can be automatically turned on, and denial is only one aspect of a total process in
coming to terms with death. Hence, when a terminal patient is thought to deny, it is
not a total "umbrella defense" sheltering him against the painful perception of approaching death. Denial is an act, or part of an act, which nullifies selectively the
meaning of a social field (Weisman and Hackett, 1966). In general, the purpose of
denying, especially in a terminal patient, is to simplify a relationship or to restore a
status quo.

From this viewpoint, the role of the physician in generating denial is clear. If the
doctor withdraws from a closer relationship with a patient, the patient is apt to make
an attempt at nullifying the void between them. He will then "deny" whatever meanings in the social field create distance between himself and those on whom he counts.
Conversely, if the doctor, or any other concerned participant in the death, can forego
the temptation to reassure the patient, total denial will not be necessary. The patient
will not need denial, and neither will the physician. As a rule, depending upon the
patient's physical state, open recognition of urgent matters of life and death will be
possible. Such a doctor-patient relationship does not require denial *by* the patient or
denial *of* the patient by the doctor. Mutual avoidance creates a distinct *void*, in which
the patient undergoes alienation and annihilation before he actually dies.

There is a widespread misconception that mutual denial promotes a better death.
What actually happens, however, is that communication is interrupted at the very
moment when openness is most desirable—at the time the prognosis becomes un-
mistakable. Patients are usually alert to whatever disturbs the people who mean most
to them. A terminal patient may, therefore, accept the widening gulf that separates
him from others. He becomes silent, and, because of silence, little can be said to him.
Interchange is reduced to banal inquiries about physical symptoms, not about inner
experience. The atmosphere becomes muted; the physician withdraws in the pious
belief that he has offered the silent patient an opportunity to talk or ask questions,
and that the patient has nothing to say. Moreover, the doctor may believe that to be
more active in inquiring about how the patient feels as a person would be too disturbing. When this impasse develops, the patient is usually given an ample dose of a sedative or narcotic, sometimes a very generous amount. The surging anxiety generated by
the imminence of death then disappears beneath a tide of narcosis.

Sometimes it is argued that proper sedation, in itself, will relieve death-anxiety, without risking the psychic distress of emotional confrontation. In the case cited as an example, however, the patient had received ample doses of tranquilizers preceding the brief psychiatric intervention, without apparent effect upon his attitude, anxiety, or depression. Moreover, his relief came too soon after the interview to be attributed wholly to the antidepressant prescribed by the psychiatrist.

Finally, the putative "distress of confrontation" is largely a misconception, even though it is the most common assumption that physicians and survivors make about the dying patient. In this case report, confrontation with death did not have to be forced upon the patient; it was all around him, permeating the circumstances, the sickroom, and the interview. His wife had sheltered him from what she feared would be a morbid precipitant of further depression. Even after his death, she maintained that he had never spoken about dying. Yet her parting words to me revealed that she had in fact known about his fear of death. Both had known; neither had spoken of it. Who was protecting whom?

Since this death scene cannot be replayed with another script, we shall not know whether the patient would have had an equally acceptable exitus without any psychiatric intervention. Nevertheless, had the psychiatrist only been concerned with offering general support and reinforcing denial, he would not have learned how much consolation and genuine support the patient had derived from music and his marriage. Actually, the psychiatrist nearly missed this information when he started to interrupt the interview at a point when he feared that the patient was tiring. His reason for interrupting was also influenced by personal anxiety about witnessing the onset of a fatal hemorrhage. Had the psychiatrist not had information about the importance of the patient's music and marriage, he would later have been more handicapped when the patient asked for "advice." He might have been limited to mouthing platitudes and encouraging the patient to believe what neither of them could really believe. As it turned out, the "advice" the patient sought during the waning hours seemed to help his mental state. While the dreaded words "death" and "dying" were not used explicitly, the doctor's attitude of thorough acceptance helped the patient to recognize and reaffirm his sense of reality for what mattered most in his earlier life.

The psychiatric care of terminal patients arouses some of the most pervasive fears of all men—extinction, victimization, helplessness, passivity, abandonment, disfigurement, and, above all, loss of self-esteem. The physician who undertakes to treat such patients, as well as the psychiatrist who intervenes in bringing about a better death, is also subject to these fears. Since he is bound to a patient who will die, the physician must also face an exacerbation of his own sense of failure, guilt, and intimations of personal mortality.

The personal misgivings, qualms, fears, misconceptions, and unwarranted generalizations of the doctor about terminal patients create many of the difficulties involved in adequately ministering to the dying. To assume that only deception, dissimulation, and denial can preserve a reasonable amount of hope is to ignore the personal plight of the terminal patient. As a result, the patient may be emotionally isolated and abandoned long before he is ready to die.

REFERENCES

Duff, Raymond, and Hollingshead, August. *Sickness and Society;* Harper & Row, 1968; Chap. 15.

Eissler, Kurt. *The Psychiatrist and the Dying Patient;* Internat. Univ. Press, 1955.

Glaser, Barney, and Strauss, Anselm. *Time for Dying;* Aldine, 1968.

Hackett, Thomas, and Weisman, Avery. "Psychiatric Management of Operative Syndromes: I. The Therapeutic Consultation and the Effect of Noninterpretive Intervention," *Psychosomatic Medicine* (1960) 22:267–282.

Kalish, Richard. *Bibliography on Death, Bereavement, and Aging;* Univ. of Calif., Los Angeles, in press.

LeShan, Lawrence, and LeShan, Eda. "Psychotherapy and the Patient with a Limited Life-Span," *Psychiatry* (1961) 24:318–323.

Lewin, Thomas. *Life and Death: Being an Authentic Account of the Deaths of 100 Celebrated Men and Women, with Their Portraits;* London, Constable, 1910.

Oken, Donald. "What to Tell Cancer Patients: A Study of Medical Attitudes," *J. Amer. Med. Assn.* (1961) 175:1120–1128.

Parkes, C. Murray. "Effects of Bereavement on Physical and Mental Health—A Study of the Medical Records of Widows," *British Med. J.* (1964) 2:274–279.

Parsons, Talcott, and Lidz, Victor. "Death in American Society," in Edwin S. Schneidman (Ed.), *Essays in Self-Destruction;* Science House, 1967.

Ross, Elizabeth. "The Dying Patient as Teacher: An Experiment and an Experience," *Chicago Theological Seminary Register* (1966) 57(3):1–14.

Weisman, Avery. "The Patient with a Fatal Illness: To Tell or Not to Tell," *J. Amer. Med. Assn.* (1967) 201:152–154.

Weisman, Avery, and Hackett, Thomas. "Predilection to Death: Death and Dying as a Psychiatric Problem," *Psychosomatic Medicine* (1961) 23:232–256.

Weisman, Avery, and Hackett, Thomas. "The Dying Patient," in *Special Treatment Situations;* Des Plaines, Ill., Forest Hospital Publ., Vol. 1, 1962.

Weisman, Avery, and Hackett, Thomas. "Denial as a Social Act," in Sidney Levin and Ralph Kahana (Eds.), *Psychodynamic Studies on Aging: Creativity, Reminiscing, and Dying;* Internat. Univ. Press, 1966.

Chapter 21

Some Aspects of Psychotherapy with Dying Persons

Edwin S. Shneidman

From the psychosocial point of view, the primary task of helping the dying person is to focus on the *person*—not on the biochemistry or pathology of the diseased organs, but on a human being who is a living beehive of emotions that include, especially, anxiety, the fight for control, and terror. And, with a dying person, there is another grim, omnipresent fact in the picture: time is finite. The situation is dramatic, unlike that of psychotherapy with an essentially physically healthy person, where time seems endless and there is no push by the pages of the calendar. One of the main points of this chapter is that just as psychotherapy is, in some fundamental ways, clearly different from ordinary talk, so working psychotherapeutically with a dying person involves some important differences from the usual modes of psychotherapy.

THREE ASPECTS OF THE DYING PROCESS

At the outset of this chapter on psychotherapy with dying persons, it is only reasonable that I delineate some issues that, in my opinion, are fundamental to understanding any list of therapeutic suggestions. There are, as I see it, some general background topics that are relevant to a keen appreciation of the "rules" for psychotherapy with the dying. The rules themselves are rather easy to comprehend in a superficial way, but their more meaningful application within the context of a stressful dying scenario has to take into account certain subtleties that lie behind the obvious and visible drama. In *Moby Dick*, death-oriented Ahab says: "All visible objects, man, are but as pasteboard masks. But in each event—in the living act, the undoubted deed—there some unknown but still reasoning thing put forth the mouldings of its features from behind the un-reasoning mask." We must look behind the apparent dying scenario if we wish to ap-preciate the powerful and poignant psychological richness inherent in the dying drama.

To be specific, I shall suggest that there are three aspects of the dying process that need to be kept in mind as one considers the dozen or so specific rules for psychother-apy with dying persons. They are (1) the philosophical (moral-ethical-epistemological) aspects of the dying process; (2) the sociological (situational) aspects; and (3) the psy-chological (characterological) aspects.

Philosophical (Moral-Ethical-Epistemological) Aspects of the Dying Process

One can begin with the assertion that, typically, death is a dyadic event, involving the chief protagonist (the dying person) and the survivors in basically an I-thou relation-ship. Toynbee (1969) has stated it succinctly:

> The two-sidedness of death is a fundamental feature of death. . . . There are always two parties to a death; the person who dies and the survivors who are bereaved . . . the sting of death is less sharp for the person who dies than it is for the bereaved survivor. This is, as I see it, the capital fact about the relation between living and dying. There are two parties to the suffering that death inflicts; and, in the appor-tionment of this suffering, the survivor takes the brunt.

And the situation is often even more complicated, involving several persons, as in the following two vignettes.

1. A physician asks me to see one of his patients. He tells me beforehand that her numerous physical pains and complaints have absolutely no organic basis. I see her and talk with her. As much as I try to eschew the use of simplistic diagnostic labels to des-cribe a complicated human being, the tag of *agitated depression* seems to describe her rather accurately. She is complaining of pain; she wrings her hands; her brow is fur-rowed; she is restless, fidgety, tearful, woebegone. She looks older than her 40 years. The story is this: her wealthy husband has a terminal disease. He may very well be dead in a few years or even much sooner. He has told her that she makes him nervous and that he cannot stand her. He has placed her in a private nursing home. She hates that nursing home and wants to return to her own home. Coincidentally, he has em-ployed a practical nurse to massage his muscular pains and also to act as chauffeur and "keeper" for his wife. At the end of my session with the wife, the nurse comes into the office to take her back to the nursing home. She is rather heavily made up, and has a rather striking figure. The picture is suddenly clear to me. The practical nurse is the husband's mistress. The wife has been evicted from her own home. "But, after all,"

says her doctor, "That poor man is dying." I discuss with him Jeremy Bentham and his utilitarian theory (see below).

2. A 70-year-old man has cancer of the esophagus. He had received a course of chemotherapy that had made him excruciatingly uncomfortable, causing nausea, vertigo, and vomiting. Several weeks later he began to show memory loss, some confusion, and uncharacteristic irritability. A thorough neurological examination disclosed a malignant brain tumor. Another course of treatment was suggested. His son—a physician (neurologist) who lived in another city but who was in daily telephone communication with his parents—asked his father's doctor to forego the treatments. To me, on the telephone, the son said: "What is the point of an unknown amount of possible good compared to an onerous treatment of absolutely uncertain benefit imbedded in a procedure that will give him a substantial amount of certain torture?" The local treating physician was incensed. The wife was in a quandary. The treating physician demanded that the patient be told "all the facts" and be permitted to make up his own mind. The physician-son retorted that his father, not being medically trained, was in no position to evaluate the facts, and more than that, his mind—specifically his brain—was no longer able to make the ordinary judgments of which he had been previously capable. As the mother's psychotherapist, I wondered at the sad game of what I called "Who owns the body?" Again, my thoughts turned to Bentham.

Toynbee (1969) raises the question of who, in the total suffering a death inflicts, is hurt the most. The two criteria are comfort and dignity—their opposites are pain and humiliation (degradation). In the late eighteenth and early nineteenth centuries, Jeremy Bentham (1748–1832), the noted English thinker, espoused a philosophy that he called *utilitarianism*, the basic tenet of which was "the greatest good for the greatest number." This was the "principle of utility": the "greatest happiness"—given the unnegotiable, dire facts—"for the greatest number is the social test of what is moral conduct."

Imagine for each of the two vignettes cited above a chart in the shape of a circle. On each chart there are four characters: on the first are the husband, the wife, the mistress, and the doctor; on the second, the father, the mother, the son, and the doctor. The second case is compounded by the fact that we do not know, from day to day, what the father is thinking or experiencing. How should the calculations of how to divide the percentages of dignity, self-esteem, well-being, comfort, sense of accomplishment, freedom from pain, and so on among the characters be determined? Who should be given the largest percentage; who the least? Should, in the first case, the wife be scapegoated and given ECT for her depression? In the second case, should the wishes of the treating physician—who may have that patient on a research protocol —supersede, in the name of science and possible help for future patients (not to mention the physician's narcissistic and professional investment in this treatment regimen), the physician-son's emotional feelings about his father's dignity, comfort, and "appropriate" death?

Far from being esoteric abstractions, these philosophic points touch on the deepest questions relating to death: who have become the high priests of death? What are the citizen's rights to death with dignity? When can a spouse or grown child say for a loved one, "Enough"? And the reader is reminded here (and this applies to the following discussions) that the author's intention is not to exhort, but rather to indicate basic background issues in the context of which the day-to-day details of therapeutic interventions are conducted.

Sociological (Situational) Aspects of the Dying Process

Inasmuch as today the majority of terminally ill persons die in institutions—hospitals or nursing homes—it is appropriate to ask: what are the constraints of the social environment on the dying person? The recent observations and reports of field sociologists such as David Sudnow, author of *Passing On* (1967) (with his intriguing descriptions of "what actually happens" in hospitals, especially in emergency rooms, and the various uses to which fresh corpses are put) and of Barney Glaser and Anselm Strauss, authors of *Awareness of Dying* (1965) and *Time for Dying* (1968) (with their enlightening concepts of "mutual pretense" and of "the dying trajectory"), teach us that a great deal that goes on in such institutions is neither in the organizational chart nor in the brochure given to visitors.

Whether or not a person is resuscitated; how much time doctors and nurses spend in a dying person's room; whether he or she will be pronounced dead on this shift or that; whether or not interns will practice surgery on the dead body—these and other occurrences are what realistic sociologists are telling us about and it behooves us to listen to them. In order to understand the dying person, we must have a keen awareness and appreciation of his or her immediate situation.

To illustrate: oily rags in a closet eventually burst into flame precisely because of the closed air of the oppressively small space. A situational analysis might be the best way to understand this phenomenon of spontaneous combustion. Similarly, one's situation—the role that one is forced to play; the expectations that others have; one's social space, such as in a hospital with its staff/patient dichotomy; the depersonalization and isolation that the very architecture of the building and the social structure of the hospital or nursing home force upon one—has an important bearing on dying behavior. The situation, which Talcott Parsons in *Toward a General Theory of Action* (1951) describes as consisting of the "objects of orientation," can have several facets that relate to dying behavior. The situation or social environment can make death more bearable and more gracious; it can also make death more isolated, more dehumanized, more fearful, and so on.

Glaser's and Strauss's concept of "the dying trajectory" deserves our closer attention. In *Time for Dying* (1968) they say the following:

> When the dying patient's hospital career begins—when he is admitted to the hospital and a specific service—the staff in solo and in concert make initial definitions of the patient's trajectory. They expect him to linger, to die quickly, or to approach death at some pace between these extremes. They establish some degree of certainty

about his impending death—for example, they may judge that there is "nothing more to do" for the patient. They forecast that he will never leave the hospital again, or that he will leave and perhaps be readmitted several times before his death. They may anticipate that he will have periods of relative health as well as severe physical hardship during the course of his illness. They predict the potential modes of his dying and how he will fare during the last days and hours of his life. . . .

At this early stage of rehearsing these aspects and critical junctures of the dying patient's trajectory, the staff may perceive a temporally determinant trajectory— its total length with clearcut stages—or an indeterminant trajectory—its stages or length or both are unclear. Although they assign as complete a trajectory as possible to the dying patient, the clarities and vagaries of the several apsects of any trajectory generate differentials in definitions among the various staff members. The legitimate definitions . . . come from the doctor. Since the definition of trajectory influences behavior, these differing definitions may create inconsistencies in the staff's care of and interaction with the patient, with consequent problems for the staff itself, family, and patient.

When ordinary, well-functioning individuals are asked what they would consider to be most important to them if they were dying, they usually list control—having some measure of say over their own treatment and management—as the most important item (followed by relief from pain, which can, in the last analysis, also be subsumed under the category of control). But we see that there are often conflicts between the dying person's fight for dignity (self-control, autonomy) and the hospital staff's desire to assign that person (i.e., the patient) to certain roles, including even the pace or rate at which those roles are to be played. In order to be a good patient, one has to die on schedule, in accordance with the dying trajectory mapped out by the staff. To die too early, unexpectedly, is an embarrassment to hospital staff; but what is more surprising (and of psychosocial interest), is that to linger too long, beyond the projected trajectory, can be an even greater embarrassment to hospital staff, and a great strain on the next of kin who may have premourned and set their mind's clock for a specific death date that then becomes painfully overdue.

Psychological (Characterological) Aspects of the Dying Process

For the terminally ill person, the time of dying is a multiscened drama, with elements of both tragic and historical pagentry. It is probably true that each person dies idiosyncratically alone, in a notably personal way, but nonetheless there are generalizations that can be made about the dying process. From a psychological point of view, the most interesting question is what are the psychological characteristics of the dying process.

On the current thanatological scene there are those who assert that there are a half-dozen or so stages that the dying person lives through in a specific order. My own experiences have led me to rather different conclusions. In working with dying persons I see the wide panoply of human emotions—few in some people, dozens in others— see the wide panoply of human emotions—few in some people, dozens in others— experienced in a variety of orderings, reorderings, and arrangements. The one psychological mechanism that seems ubiquitous is denial, which can appear or reappear at any time (see Avery Weisman's *On Dying and Denying*, 1972). Nor is there any natural law that says an individual has to achieve a state of psychoanalytic grace or any other kind of closure before death sets its seal. In fact, most people die either too soon or too late, leaving behind loose threads and fragments of unattended business.

My own notion is more general in scope, more specific in content. In spirit it derives from the work of Adolph Meyer and Henry Murray. My hypothesis is that a *dying person's behavior will reflect or parallel that person's previous behavior as it evinced itself in response to situations of threat, stress, or failure*. There are certain basic characteristics common to all human beings. One is that individuals die more or less as they have lived, and how they die is influenced as well by those aspects of personality that relate to their conceptualization of their dying. To put it oversimply: the psychological course of the cancer mirrors certain deep troughs in the course of the life—oncology recapitulates ontogeny.

What is especially pertinent is how an individual has behaved at some of the most stressful, least successful, periods-of-failure times in his or her life, whether those incidents related to situations of stress in school, job, marriage, separation, loss, or whatever. The hypothesis further holds that an individual's previous macrotemporal patterns and coping mechanisms will give clues as to his patterns of behavior when he is dying—whether he will fight his illness or surrender to it, whether he will despair or deny and so on—as he becomes increasingly aware of his life-threatening situation and finally convinced of the imminence of his own death.

One example of this hypothesis—that people die pretty much as they have lived in terms of how they have reacted to the stressful periods of their lives—would be a dying person's tendency to premourn himself, that is, to bemoan his own fate as if he were already dead, to pull away from life, to decathect, to deinvest, to inure himself for his own departure. Specifically, parallels might lie in the patient's previous patterns of premourning, that is, if the dying person has ever had, earlier in his or her life, the tragic occasion to have premourned a loved one, say, his or her child who was dying over a course of time (of, for example, leukemia), and has experienced at that time a period in which there was some pulling away, deinvestment, a protective letting go before the actual death of the child, then one might look to the details of that earlier experience for subtle indications as to what the current patterns and details will be in that individual's premourning of his currently impending death.

PSYCHOTHERAPY WITH THE DYING: ITS UNIQUENESS

I believe that working intensively with a dying person is different from almost any other human encounter. In one of my recent books on death (1976), I attempted to explicate some of the important differences between *conversation* (or ordinary talk) and a *professional exchange*. The main point to be made was that when a clinical thanatologist (physician, psychologist, nurse, social worker, or any trained person) is working with a dying person, he or she is not just talking. This is not to say that there is not an enormously important place for mere *presence*—which, after all, may be the most important ingredient in care—or for sitting in communicative silence, or for seemingly just talking about what may appear to be trivial or banal topics.

Working with the dying person is a special task. A person who systematically attempts to help a dying individual achieve a more psychologically comfortable death or a more appropriate death—given the dire, unnegotiable circumstances of the terminal disease—is either a psychotherapist or is acting in the role of a psychotherapist. That role cannot be escaped. This is not to say that many others—relatives, dear friends, church members, neighbors—cannot also play extremely important roles. But the distinction between a conversation and a professional exchange is crucial. More than that, I now believe that working with dying persons is different from working with any other kind of individual and demands a different kind of involvement; and I am willing to propose that there may be as important a conceptual difference between ordinary psychotherapy (with individuals where the life span is not an issue) and psychotherapy with dying persons as there is between ordinary psychotherapy and ordinary talk. In the chart below, I have attempted to limn out what I feel are some of the important nuances of these differences.

	In a conversation the focus is on:	In a professional exchange the focus is on:	In a thanatological situation the focus is on:
Content	1. Substantive content, i.e., the talk is primarily about things, events, dates—the surface of the world.	1. Affective (emotional) content, i.e., the exchange focuses (not constantly, but occasionally) on the feelings and the emotional tone of the patient, sometimes minimizing the facts.	1. The topics of death and dying. It is not the clinical thanatologist who introduces these topics. The dying person will, if permitted, bring them up, because those topics are understandably uppermost in the patient's mind, except when they are denied. The important point to be noted is that when these topics do come up, as they almost invariably do, the thanatologist does not run from them, or from the patient.

	Conversation	Professional exchange	Thanatological situation
Level	2. Manifest level, i.e., conversation focuses on what is said, the actual words which are uttered, the facts which are stated.	2. Latent level, i.e., the professional person listens for what is between the lines and below the surface, for what is implied, not expressed, for what may be unconsciously present.	2. Both manifest and latent levels. The manifest levels may come to include topics around death: burial arrangements, disposition of belongings, etc.; the latent meanings of many of those overt arrangements may involve the wishes for continued control, for extension of life, and for certain kinds of immortality. In the dying scene there are both coded messages and statements of breath-taking candor.
Meanings	3. Conscious meanings, i.e., dealing with the other person as though what was said was meant and as though the person were a "rational man" and "knows his own mind."	3. Unconscious meanings, i.e., listening for unconscious meanings and latent intentions (e.g., double-entendres, puns, hidden meanings, latent implications, etc.).	3. The distinction between conscious and unconscious meanings is complicated in the dying scene by the very irrationality of death itself. It is difficult to be rational about the end of one's own life and ceasing to be. The clinician listens, tries to comprehend, and is sparing with interpretations, knowing that comfort and peace of mind are more important than new insights when one is racing the clock.

	Conversation	Professional exchange	Thanatological situation
Abstraction	4. Phenotypic, i.e., concern with the ordinary, interesting details of life, where what is talked about is the same as "what is meant."	4. Genotypic, i.e. search for congruencies, similarities, commonalities, generalizations about the patient's psychological life.	4. When the thanatological interchange is genotypic, it focuses on the other comparable periods of the dying person's life: episodes or instances of stress, threat or failure, other "little deaths" or endings, previous patterns of premourning. Of course, earlier times of triumph, success, and happiness are neither neglected nor depreciated. In all this, the patient sets the pace.
Role	5. Social role, i.e. an exchange between two people who are essentially equals (like neighbors or friends, etc.) or who depend on the prestige of age, rank, status, etc., but who have an equal right to display themselves, to ask each other banal or intimate questions, neither being the patient.	5. Transference, i.e., the exchange is between nonequals; between one person who wishes help (and tacitly agrees to play the patient's role) and another person who agrees to proffer help (and thus is cast in the role of physician, priest, father, magician, witch doctor, helper). Much of what is effective in the exchange is the patient's transference onto the therapist.	5. The most important difference lies under this rubric. If one choses to work intensively with a dying person, then one can deliberately attempt to create a situation of rather intense and deep transference from the patient to the therapist (and, along with it an intense countertransference from the therapist to the dying person). It is unlike any other situation. The stark reality is that the patient will die soon, so that ethically speaking, the therapist can afford quickly to become a key, significant figure in the dying person's life.

SPECIFIC CHARACTERISTICS OF WORKING WITH THE DYING

I believe that every physician should be a clinical thanatologist, at least once (preferably early) in his or her career, and thus deal intensively (5 or 6 days a week, for an *hour* each day) with the personal-human-psychological aspects of a dying person. This means sitting unhurriedly by the bedside and coming to know that dying person qua dying person—over and above the biochemistry, cytology, medicine, and oncology of the case. This also means not avoiding the dying and death aspects of the situation, but learning about them, sharing them, being burdened by them (and their enormous implications)—in short, sharing the intensity of the thanatological experience.

The therapist's reward for performing this difficult task, that is, treating one person intensively as a paradigm of how one might optimally (if there were unlimited time and one had infinite psychic reserves) treat every dying person, is an enriching experience that will illuminate all the rest of one's practice and will enable the busy physician to be much more effective in the necessarily briefer encounters with all his patients, terminal or otherwise. The proper role of the physician in the twentieth century is not only to alleviate pain and cure the sick but also, when the situation requires it, to help people die better. And how can the physician really know how this may be done unless he or she makes the time to experience intimately at least one or two intensive dying episodes?

The following is a list of some of the specific characteristics of working with *dying* persons, as opposed to those who are "only" critically ill, sick, diseased, injured, or disturbed. These characteristics are the building blocks of a new specialty—of import to all care givers and not limited to physicians—called *thanatology*.

What is special and different about thanatological work?

1. *The goals are different.* Because the time is limited, the goals are more finite. The omnipresent goal is the psychological *comfort* of the person, with, as a general rule, as much alleviation of physical pain as possible. For a person who is terminally ill, addiction is not an issue, yet many physicians are niggardly or inappropriately scrupulous about the use of pain-relieving substances. We have much to learn from Dr. Cicely Saunders, founder of St. Christopher's Hospice in London, about the humane uses of morphine, alcohol, and other analgesics (1976). Deep insight is not the goal of psychotherapy with the dying. There is no rule that states that an individual must die with any certain amount of self-knowledge. In this sense, every life is incomplete. The goal, as one fights the clock and the lethal illness, is to *will the obligatory*; to make a chilling and ugly scene go as well as possible; to give psychological succor; to permit the tying-up of loose ends; to lend as much stability to the person as it is possible to give.

2. *The rules are different.* Because there is a foreseeable, although tentative, death date in the future—it can be a matter of months or weeks—the usual rules for psychotherapy can be modified. The celerity with which the relationship between therapist and patient is established, as well as the depth of that relationship, is totally appropriate for a dying person, while for an ordinary patient it might appear unseemly and even border on the unprofessional. But the love that flows between patient and therapist (and therapist and patient) when the patient is a dying person can be sustaining,

even ennobling. One might ask what would happen if the patient were to have a remission, even recover. That is an embarrassment devoutly to be wished; in that rare case, the therapist would simply have to "renegotiate" the "contract" or understanding between the two of them. But, in general, intensive work with a dying person permits a degree of transference and countertransference that ought neither to be aimed for nor tolerated in perhaps any other professional relationship.

3. *It may not be psychotherapy.* Obviously, working with a dying person should, for that person, be psychotherapeutic. (Anything that might be iatrogenic should be avoided.) But the process itself may be sufficiently different from ordinary psychotherapy that it might very well merit a label of its own. The labelling is not of the primary significance. What is important is that the process be flexible, which is somewhat different from eclectic, and be able to move with the dying person's changes in needs, shifts of mood, efforts toward control, detours into denial, and so on. Psychotherapy with a dying person incorporates elements of traditional psychotherapy, but it also is characterized by other genres of human interaction, including rapport building, interview, conversation, history taking, just plain talk, and communicative silences. There is no movement toward goals such as termination of therapy; there is rather a process that goes on until it is interrupted by death.

4. *The focus is on benign intervention.* In thanatological work, the therapist does not need to be a *tabula rasa,* nor does he or she need to be inactive. There can be active intervention, so long as it is in the patient's interest. These interventions can take the form of interpreting, making suggestions, advising (when asked to), interacting with doctors and nurses in the hospital ward, interacting with members of the family, arranging for social work services, acting as liaison with clergy, and so on. The notion that any intervention on the part of the therapist is an incursion into the patient's rights and liberties is here rejected as an obtuse idea that does not distinguish between benign and malign intervention. The clinical thanatologist can act as the patient's ombudsman in many ways—on the ward, in the hospital, and within the community.

5. *No one has to die in a state of psychoanalytic grace.* If the Jehovah or "savior" complex that is understandably present in many psychotherapists is laid aside, there still remains in the motivational system of any effective therapist an underlying concern with "success." In the case of the dying patient, the therapist must realign his notions of what he can realistically expect to achieve and do for that person. It is a process that no matter how auspiciously begun or effectively conducted always ends in death. We hear phrases like *death work,* but we need to appreciate the fact that very few individuals die right on psychological target with all their complexes and neuroses completely worked through. The therapist needs to be able to tolerate such incompleteness and lack of closure. No one ever untangles all the varied skeins of one's intrapsychic and interpersonal life; to the last second there are psychical creations and recreations that require new resolutions. Total insight is an abstraction; there is no perfect state of mental homeostasis.

6. *"Working through" is a luxury for those who have time to live.* It follows from the above that people die either too soon or too late, and leave behind them loose threads and unfinished business. The goal of resolving life's problems may be an

unattainable one; the goal of an "appropriate death"—Avery Weisman's (1972) felicitous concept—of helping the dying person to "be relatively pain free, suffering reduced, emotional and social impoverishments kept at a minimum . . . resolving residual conflicts, and satisfying whatever remaining wishes are consistent with his present plight and with his ego ideal" may be more attainable. The best death is one that an individual would choose for himself or herself if that choice were possible. Very few important psychological complexities are completely worked through by the time of death. There is much merit in willing the obligatory. The dying person can be helped to put his or her affairs in order, although everyone dies more or less in a state of psychological intestate.

7. *The dying person sets the pace.* Because there are no specific substantive psychological goals (of having this insight or coming to that understanding), the emphasis is on process and on the thanatologist's continued presence. Nothing *has* to be accomplished. The patient sets the pace. This includes, even, whether or not the topic of death is ever mentioned, although, if permitted, it usually will be. The therapist will note the usefullness of *the method of successive approximations*, in which a dying person may say, over the course of many days, I have a problem, an illness, a tumor, a malignancy, a cancer, a terminal metastasis. This is not a litany that needs to be recited. Different individuals get in touch with their illnesses at various points of candor. Any one of these points is equally good, so long as it is comfortable for that person.

8. *Denial will be present.* We have already characterized the notion of a half-dozen stages of dying as a simplistic one. In the most popular explication of this approach, denial is listed as the first stage ("No, it can't be me!"). But our disavowal of the idea of a few stages of dying should not lead us into the error of neglecting the importance of the psychological mechanism of denial itself. Denial is not a stage of dying; it is rather a ubiquitous aspect of the dying process, surfacing now and again (at no predetermined regular intervals) all through the dying process. It is only human even for the most extraordinary being occasionally to blot out or take a vacation from his knowledge of his imminent end. It is probably psychologically necessary for the dying person intermittently to rest his own death-filled train of thoughts on a sidespur, off the main track that leads only to blackness and the unknown. This means that the clinical thanatologist must be prepared for the dying person to manifest a rather radical change of pace, and, for example, suddenly to start talking one day about leaving the hospital and taking a trip. If the therapist will only go along with this transient denial, the dying person will, as abruptly as he began it, abandon it and return to the reality of the present moment.

9. *The goal is increased psychological comfort.* The main point of working with the dying person—in the visits, the give-and-take of talk, the advice, the interpretations, the listening—is to increase that individual's psychological *comfort*. The criterion of *effectiveness* lies in this single measure. One cannot realistically be pollyannish or even optimistic; the therapist begins in a grim situation that is going to become even grimmer. The best that he can hope to accomplish is to help the ill person in whatever ways it takes to achieve the patient's increased psychological comfort. However, hope should never be totally abandoned.

10. *The importance of relating to nurses and doctors on the ward.* Whether the dying work is done in a hospital or in some other place it cannot be conducted as a solo operation. (It would be difficult to be a clinical thanatologist in a private practice.) It is of key importance that other personnel on the ward be kept informed of the dying person's state, condition, and needs, and, in addition, that they be made aware of the guiding concepts that underlie this special therapeutic exchange. Like clinical research on a ward, thanatological work often does not go well without the cooperation of the chief nurse. It is understood that no one approaches a patient as a *patient care specialist*—the euphemism for clinical thanatologist—unless he or she has been asked to do so by the physician in charge of the case. Then such a person, who has already been introduced to the patient by the responsible physician, acts as any consultant would act. The difference is in the frequency and duration of the visits; they should be daily and last approximately an hour, the importance of which has already been stressed.

11. *The survivor is the victim—and eventually the patient: the concept of postvention.* Arnold Toynbee (1969) wrote eloquently on his view that death was essentially a two-person event and that, in the summation of anguish, the survivor bore the brunt of the hurt. All that has been said above should now be understood in the context of advocating that almost from the beginning of working with the dying person, the clinical thanatologist ought to become acquainted with the main survivor-to-be, to gain rapport with that person, and to have an explicit understanding that he or she will see the survivor in the premourning stages and then for a while, at decreasing intervals, for perhaps a year or so after the death. *Postvention*—working with survivor-victims—ought to be part of any total health care system. It is not only humane; it is good medical practice, for we know, especially from the work of Colin Murray Parkes (1972), that a population of survivors (of any adult age) is a population at risk, having markedly elevated rates of morbidity (including surgeries and other hospitalizations) and mortality (from a variety of causes of death) for at least a year or so after the death of a loved one. Postventive care relates not only to the loss that the survivor has suffered but also to other aspects of functioning under stress that that mourner may be experiencing.

12. *Just as the role of transference is paramount, the place of countertransference bears careful watching and a good support system is a necessity.* A terminal person's dying days can be made better by virtue of the joys of transference onto the thanatological therapist. The therapist, if willing and able, should work for an intense transference relationship. But there is a well-known caveat: where there is transference, there is also countertransference—the flow of feeling from the therapist to the patient. The therapist invests himself in the patient's welfare and is thereby made vulnerable. When the patient dies, the therapist is bereaved. And during the dying process the therapist is anguished by the prospect of loss and the sense of impotence. Dealing with dying persons is difficult work. The therapist would be well advised to have good support systems in his or her own life—loved ones, dear friends, a congenial work situation, and peer consultants.

It is also important to remember that a physician needs to take vacations from death. A gynecological oncologist, for example, might intersperse his practice with obstetrical cases, and thus deliver babies as a balance for treating those patients who are dying of cancer of the uterus. And, as a further suggestion, a physician in oncological practice should not fail to seek out psychological or psychiatric consultation for patients if they are significantly depressed or otherwise disturbed about dying and for himself as well if he feels that his own equanimity has been disturbed. This type of psychotherapeutic help might well be made a routine part of a physician's dealing with dying persons, lest the physician fall prey to the predictable consequences of the unusual psychological stresses that come from working constantly around and against death.

A DYING PERSON: AN ILLUSTRATION

What follows are some excerpts from one tape-recorded session with a 22-year-old man who was dying of leukemia. He was an only child, unmarried, largely estranged from his mother; his father had died many years before. This session occurred about a week before his death, some 6 weeks—during which time I saw him each weekday—after I had first been asked to see him by his hematologist because of his difficult and cantankerous behavior in the hospital. (He had cursed some of the young nurses, and, worse, had thrown a bedpan across the room.) On my initial visit to his room, I walked in, introduced myself, put my hand gently on his, and said that I had heard that he had been misbehaving himself. He burst into tears and I knew that I had a patient. In this particular session, the hour began with his words, spoken slowly and in a low voice.[4]

P: I'm giving up. I want it to be over. I don't expect any miracles anymore. The sweating and the fevers just get me down. And yet I feel good. It's going to be a slow process. Maybe not so much a painful process, but a slow process. I'd like to get out. And then I'd also like to sleep and die. I mean I don't know what to say. I'm just tired. I woke up this morning. I was really frightened. I was saying, dear God, dear God what am I going to do? Dear God, dear God doesn't answer. Waiting like this.

S: Were you really frightened, terrorized?

P: Yeah, I was really frightened.

S: What did that fear feel like? What was it fear of?

P: Oh, the unknown and another day, another day. Something else to keep me going. (Coughing) Dr. Shneidman, if there was a way I could end it now, I would do that. It's taking so long. I don't have much patience I guess.

S: That's true. That's true this is a trial for you in many ways, including that one.

P: Including patience you mean?

S: Yes. I don't think in your life you had a period when you had to be so patient.

P: How do you do it?

S: There's no easy way.

P: I'm scared. You said you'd say what death was.

S: Pardon me!

P: You said you'd say what death was. You said it was something that I wouldn't know anything about.

S: Yes.

P: If I could only be sure that it would be peaceful. Will it be peaceful?

S: I can guarantee it.

P: Because that's so important. It's almost more important than anything else, that it be peaceful. My mother still wants to believe that maybe something can happen.

S: In what ways have your relationships with your mother changed in the last several days?

P: I've loved her. I let myself love her. (Weeping) Without any ties. I let myself love her without feeling that she was going to emasculate me. I've let her love me. [In a subsequent session he said "You let me do this."] I've let her be a mother. She's been so beautiful. I get more comfort from her than from anybody else.

S: That's beautiful. Do you think it took your being sick for that to happen?

P: I don't know. I know for me it has because now there's no reason to be wary of her castrating tendencies because she really means well for me. And she brings me such comfort, and she's so selfless. Crying's not supposed to help. It hurts when you get a fever and you sweat a lot, which is what I do . . . .

S: What would you do differently?

P: That's a hard question because I don't know if I can be honest. I mean I could say one thing now and if it happened, do something else. I suppose I'd be very wary about all health things and I suppose I'd be very slow to get started again, but I think I would know myself a little better, a lot better. I think I would look upon myself as a much better person. I think I'd be less concerned about my physical appearance, although I don't think I would ignore it. I think I'd be less selfish and less into security for myself, it being very important then. I think I'd be more concerned with trying to get the most out of every day.

S: Would you tend more to creature comforts, your own environment, what you looked at, what you touched and smelled and saw and heard.

P: I've always been a little like that. I suppose I'd always want to have a comfortable environment, but I know that small, irritating things wouldn't be small, irritating things to me. I could take things a lot better. I know I could. And if there is a God, if there is somebody that I knew I could pray to that maybe could perform this miracle, I'd be most thankful and I'd show it in every way I could. (Coughing) It's so farfetched, so unreal. I don't have a chance. I want to live so much. I don't want to die now. I'm half there and I'm half here, maybe more than half there, because I don't get any encouragement anymore about living from the doctors. Right now, the big thing is just doing as good a job as possible to keep me alive for as long as possible, which is something I really don't want to do. Because if it's over, shouldn't it be over? Shouldn't I be out of the way? My mother keeps saying take each day as it comes. It's very difficult, extremely difficult. I had a lot of trouble doing that before. I'm having even more trouble doing it now.

S: Is there anything in life that prepares one for the kind of thing you're going through?

P: Well if there is, I never experienced it, because I certainly am not prepared for it. The nurses give nice care. They've been very nice. So many people have said how much I touched their lives.

S: I'm sure that's true.

P: All kinds of people, young, old, my contemporaries. I never knew it.

S: How does all that make you feel?

P: I went to bed last night after listening to it, hearing it, and talking about it. I went to bed last night feeling good, and it was very comforting. But then I woke this morning and I was in this terror. It's like I need constant reassurance that I've been a good person and that there's someone there to love me. I guess I don't call that much of a success.

S: How do you mean?

P: I suppose if I'd been that way, I would be much more capable of taking this thing.

S: With more stoicism and equanimity?

P: Yeah. Maybe even fighting it better. I haven't fought it very well. It's almost as if I've wanted to die, from the time I got it. Not wanted to die, but knew I was going to die.

S: Sort of gave in to it?

P: Yeah ... I remember a few months ago they did a blood test and a bone marrow test and then the doctor gave me a shot that turned out to be Valium and then he told me I had leukemia.

S: How did he tell you? Did he preface it in any way?

P: I think he told me, he told me in a way that was like we caught it at a good time, that we really have a good chance, that they wanted me to go to the hospital.

S: What were your reactions?

P: I called my mother right away.

S: What went through your head? Did you know what that diagnosis meant?

P: (Coughing) I recognized the seriousness, but I was in a state of shock.

S: What did you say to your mother?

P: I told her I had leukemia.

S: What was her reaction to that?

P: She cried ... but I really thought I was going to be cured. I mean they told me I was. They told me I had a really good chance. And they've tried everything. Now a perfectly good person with an awful lot to give is going to die. A young person is going to die. The death is going to be senseless.

S: You say it in such a shatteringly objective way about yourself.

P: It is a senseless death. I've asked the same question, why me? I don't get any answers. I suppose if somebody has to get it, it's just a disease and there's statistics and somebody has to get it, so maybe a friend of mine who's sailing along very nicely now thinking how sorry he is for me is going to get killed in an auto accident, because somebody has to get killed in an auto accident.

S: That's an interesting idea, like there's so much misery and so much death and it has to be distributed.

P: Yeah. I wish I could sleep, get some rest, but I dwell so much on it, on the dying. But if I get out I don't want to sleep. I want to get out. I want to do some things, just some things, maybe have a French meal, go to a movie, sleep with my lover again. In a way though it might make it more difficult. But why not? Why shouldn't I do it? Why shouldn't I walk outside again? I wonder how much I've missed. Now it's irretrievable. Do you think it's a good idea, even if I'm not a hundred percent right, if the doctors say it's okay for me to go out, do you think it's a good idea for me to go?

S: Naturally. Don't you? What do you mean even if it's not a hundred percent right?

P: You know, I'm still sweating. I think it's part of the leukemia. My throat still bothers me a bit, my stomach still bothers me a bit.

S: Well I'll put the question back to you, What do you think?

P: I almost think that almost anything is better than just lying here in this bed. I hate to be a burden to people on the outside but I'll never be completely well . . . I'm really at a low point.

S: I know, and a difficult one.

P: A really low point. . . . Do *you* fear death?

S: Yes, of course, but I think I'm more afraid of the incompleteness of my life. Why do you ask?

P: I was just wondering about somebody who is more or less a specialist in the area of death, how he felt about it.

S: Well, I'm as mortal as anybody, as human as anybody. There are different levels of me just as there are different levels of you.

P: (Sigh) I feel peaceful now.

S: I'll come to see you on Monday, around 11 o'clock.

P: I hope I'll be here.

S: If you leave the hospital, please call me and let me know.

P: I mean I hope I'll still be here physically.

S: It's a sine qua non. See you.

At the beginning, when I first began to see this young man, his mother had taken a prejudiced (before she met me) dislike to me. Her principal grievance was that her only baby was talking to me, but not to her. But during her son's dying process, she and I began to meet. I listened to her and gave her emotional comfort; she came to trust me and to look forward to our sessions. After his death—in a departure from my usual form—I went with her to the funeral and stood beside her and supported her arm at the graveside. At her wish, I have continued to see her, intermittently, over the past few years. In these sessions, we talk about her grief and her resurgent feelings about her late son. We are brought together by our admittedly unequal yet common loss.

BIBLIOGRAPHY

Glaser, Barney G. and Anselm Strauss: *Awareness of Dying*, Aldine, Chicago, 1965.
—— and ——: *Time for Dying*, Aldine, Chicago, 1968.
Hinton, John: *Dying*, Penguin, Baltimore, 1967.
Murray, Henry A.: "Toward a Classification of Interaction," in Talcott Parson and Edward A. Shils (eds.), *Toward a General Theory of Action,* Harvard, Cambridge, Mass., 1951.
Parkes, Colin Murray: *Bereavement: Studies of Grief in Adult Life*, International Universities Press, New York, 1972.
Parsons, Talcott and Edward A. Shils (eds.): *Toward a General Theory of Action,* Harvard, Cambridge, Mass., 1951.
Saunders, Cicely: "St. Christopher's Hospice," in Edwin Shneidman (ed.), *Death: Current Perspectives,* Mayfield, Palo Alto, Calif., 1976.
Shneidman, Edwin S.: *Deaths of Man,* Penguin, Baltimore, 1974.
—— (ed.): *Death: Current Perspectives,* Mayfield, Palo Alto, Calif., 1976.
——: "Aspects of the Dying Process," *Psychiatric Annals,* 7(8): 25–40, August 1977.
Sudnow, David: *Passing On,* Prentice-Hall, Englewood Cliffs, N. J., 1967.
Toynbee, Arnold et al.: *Man's Concern with Death,* McGraw-Hill, New York, 1969.
Weisman, Avery D.: *On Dying and Denying,* Behavioral Publications, New York, 1972.

Chapter 22

A Little Myth
Is a Dangerous Thing:
Research in the Service
of the Dying

Richard A. Kalish

As the stream of books and articles on death, dying, and bereavement swells to a river and then to a flood tide, health care professionals are increasingly considering new forms of medical care and psychosocial treatment for those who are dying. Most of the books and articles published to date contain immense amounts of advice; although some of the advice is platitudinous or redundant, a great deal of what is said either seems to make good sense or effectively challenges accepted assumptions that determine what type of care is offered. However, a major shortcoming of these publications is that they do not make available research criteria or clinical data that would enable professionals to evaluate the applicability of the advice.

There are many justifiable questions about our current knowledge of death and dying. What do we know about caring for the dying person and what is the basis for our knowledge? Is *denial* the first natural step in the dying process? Must a dying person experience and overcome denial to die an "appropriate" death? Do most dying people want to die at home? Are older people more afraid of death than younger people? Do dying people want to talk about their plight, and, if so, to whom?

Most advice on the issues raised by these questions implies that there is substantial data on the needs and attitudes of people who are terminally ill, but is there? In this chapter, I will discuss the research base of a number of the issues related to working with dying patients.

Different people define research differently. For some, only the most rigorously conducted, well-designed study, complete with appropriate experimental or statistical controls, constitutes research; for others, a run of 22 clinical cases observed by a competent specialist qualifies. For the purposes of this study, research includes the gamut of investigative approaches. However, I will briefly describe the methodologies of the studies under discussion so that you can decide whether they meet your criteria for reliable research.

STAGES OF DYING

The stages of dying described by Elisabeth Kübler-Ross (1969) are well known. She developed her theory about the successive psychological states of terminally ill patients from her own clinical insights supported by discussions with about 200 terminally ill and critically ill persons (Kastenbaum, 1975), but her sudden surge to international fame and her personal charisma have tended to detract from a careful analysis of the heuristic value and psychosocial validity of the stages she defined.

A careful evaluation of Kübler-Ross's *stage theory* should not hinge on these extraneous factors. Rather, it is necessary to resolve four main issues. First of all: Do the stages actually occur? Or, to refine that question: How, if at all, do they occur for which, if any, terminally ill patients? Why do they occur for these individuals? Because so many hundreds of thousands of physicians, nurses, and patients know Kübler-Ross's work, do the stages become self-fulfilling prophecies? What happens when they do not occur? To what extent are they influenced by our particular system of medical care, or by our particular approach to child development that influences attitudes toward self, sickness, dying, death, and the continuation of existence (you may prefer the word *soul* or *self*) after clinical death?

The next global issue is whether Kübler-Ross's stages are adaptive. Is *acceptance* an appropriate feeling for some, many, or all dying persons? When does (or should) acceptance occur? Is the change from acceptance to *anger* actually a regression to be avoided by improved psychosocial care? How do (or should) health professionals intervene to move a dying person through the other few stages to acceptance?

Third, what does it mean when the stages do not occur? Does this lack reflect an inadequate health care system? Or does it reflect individual or cultural and subcultural differences among patients? Closely related to these questions is the question of whether family, friends, and professionals should encourage the stages to occur, which is tied to the previous matter of whether and for whom these stages are adaptive.

A fourth problem concerns the universality of the dying process. Kastenbaum (1975) points out that Kübler-Ross's theory does not sufficiently account for the nature of various diseases, sex and age differences, ethnicity and other subcultural backgrounds, personality or cognitive styles, or the sociophysical milieu. He further states that

Clinical research concerning the dying process by other investigators does not clearly support the existence of the five stages or of any universal form of staging. A recent review of the literature, scant as it is, finds no evidence for five predictable stages of psychological adaptation. Other investigators' data "show the process of dying to be less rigid and even stageless. There is some consensus among all researchers that terminal patients are depressed shortly before they die, but there is no consistent evidence that other affect dimensions characterize the dying patient" [this quotation from Schulz and Aderman, 1974]. We must add that this negative conclusion is based upon studies conducted by various clinical investigators with equally various populations, techniques, and objectives, none of which were to make critical tests of stage theory.

Application of the stage theory of dying to medical practice places physicians in a bind, particularly given the extreme popularity of Kübler-Ross and her work, and the lack of systematic research that substantiates or contradicts that work. The problems of physicians are exacerbated by the immense following Kübler-Ross has among hospital nurses. Health professionals have the delicate task of sailing a safe course between the Scylla of being stampeded by the impact of Kübler-Ross's work and personal charisma, and the Charybdis of refuting a concept that has gained a wide following and that appears to have substantial heuristic value, at least to some medical personnel.

All four of the issues generated by Kübler-Ross's theory of stages are amenable to empirical testing. Preliminary, but still very useful, data could be obtained by physicians in private practice, who might find some way of working together to systematize and record their observations of dying patients. Evaluation of such observations would help spotlight the extent to which the five stages occur.

COMMUNICATION WITH THE DYING

There is some research on communicating with the terminally ill, including both quantitative and qualitative studies of various aspects of the problem. I will discuss three facets of this issue, using research based on (1) the statistical analysis of a survey and (2) on the rigorous analysis of nonquantitative data.

1. *Who wants to know?* In 1970, I directed an interview study of 434 persons in the greater Los Angeles area. One-fourth of the respondents were black, one-fourth were Japanese American, one-fourth Mexican American, and one-fourth Anglo; roughly equal thirds were 20 to 39 years old, 40 to 59, and 60 years and over. All interviews with Japanese-American and Mexican-American respondents were conducted by bilingual interviewers, and all participants were interviewed by individuals of their own ethnic group. We built in reasonable controls to equalize socioeconomic differences (Kalish and Reynolds, 1976).

The interviews lasted an average of 65 minutes and included the following questions. "Now I am going to ask you some questions about a few situations we have invented. First, imagine that a friend of yours is dying of cancer. He/she *(make the friend the same sex as the informant)* is about your age. His/her family has been told by a physician that he/she will die soon. Should your friend, the patient, be told?"

Of the black respondents, 60 percent said yes; 49 percent of the Japanese Americans, 37 percent of the Mexican Americans, and 71 percent of the Anglos also replied affirmatively. Some members of each ethnic group asked for additional information. Between 5 and 12 percent of each group stated that it would depend; the others responded negatively. of the men, 55 percent answered yes; 52 percent of the women did the same. Of the younger adults, 59 percent said yes, whereas 56 percent of the middle-aged and 42 percent of the older interviewees replied in the affirmative.

Of those who responded affirmatively, we then asked "Who should tell him/her?" Between 55 percent and 70 percent of each group specified the physician; from 16 percent to 30 percent named a family member; a very small number referred to the clergy. Sex and ethnic differences were minimal, but those in the middle-aged group were most likely to mention the physician, whereas those 20 to 39 years of age more often indicated a family member.

Finally, we asked, "If you were dying, would you want to be told?" More than 70 percent said yes in every category, except for Mexican Americans, among whom only 60 percent agreed. No other sex, ethnic, or age-related differences emerged.

The point in citing all these figures is to suggest that we can learn what it is that most people *say* they want; we can learn how large a minority of persons requests something else; and we can gain some understanding of how social roles influence choice.

The results of our study reveal that more people say they would want to be told they were dying than feel others like themselves should be told. And second, most people entrust the physician with this responsibility.

Applying these results is, of course, not simple. We might decide, for example, that physicians should be provided with more support and more encouragement in providing the terminally ill with an explicit understanding of the meaning of their medical condition. Or we might decide that physicians (at least those who feel uncomfortable with this role) should be encouraged to engage other health professionals for the task, while simultaneously providing a public education program that legitimizes the fulfillment of this responsibility by these other experts. Or perhaps we would encourage patients to ask physicians more directly about the life-threatening nature of their health conditions. And there are other possibilities.

In the second study I wish to discuss, Dr. Barney Glaser and Dr. Anselm Strauss (1965) applied *grounded theory* (a rigorous nonquantitative social research methodology) to an analysis of how dying persons are affected by the extent of their awareness of their own terminal condition. Glaser and Strauss described the various types of awareness as *closed awareness* (the patient does not recognize that he or she is terminal), *suspicion awareness* (the patient suspects terminality and attempts to learn more, while the staff parries these attempts and tries to keep the context closed), *mutual pretense* (both patient and staff know of the prognosis and can communicate openly in terms of the prognosis), and *open awareness* (all involved know and can, when they wish, discuss their awareness with each other). These researchers made a similar analysis of family members. Although Glaser and Strauss tend to avoid passing judgment, there is little doubt that they interpret their evidence as supportive of the development of an open awareness in most circumstances. Their findings based on a qualitative approach confirm the results of my quantitative approach: people say they want to know and seem to fare better when they do know.

2. *The where and when of dying.* There are other considerations on which we have a modest body of research evidence. For example, investigators have asked people where they wished to die, and the answer was fairly clear: at home. Whether the respondents were men or women, young or middle-aged or old, black or Mexican American or Japanese American or white, more respondents stated they wished to die at home than stated they wished to die anywhere else (Kalish and Reynolds, 1976).

The next logical question is, Where *do* people die? The answer is even clearer, because we can look at the records instead of having to ask people. Today, people in our society die in hospitals. Studies in both the United States and England have established that most people die in general hospitals (Cartwright, Hockey, and Anderson, 1973; Lerner, 1970).

If most people say they want to die at home and end up dying in hospitals, what is going on? The answer is obvious to the point of absurdity: people are not dying where they wish to die. Some die from a condition that requires hospital attention, or so quickly that the very notion of dying at home was not even a vague possibility. Others die in hospitals because they have no one to take care of them at home, finances will not permit home care, space at home is insufficient, or they have been institutionalized for a period of time and home no longer exists outside of institutional walls. But a third group (we can only guess at its size) does not die at home because health professionals do not offer that possibility as a reasonable option to family members, and community agencies do not offer the kinds of supplemental help that would make home care possible.

The fact that relatively few people ask to die at home is not truly relevant because so many terminally ill people are under the impression that dying at home is not a real option for them. (There is another researchable notion slipped into that sentence. What proportion of dying people are in fact under the impression that dying at home is not a real option and what proportion of these people would prefer to die at home if there were some form of supportive services?)

A fairly recent development in health care has attempted to respond to some of these concerns. The hospice movement, initiated in England, is now expanding in the United States and Canada, as well as in continental Europe. The outpatient care of hospice programs is permitting more and more people to die at home.

Research on this issue, however, has done more than point out that most people wish to die at home. It has also pointed out that many people do not want to die at home. More middle-aged people want to die in hospitals than either young or old people; more women want to die in hospitals than men, although differences between the sexes are slight (Kalish and Reynolds, 1976). Perhaps women are more likely to ask to die in hospitals because they are less likely to have spouses available to care for them; perhaps people between the ages of 40 and 60 wish to die in hospitals because they have greater faith in modern medicine or because they wish to avoid inconveniencing those who would care for them. There are many other possible reasons for these differences in attitude. The research has not yet clarified the basis for the discrepancies, but subsequent research could easily do so.

Health care practitioners inevitably play an active role in determining where patients die. They take an equally active part in determining when death occurs, although this question is much more fraught with moral, psychological, and professional ethical considerations. The recent "death with dignity" legislation now in effect in California has taken this issue out of the realm of theory and made it a practical matter for every medical decision maker, which includes almost every practicing physician.

In our study of 434 persons in the greater Los Angeles area (referred to above) we included the following question, "Do you feel people should be allowed to die if they want to?" Just a shade under half of the respondents said yes; most of those who answered in the affirmative used a person who was dying anyway or who was in very great pain as a point of reference. About 6 percent of the entire group of 434 carefully selected persons stated that "wanting to" was sufficient reason to be permitted to die (Kalish and Reynolds, 1976).

That these respondents were almost evenly split on whether people should be allowed to die when they wished (the interviews were conducted 6 years before the 1976 death with dignity bill was brought up in the legislature) indicates that this is a very delicate matter. The research merely underscores the ambivalence felt within one community, an ambivalence that is most definitely mirrored in many other communities.

3. *Psychotherapy with the dying.* The criteria for evaluating the effectiveness of psychotherapy in general are still being debated, so that it would be remarkable if a good study of counseling or psychotherapy with the terminally ill were available. None is. However, two sets of reports from psychotherapists who worked with dying persons and systematically observed the effects of their programs have been published. Nearly 2 decades ago, LeShan was a psychotherapist with terminally ill, nonelderly cancer patients in a New York City hospital. He recorded his experiences in dramatic fashion. Not unexpectedly, he evaluated the program as successful, but included the advice that no psychotherapist should ever spend more than 25 percent of his or her time with the terminally ill (LeShan, 1969; LeShan and Gassman, 1958; LeShan, personal communication, 1968). Le Shan focused his efforts on mobilizing the dying person's will to live, because he found that concentrating on the fear of death was a treatment that did not ensure successful therapy. Thus, rather than preparing his patients for death, he emphasized their inner strength and the power of their own resources in order to encourage and enable them to live their lives as fully as possible in their remaining months.

The second group of papers describes the use of LSD with terminally ill patients. Pahnke, Grof, and their associates have discussed individuals displaying dramatic improvement in affect and zest for life as a result of closely monitored LSD sessions (Pahnke, 1969; Pahnke and Richards, 1966; Richards, Grof, Goodman, and Kurland, 1972). The financial costs (in professional time) of these treatments was considerable, and the apparent peace and calm that I and others have observed in patients undergoing more traditional medical therapy at St. Christopher's Hospice in London suggest that more traditional care also produces substantial results. These observations indicate that further research is necessary to assess whether the effectiveness of the LSD treatment resulted in large part from the intensive interpersonal caring relationship that accompanied the experience or from the LSD experience itself. Although difficult to undertake, an investigation of this issue would be extremely valuable.

Because all available research on counseling and psychotherapy with the dying is still restricted to the description, all we are able to say is that dying people benefit (just like everyone else) from caring relationships. There is nothing really new about that. However, dying people are often in a situation where caring relationships are not forthcoming; the research evidence underlines the importance of showing concern and affection for terminally ill patients, reminding us that the fact that they are dying should not preclude them from receiving the close attention and care accorded healthier patients who are more likely to recover.

THOSE WHO SURVIVE

It would not be appropriate to discuss these matters without at least a brief word about the care of the survivors, who are known to be highly prone to morbidity, illness, and death. These persons are often ignored by physicians and other health care professionals, until they appear with symptoms; and we know that if the prerequisite of the personal attention of a physician is having symptoms, then people will have symptoms.

The research evidence reveals that nonelderly, recently bereaved widows suffer a rise in medical complaints (see Parkes, 1972), which may reflect the stresses and strains of providing extensive patient care (e.g., lack of sleep, erratic eating habits, limited opportunity for social relationships), that is, the limitation on or lack of normal living. Symptoms of bereavement can also reflect the physiologically based changes that Erich Lindemann (1944) described in his classical article on grief, changes that cause choking, shortness of breath, lack of muscular power, and so forth. Or there may be more subtle forces at work (subtle only because we do not yet understand them). I would speculate, for example, that the relationship between stress and the onset of breast cancer may, if adequately investigated, turn out to be both statistically and medically significant. If so, it would mean that a biochemical response to psychosocial stress can precipitate the illness.

In studying survivors, I would look with particular interest at one group: those with primary responsibility for both the physical care of the dying person and the decisions related to that care. The daughter who cares for her dying mother has experienced quite a different set of stresses, relationships, feelings (e.g., guilt and absolution of guilt), and roles (e.g., gatekeeper of information and communication) than the daughter who visited regularly or the daughter who visited irregularly. Mourner type one is not mourner type two is not mourner type three, any more than dying person type one is dying person type two is dying person type three.

CONCLUSION

In conclusion, I would like to point out that we certainly need good rigorous and creative (those terms need not be contradictory) research on death, dying, and bereavement. Many of you are in a position to add significantly to our knowledge of these concerns. Although the literature is filled with advice on how to die and how to work with the dying, there is an absence of solidly based analyses of good qualitative and quantitative clinical data. Many of you have insights, based on 30 consecutive cases of emergency room deaths, based on attempts to change hospital policy, based on innovative courses in medical school, based on inservice training of paraprofessionals, based on epidemiological data collected while you were in Pakistan.

Those of us who are not health clinicians need your insights more than we need another exhortation to love and honor. You are in an excellent position to develop the ideas on which we can develop our research projects. We hope you will read some of our research, theory, and speculation, as we try to read some of your clinical and policy papers. Sometimes we who focus on research develop a mythological devotion to the truth inherent in our data, and we need clinicians to disrupt our stereotypes in the same way that we often try to disrupt theirs.

BIBLIOGRAPHY

Cartwright, A., L. Hockey, and J.L. Anderson: *Life Before Death*, Routledge & Kegan Paul, London, 1973.

Glaser, B.G. and A.L. Strauss: *Awareness of Dying*, Aldine, Chicago, 1965.

Kalish, R.A. and D.K. Reynolds: *Death and Ethnicity: A Psychocultural Study*, University of Southern California Press, Los Angeles, 1976.

Kastenbaum, R.: "Is Death a Life Crisis? On the Confrontation with Death in Theory and Practice," in N. Datan and L.H. Ginsberg (eds.), *Life-Span Developmental Psychology: Normative Life Crises*, Academic Press, New York, 1975, pp. 19–50.

Kübler-Ross, E.: *On Death and Dying*, Macmillan, New York, 1969.

Lerner, M.: "When, Why, and Where People Die," in O.G. Brim, Jr., H.E. Freeman, S. Levine, and N.A. Scotch (eds.), *The Dying Patient*, Russell Sage, New York, 1970, pp. 5–29.

LeShan, L.: Personal communication with the author, 1968.

———: "Mobilizing the Life Forces," *Annals of the New York Academy of Sciences*, **164**:847–861, 1969.

——— and M. Gassman: "Some Observations on Psychotherapy with Patients Suffering from Neoplastic Disease," *American Journal of Psychotherapy*, **12**:723–734, 1958.

Lindemann, E.: "Symptomatology and Management of Acute Grief," *American Journal of Psychiatry*, **101**:141–148, 1944.

Pahnke, W.N.: "The Psychedelic Mystical Experience in the Human Encounter," *Harvard Theological Review*, **62**:1–32, 1969.

——— and W.A. Richards: "Implications of LSD and Experimental Mysticism," *Journal of Religion and Health*, **5**:175–208, 1966.

Parkes, C.M.: *Bereavement: Studies of Grief in Adult Life*, International Universities Press, New York, 1972.

Richards, W., S. Grof, L. Goodman, and A. Kurland: "LSD-assisted Psychotherapy and the Human Encounter with Death," *Journal of Transpersonal Psychology*, **4**:121–150, 1972.

Saunders, C.: "The Moment of Truth: Care of the Dying Person," in L. Pearson (ed.), *Death and Dying*, Press of Case Western Reserve, Cleveland, 1969, pp. 49–78.

Schulz, R. and D. Aderman: "Clinical Research and the 'Stages of Dying,' " *Omega*, **5**:137–144, 1974.

Chapter 23

In Control

Robert Kastenbaum

It is what the patient wants. And the physician . . . the nurses, the relatives. It is what janitors want as they mop the floor and hospital administrators as they pick up the telephone. Should psychiatrists or social scientists appear on the scene, then we just have a wider assortment of people seeking the same goal if by different means.

Everyone affected by the dying situation wants to stay in control. This is not the only desire of people in this situation, but it is a need that must be attended to if other goals are to be met. If one's sense of control is not seriously threatened, then the feeling of being out of control does not become an issue, and the individual is free to use all of his or her resources to attend to other needs, such as providing care and comfort to those involved. But if those affected by a dying situation do not have a firm sense of control (and dying *is* a situation; it is not just an internal process that takes place within the stricken individual), then they lack a secure home base for their interactions with others.

Let us now explore what it means to be in control in situations where death threatens. I will focus on medical and, in particular, hospital situations, although some of the dynamics analyzed can be found in other life-threatening situations as well.

HOW WE TRY TO STAY IN CONTROL

Here are a few illustrations of some of the many specific ways by which people try to stay in control in the dying situation. The examples cited are from the perspective of the patient, the physician, the nurse, and the patient's relative. A more detailed survey might also include examples from the perspective of the hospital janitor, the clergy, the hospital administrator, the psychiatrist, the social worker, and the social scientist, but such a survey is beyond the scope of this chapter.

The Terminally Ill Patient

Mrs. L. has been fighting a losing battle with cancer for almost 2 years. She is now hospitalized for what might be the last time. Although she seems to be clearly on a downhill trajectory, Mrs. L. is not seen as "acutely dying" by hospital personnel.

There are a number of small ways in which she is making herself unpopular. Mrs. L. is fussy about her food, and complains about the way it is prepared and served. She also pesters nursing personnel with requests throughout the day, including questions about time (What time is it? Shouldn't the doctor be here already? etc.). Staff members work fast when they are with her to minimize the possibility of their being drawn into conversations about her personal life. Mrs. L. has a way of turning a straightforward comment (or no comment at all) into an autobiographical monologue.

This seemingly ordinary behavior represents a desperate attempt on the part of Mrs. L. to reinstate her sense of control. Mrs. L. has already lost much. Her physical attractiveness has been ravaged by months of draining illness and by the side effects of treatment. What made her a valuable person in her own mind was chiefly her role in the family constellation, that is, her role of wife, mother, and grandmother, of dedicated and successful homemaker, and of active, open-hearted neighbor. Much of life as she has known it now seems remote or gone forever. She has little day-by-day control over the life of her family; even her body seems to belong more to the doctors and to the nurses than to herself. She cannot control where she is, or even who walks into her room when. What is there left for her to control?

If they would serve her tea as she likes it when she really wants it, this would bring a few minutes of the day into alignment with the rest of her life. *If* the medical and nursing staff knew *who* she was and appreciated her as a person, then she could more readily think of herself as something more than a diseased and failing body. *If* she at least could predict or count on visits from physicians and other important people, then she would feel like she had a bit of mental control over the situation. Like many patients, she has already all but given up the effort to share control of her own life with the physician. But she has not given up little strategies for trying to have somebody do something her way!

The Physician

Three physicians are touring the ward together. They pause at the doorway of one room and continue a vociferous discussion among themselves. When they do enter the room, they spend less than 5 minutes within the patient's radius. During this time the physicians continue to direct their eye contact and their comments to each other. There are no introductions, explanations, or other amenities offered to the patient— and no opportunity for the terminally ill person to express questions or other needs.

Occasionally a lone physician ventures into the room, but usually comes and goes without establishing personal contact with the patient. The physician seems preoccupied with more important matters and has no time to waste.

Behavior patterns of this kind also represent a need to stay in control. That need is more readily perceived by patients and relatives than many physicians realize. It is obvious that physicians locked into such patterns of noninteraction are avoiding significant contact with the terminally ill, even if the physicians do not recognize this themselves. The physician is seldom around when his patient finds it necessary to apologize for his doctor's behavior. "Oh, Doctor T. is all right. He's a good man. But I guess some days he just can't face any more losers like me."

The physician's need to maintain control in a situation by minimizing personal contact with other people is often seen as a weakness by patients, relatives, and other health care staff. In most instances people really do want the physician to exercise a strong measure of control in the situation. Therefore, they will try to find excuses for the physician's inability to behave the way mature and humane people do with each other.

The physician not only has much less to lose in the situation than the person whose entire life is in jeopardy, but also has many more ways of exercising control. The physician can—and does—come and go of his own volition. He has that personal control over his own life that the patient has been forced to yield to the disease and the treatment process. Furthermore, he has a high measure of control over the behavior of others in the situation, including staff, relatives, and patient. He can, in addition, call in consultants, or supportive diagnostic and treatment services, and he can make arrangements for coverage when he will not be available. The patient cannot find anybody else to take over his dying for him for a few days, and is often in the lower ranks of the hospital's power hierarchy.

Sometimes, as in the previous example, a patient's diagnosis of a physician's behavior may be right on the button. Dr. T. has, in fact, had an exceptionally tough day and does not feel up to any more encounters with terminal illness for a while. It would be a truly wise Dr. T. who was able to recognize that his own up-against-the-wall feeling and his fear of losing control is but a pale shadow of the feelings his patient may be experiencing day after day.

The Nurse

Nursing personnel are being asked to report and reflect on some of their experiences with terminally ill patients. The most recent experience for one LPN was "a little Greek man. He was cute. He was just a terrific little guy. He had a great big smile on his face and then he died. Cute as a button. Always wobbly. He was just a doll."

An RN, speaking of another patient, reflects that "I never felt sorry that he died. He was well up there in age and I imagine he did suffer to a certain extent. But I knew he was prepared. Everything was done for him. The priest had seen him. I really never felt real bad about it."

Speaking of the prospect of their own deaths, one nurse stated that, "If I'm going to die, then that's the way I want to go, sitting in a chair and just pass away. I think it's the only way to go if you're going to go." Another gave a response that seems to be rather typical of Americans in general: "I don't want to be a burden. I'd rather be dead than have to depend on somebody else for everything."

What are the staying-in-control strategies here? The "little Greek man" was described with affection. This is not the physician's defense of brusque, impersonal behavior. Nursing personnel, especially those who work with chronically ill, hospitalized patients, spend appreciably more time at the patient's bedside than most physicians do. Nurses and patients are part of the same scene long enough to develop personal feelings for each other. By allowing herself to care for "the little Greek man," the LPN gave up the possibility of staying in control of the situation by acting in an aloof, so-called professional manner. But her caring exposed her to the pain of grief when he died. In this instance, protection is devised by reducing and simplifying the patient. "Cute" is an expression that minimizes depth, complexity, maturity, sorrow. In fact, the patient is "just a *doll*," not a person as real as you or I. The LPN perhaps could have maintained a warm, affectionate relationship with the patient that brightened his last months. But to stay in control of the situation, it is doubtful that she could have let herself see him straight-out as a human being who was soon to lose his life.

Focusing upon the terminally ill patient's advanced years is another common way of staying in control of one's own feelings. The death is then seen as less important than that of a young person. This, of course, is strictly the outsider's view. The old person's life, being the only one he has, may still be very important to *him*; and it may be very important to others as well. But if it is possible to minimize the scope and quality of the person's life for any reason, then it is possible to find comfort in the belief that not much has been lost through death.

The RN who "never felt sorry that he died" reveals much about herself by her short statement. She does not want to be emotionally devastated by the patient's death. On the other hand, she does not want to be seen by herself or by others as a cold person. The case she reports is one that neither disturbed her nor made her feel guilty because her response was so minimal. In this situation, it appears that others helped the nurse keep her own control by maintaining control themselves. The patient was prepared; that is, he had himself under control. The priest had provided the ritual and support of his religion. Medical and nursing care had been attentive. With so many people taking responsibility for their particular areas of concern, the nurse could concentrate on her own role and her own feelings. Her ability to stay in control was not placed under heavy stress.

The two nurses who were quoted about their own deaths were firm in their preference for dying quickly ("*If* I'm going to die . . . "). This is a general attitude in our society, and is by no means limited to nursing personnel. The prospect of losing control, of having to be dependent on somebody else, seems to frighten many people more than the prospect of death itself. And, if that is how a staff member feels about his or her own life, it is easy to assume that patients must feel the same way. Because communication between staff and terminally ill patients often leaves much to be desired, this assumption may not be readily checked against reality. A patient's death is accepted by staff with more equanimity when it is assumed that he or she would rather be dead than live in a burdensome and dependent manner. By interpreting death as a more desirable outcome than dependent survival, staff can more easily maintain a sense of control. Death, in other words, has not challenged the staff's competence or undermined its values; matters have worked out just as they should have.

The Next of Kin

Relatives may be either very prominent or hardly involved in the dying situation. Let us consider just one type of configuration, a type that seems to be fairly common today. The terminally ill person is an elderly man. The true next of kin is his wife. She is elderly and semi-incapacitated herself, and the staff finds itself having more contact with a middle-aged daughter. She acts as the spokesperson for the entire family. But in the last few days of the old man's life there is a flurry of contact from other children, some of whom live far away, and from a brother whom the dying man has not seen in years. Each of these relatives has a separate interest and area of concern. They all seem to have different expectations about what should be happening and who should be making what decisions. The staff, preoccupied with its specific responsibilities to this and other patients, cannot provide a united front to hear, evaluate, and respond to these various concerns and pressures.

There is a tendency to channel information through the family member the staff has become best acquainted with over a period of time, as well as to be receptive to that person's requests. But she appears to be asking for a great deal of control over the situation. She wants to know all the medical information first (even before the dying man himself). In fact, she insists that nobody on the staff tell him how serious his condition is, and that anybody in the family who is untrustworthy in this regard should not be allowed to visit with him. She is strong and persistent in her views—which also include what should and should not be done in efforts to prolong his survival.

In this type of situation it is difficult for the staff to respond in a balanced and flexible manner. The physician or nurse may have come to know this next of kin well enough to appreciate the strain her father's illness and approaching death have put her under. They see that she has intensified her need to seem in control of as many details as possible in order to protect against her feeling of impending inner collapse. With the investment of some time, sensitivity, and intrastaff communication, ways are found to support her general sense of control without reducing the treatment and management options the staff believes must remain within its domain. The staff is willing to help her keep her own anxieties within reasonable bounds and to consider her suggestions and requests. But the staff is not willing to take her side in an intrafamily power struggle, nor to permit her to control everybody else's behavior in the situation.

But staff reaction is not always this judicious. Irked by the next of kin's demands, medical and nursing personnel may make themselves unavailable to her or give her no satisfaction in what dealings they do have with her. This is likely to intensify her need for control and lead to increased hounding of the staff or other unwelcome control-seeking strategies on her part. In the other extreme, the staff might accept most of her requests as though they represented the entire family—and the patient as well.

In so doing, the others are virtually shut out. Either alternative is apt to be rigid and arbitrary. Staff and next of kin, locked in a struggle for control, are likely to find ways in which to harass and punish each other. The patient himself may almost be lost in the process.

I have seen patients become increasingly isolated by such power disputes and uncertainties. One woman, for example, entered a hospital with a terminal prognosis that apparently had not been communicated to her. Her community physician, acting upon the expressed wishes of the family member best known to him, asked that the prognosis not be revealed to this patient. But the physician responsible for her inhospital care believed that she ought to be told the truth and have an opportunity to prepare herself for death, and was supported in this view by two other members of the family. For almost a week, this woman existed within the hospital as a nonperson. Nursing personnel felt so uncomfortable about being near her ("What if she asks?") that, inadvertently, they tended to stay clear of her bed. Contacts were perfunctory and only occurred when the bare minimum of service had to be provided. This was not the usual practice in this hospital, so the departure from customary standards created additional tension among the members of the staff. Furthermore, the patients in the beds nearest this woman also suffered from the same isolating treatment that she was receiving. Whoever approached this area of the ward felt concern that his or her ability to stay in control of the situation would be severely challenged.

Yet this situation proved fairly easy to resolve, once the staff clearly recognized what was happening. One staff member was entrusted by the others with the responsibility for developing rapport with the new patient. As the rapport developed, the staff member said as much or as little as was advisable to help the patient adapt to her situation; the rest of the staff was supportive. Just the decision to adopt this plan of action led to a relief of tensions and the provision of normal services to the patient. And, as it turned out, the patient already had a strong partial recognition of her prognosis. Over a period of several weeks *she* told the staff member what was happening to her, and expressed a few personal wishes that were respected by the staff. The direct issue of what to tell her never came up. Essentially, the patient had been given the opportunity to control as much of her life as she cared to, within the limits of her illness, and the staff was then free to exercise its own good judgment in looking after the rest of her needs.

CONSTRUCTIVE CONTROL: A FEW SUGGESTIONS

Staff members as well as patients are often among the sufferers in the terminal illness situation. The most sensitive staff members are often the most likely to become emotionally depleted, that is, to experience a kind of emotional exhaustion, a state of being drained that itself increases the likelihood of further stress. The drained staff member is more apt to make errors on and off the job, to be prone to accidents, to fall prey to illness, and to encounter problems in personal relationships because normal emotional resources have been reduced to such a low point. Reactions to grief and loss also take a toll. Although "professionalism" protects against grief, a particular patient's death at a particular time in a staff member's life may penetrate the defenses and cause the type of emotional pain we usually associate with death in our personal lives. Additionally, there is self-imposed suffering when a staff member suspects that the situation has not been managed properly. Physicians and nurses second-guess themselves or each other. The outcome can disturb staff morale by causing a particular physician or nurse to be scapegoated, which jeopardizes the communication network through the arousal of anxiety, guilt, and anger, and thus makes everybody suddenly appear more touchy, formal, and intolerant of each other.

The staff's anguish often remains "illegitimate." They are not supposed to be suffering. They do not have the "right" to suffer in the same way as terminally ill patients and their families do. Because little of their training and experience prepares professionals for the distress they feel in caring for the terminally ill, this phenomenon of staff suffering is not openly expressed or acknowledged, which makes it even more difficult to bear. When the staff seeks to stay in control, then, it is not only a matter of controlling what is outside, i.e., the patient's situation, but also what is inside, i.e., the staff member's emotions.

Professionals sometimes fiercely resist acknowledging the distress that they themselves feel in the terminal care situation, and act as though this distress represents an unforgiveable weakness of character. Such resistance may also stem from a reluctance to recognize how many of our thoughts and actions are designed to retain control. We all know physicians who are so well practiced in control-seeking maneuvers that these maneuvers themselves appear to be out of control; for example, the physician who simply does not hear what is being said to him because he has already instituted a familiar, almost automatic set of responses intended to narrow and neutralize the situation. Control mechanisms that are not responsive to a particular situation, that do not even wait for the situation to develop in its own way before snapping into place, themselves become part of the problem.

The first steps toward developing more effective control for all concerned in the terminal care situation are difficult to take. Most people are not apt to realize that they too share in the "white knuckles" syndrome, and that some of their strategies for staying in control may be contributing to the tension. Nevertheless, let us explore a few of the simpler ways through which the valid objectives of staying in control can be achieved without introducing new stress and distortions.

A Legitimate Aim

Perhaps the first step is simply to recognize that the need to stay in control is proper, normal, and legitimate. Although this is an obvious proposition it is worth stating explicitly. The physician, the patient, and others in the terminal care situation sometimes behave in ways that threaten to "steal" control from each other. It is easy to fall into the pattern of *attacking* a person's need for control or to behave as though it is "either him or me," when the larger reality is that everybody has a legitimate need for staying in control, and nobody will be successful all the way (death being death). It is more useful to discover ways by which each person can maintain a reasonable and appropriate sense of control that does not undercut anybody else's attempt to meet his or her own need for control. Even if a physician, nurse, patient, or relative is behaving in what seems to be a wildly inappropriate way, his or her legitimate need for a

sense of control deserves respect. It is a question of matching the individual's need to
the appropriate attitudes and actions.

Control by Options and Choices

What happens when control does fail? What precisely do we guard against when we
seek to maintain control? The answer probably has something to do with a sense of
helplessness. Some psychoanalysts and existential thinkers would describe it more
dramatically as *catastrophic anxiety*, but helplessness will do. I remember a great hulk
of a man who was lying in bed with tears in his eyes and his fists clenched. He had
been silent for at least 3 days. "You feel so damned helpless you could cry," I ventured. "Damned right!" he replied, and that was the beginning of a supportive relationship between the two of us. Any individual in the situation—physician included—
may at a particular time have only one or two maneuvers or defenses existing between
him- or herself and a state of infuriating, unacceptable helplessness. Let us remind ourselves of a few of the simple, unexotic, inexpensive strategies that can be used to provide more alternatives to the state of perceived helplessness.

A policy of *behavioral options* can be instituted early in the course of treatment.
The sooner this policy is established, the more likely it is to remain effective when the
illness has reached an advanced state. The physician is usually the central figure here,
although the nurse, the relative, and others may be important as well. The physician
makes it clear that certain components in the treatment regimen must be followed just
so. But there remain a number of choices for the patient to make. At first these can be
spelled out in general terms with a few specific illustrations. Later, as the patient continues to succumb to the illness and experiences decreasing control over his or her life,
the remaining choices are highlighted more clearly. If this general approach is well
developed, then even when the patient is limited to the restricted environment of the
hospital bed, there will still be both some sense and reality of choice remaining.

The particular behavioral options are apt to vary from person to person, depending
upon the individual's lifestyle and the specific circumstances of his or her illness. At
early points in the terminal trajectory the individual may retain options about such
broad classes of behavior as working and traveling. For example, there may be several
months during which the patient could continue to work full time, but he or she might
want to consider the option of gradually reducing, without giving up, work in order to
take a long-delayed trip, or to attend to other personal or business interests. Later the
options remain important even though their scope may be sharply reduced. Diet and
medication are two typical examples. Must the patient really be on a standard and
stereotypical diet? For certain illnesses the answer is yes. But this is often not so. It
is habit and convenience that take dietary choice away from the patient—as well as the
need of others to exercise their own control and thereby quell their own inner anxieties. Food has a personal meaning for each individual. In a way, how the question of
a patient's food is resolved is a test of the institution's and staff's intention to love,
support, and care for the patient in his or her time of need. The removal of choice in
this area can cause the patient to surrender any desire to participate in his or her own
care. An important survival link—eating—has become more a part of the system than of
the person's own relationship with the world. The patient's continued interest in food,

in bodily replenishment, and in breaking the day's monotonous routine by means of an attractive meal can contribute to the preservation of what is commonly called the *will to live*. This phenomenon is difficult to define operationally, but seems to have a solid basis in reality. The complexities of researching "will to live" do not for a moment suggest that the phenomenon be neglected in clinical practice. Such small behavioral options as allowing patients with guarded prognoses the luxury of a mug of beer or a glass of sherry (in appropriate stemware) can seemingly rekindle some patients' interest in life and survival.

Medication also involves a delicate balance between outer and inner control. The purpose of medication is often to enable the patient to experience more freedom from disturbing and disabling bodily states: in other words, a preservation or restoration of control. Yet the medication is prescribed and administered by health personnel who have knowledge, skill, and control on their side. The staff's willingness to appropriately share medication control with the patient can do much to keep the terminally ill individual feeling like a participant rather than simply a recipient (at the extreme, a victim) of treatment. Whenever it is realistic for the patient to determine timing or dosage, or to decide between two medications that differ, for example, in side effects, it is often advisable to make such options available to the patient. The rules for sharing medication control with the patient can shift as the stage of illness changes, but *some* kind of patient option may remain possible throughout the illness. Sometimes the choices are of major personal significance; there are some people who prefer to bear pain instead of suffering any diminution of awareness, and others who are demoralized by one kind of side effect but who can tolerate other side effects well. Yet, apart from the specific differences between behavioral options concerning medication, the most important aspect is often simply the sense of participation the patient gets in the process, the feeling that he or she is retaining partial control in a situation that is threatening to get out of the patient's control completely.

Consider briefly two other areas of behavioral options. How much and what kind of activity should be permitted for the terminal inpatient? We may now be speaking of a very limited range of behavior: going to the bathroom as contrasted with the bedpan; staying in bed as opposed to walking about a little; getting one's self dressed in street clothes occasionally versus staying in the hospital gown, etc. Physicians sometimes issue orders that would control even such small behaviors as these, in other words that would *remove* both the self-control of the patient and the behavioral option of the nursing staff. When there is no absolutely compelling medical reason to specify every detail of the patient's activity, it is better to leave such decisions up to the nurse in her capacity as the patient's mediator. Good communication between medical and nursing staff will insure that the nurse's decisions reflect the physician's overall treatment objectives. But the nurse, who spends more time with the patient and who knows more about his or her energy and needs at any given moment, is frequently in a better position to decide what options should be passed on to the patient, which not only maintains a little more flexibility and room for personal preference in the terminal care situation, but also strengthens the nurse's sense of control. With appropriate and legitimate powers vested in her by the physician, the nurse will not have to "usurp" control, nor be trapped between the patient's requests and the somewhat remote orders of the physician. There is an additional advantage here. A person who functions in the nurse's position has many opportunities to become sullen and passive. This does not necessarily have anything to do with what the person is like as an individual; rather it reflects on a role in which there is often not enough legitimate power available. One of the most destructive elements in some terminal care situations centers on nursing personnel who are deprived of most options for influence and control, and who, as a result, acquire a brusque and aloof professionalism that is far removed from their personal qualities of sensitivity and caring. The physician who is secure enough to relinquish some of his or her own unnecessary control and place it in the capable hands of the nurse may thereby infuse the entire situation with more naturalness and warmth. The physician usually has enough other decisions and control maneuvers to make that are directly within his realm of competence; he can well afford to trust nurse, patient, and perhaps relatives in such areas as deciding options for daily activity.

Visiting is another area of behavioral options that is considered significant by both patient and family. The drive to help the patient retain some semblance of self-control often runs into special difficulties here. Hospital rules are notoriously inflexible. The terminally ill person and those close to him or her find themselves caught between two extremes: trying to manage total care in a home environment or almost completely surrendering personal contact by accepting admission to the hospital. The hospice model for terminal care and some of the palliative care ward variants provide alternatives to rigid and restrictive visiting regulations and, indeed, some cultures have never fully embraced the Western system of virtually excluding family support inside hospital walls. But many of the terminally ill today find themselves in traditional health care settings that bend little to the interpersonal support needs of patient and relatives.

Recent studies document what good observers (including a number of physicians) have known for years: that the continuation of interpersonal support by family and friends can make a critical difference in the patient's adaptation to illness and length of survival. Yet physician, patient, nurse, and relative may all run up against the stone wall of administrative rules and regulations even when the administration agrees that current visiting policies should be liberalized and adjusted to suit the individual case. Here is a very specific are in which determined physicians can improve the well-being of their terminally ill patients and at the same time reduce some of the pangs of grief for survivors-to-be. The hospital really does not need to exercise so much control over who may visit a patient when. The consequences of institutional overcontrol are much more severe for the patient and his or her family than the mostly fantasied consequences of sharing control with those involved in the dying process are for the institution. Where, however, are the physicians who will stand up against such counterproductive visitation restrictions?

These are just a few types of behavioral options that could more often be made available to people directly involved in the dying experience and in terminal patient care. Many other examples will occur to the physician who reflects upon his or her own experiences.

Education and Information

People generally feel less helpless (more in control) when they can *do* something in a difficult situation. But sometimes there is really very little that can be done. At such times the danger of collapsing into a state of profound apathy or helplessness can still be reduced by enhancing the individual's sense of mental control. We are all familiar with certain extreme mental devices that people may sometimes use in order to stay in control, for example, psychotic flights from reality, sudden lapses into senility, fanatic espousal of doctrines that appear quite removed from the rational order of things. We have also seen those desperate, although less extreme, situations where an individual clings to any treatment, doctrine, or "miracle" cure, no matter how ridiculous or unproven, that holds out even the slightest hope of recovery.

But why should people be forced to extremes in seeking mental control over suffering and terminal illness? Health personnel often fail to provide reasonable alternatives. The physician and the nurse control their own feelings of impending disorganization or helplessness by calling on their knowledge and expertise. This is certainly one of the more constructive and realistic strategies available. It can be made more available to patients and their families as well. Patient education (and family education) about the nature of the illness and its treatment can be helpful in at least two ways. While there are still things to be done, the informed and involved patient-relative team can help to maximize the effect of the treatment effort. The patient is easier to care for because he knows what to expect. He feels more like a participant in the treatment process because, in fact, he is performing some of the actions himself. But even when the range of doable things is decreased, knowledge and informed expectation can help reduce fear of the unknown and head off needless or exaggerated concern over relatively minor symptoms or treatment. A tendency on the part of the patient to blame himself for lack of competent functioning, or to blame others for inferior or inadequate care can be alleviated by providing the patient with accurate information. Do physicians realize how many patients torment themselves with the thought they are somehow failures or morally weak when, in fact, they are simply experiencing problems typical of their stage of illness and treatment? By cuing a patient into the details of his condition over time, health care professionals can often spare the patient the extra burden of suffering and anxiety—the burden that is in addition to the burden of the illness itself. Naturally, communication of appropriate information in a useful way requires a good relationship between health personnel and patient. Hitting the patient or relative with the hard facts of a case all at once is not the answer. What is required instead is an ongoing process by which the physician helps the patient and relative remain knowledgeable.

Keeping the communication network open (and checking frequently for possible misunderstandings) will help minimize the occurrence of those heart-stopping moments of sudden, disasterous news that so many patients and relatives dread. The crisis of to tell or not to tell will not happen nearly as often. The resourceful physician will recognize all the talent available to him on his treatment team. Some types of information may best be communicated to the patient by nurses, technicians, consultants, or other patients who have mastered these situations themselves.

The patient who is forced or encouraged to dwell in ignorance about the course of his illness is more apt to sink into apathy or helplessness, or to take flight in extreme mental-control maneuvers. Any of these responses distress relatives and staff. It is also true that knowledge can be painful as well. What is needed, then, are education programs sensitive to the needs of patients and their families and a way of sharing professional knowledge with those personally involved in the dying situation so that the terminally ill might develop the maximum sense of mental control possible within the limits of their own capabilities and of existing medical knowledge.

LETTING GO

We can control only up to a point. Sooner or later we must let go. Many of us undergo this necessary and sometimes painful process at various times in our lives, for example, the parent who must let go of his or her child. Because our culture emphasizes control, we receive much more practice and encouragement in building up systems of power and influence than we do in perfecting the art of letting go. This general bias against letting go is worth keeping in mind. Otherwise we might too readily conclude that the terminal care situation is unique in this respect. It is closer to the truth to regard letting go when one is on the brink of death as but one critical arena that challenges our absolute and compulsive need to stay in control. Many previous cultures—and some current ones as well—have devised lifestyles that depend less on the illusion of control, or, at least, on the illusion of personally oriented control.

To put it differently, many of us are bad losers, and death in our contemporary society is often interpreted as total loss. There is a distinctly practical side to this proposition. The psychology of learning and conditioning tells us that in times of stress we are most likely to fall back upon our most overlearned responses. We have been practicing to stay in control all of our lives (at least, this may be said of people with the competitive educational and occupational successes of the physician). The stress of the dying situation potentially arouses in everyone involved a massive response to control, control, and control again. If one cannot control by changing the outcome, perhaps one can control by controlling the behavior of others, by leaving the scene, or by employing a well-rehearsed strategy to control one's own thoughts and feelings.

The point can be clarified by focusing on one type of person who becomes a physician, although this type of person can pursue other careers as well. This is the tightly wound, time-grasping, achievement-oriented individual whose personality appears to be the very incarnation of the so-called Protestant work ethic. He functions best in harness. He may be superlative under work pressure. But those moments when just letting go is what body and mind seek may be denied him. It may be hard for him to fall asleep because this is a kind of letting go. Sports and recreational activity may be transformed into intense competitive actions rather than used for spontaneous release. Sex, even good old sex, may take on a grim, driven quality in which he does not truly surrender the taskmastering ego. Now, do we honestly expect such a person to be very good at letting go when a patient approaches death? Do we expect such a person to help others let go? We do not want to mistake abrupt abandonment for letting go. If

by letting go we mean to imply something characteristic of release and natural relinquishment, of accepting the limits of control without either rage or disorganization,
then we may be waiting a long, long time for such a physician to let go.

If the patient has these same personality characteristics, then the final scenes of his
or her dying situation may be singularly frustrating for all involved.

However, even if neither physician nor patient are this type of person, the dying
situation itself tends to intensify the difficulty we have with letting go. We seldom, if
ever, think of helping each other *rehearse* for letting go, and we waste opportunities
to do so. It becomes so much more convenient for us to employ mechanical or chem-
ical techniques, to make decisions by turning off the machines or by withholding
life-sustaining procedures, or by "snowing"* the patient. This is in keeping with the
accepted procedures of inhospital terminal care, and has little to do with encouraging
the mutual letting go of staff, patient, and patient's family.

Yet letting go is not necessarily that difficult. Many patients still find ways of letting go even in environments that offer them very little support in this. Religious faith
comes to the rescue for some, but this is not an automatic solution by any means.
Some religions only increase the dying patient's anxiety and despair; others do not
seem to reach the person when he or she is most in need. We must therefore try to
understand *why* faith does sometimes contribute so much to the serenity of a person's passage from life to death. Such an understanding will help us to create an environment in which letting go is made easier for all dying patients, whether they hold
to a codified religious belief or not.

The ways by which faith works may be at least partially amenable to careful observation and research. The question itself is relevant to terminal care and is necessary
even if it makes some of us uncomfortable because of its nonrational or nonscientific
overtones. I have just one suggestion to offer in this regard.

Perhaps faith works because it allows a person to relinquish the obligation of staying in control beyond a reasonable point without demolishing the core assumption
that there is still an enduring intentionality in the situation itself. The physical reality
of a failing body makes it clear to the dying patient that he or she cannot hold on
much longer. How satisfying it would be to just let go. One possible image of this
process is that of the self, finally unburdened of its obligation to cope and need to
control, assuming the shape of an incredibly light sphere. This transformed self may
be visualized as a bubble that floats off, while, at the same time, retaining its shape
and integrity. The resemblance between this image and the ancient conception of soul-
birds and other such deathbed emanations is obvious, and I will not apologize for it.

The person is able to let go because he or she feels that there is still a responsible
and purposeful force at work in the total situation. Some people see this force within
the context of a particular religious faith. A terminal care environment that offers
symbolic support for such beliefs probably facilitates the letting go process. But if
this analysis approximates the truth at all, then a conventional religious faith is not
absolutely required. It may suffice for a patient to feel a strong sense of bondedness
and trust in the environment. The dying person can let go because others are there,

---

*i.e., rendering the patient unconscious by the use of drugs—without informing him or her.

because the world has proven itself a dependable and comforting place. One dying man spoke to me of making "a soft landing."

This discussion may seem to be taking us far afield from the realities of clinical practice. Not so. For a person to feel free enough to give up no longer rewarding efforts at self-control, he must have something to go on. This translates, at least in part, into the entire pattern of detailed care that has been provided: the medications that came on time, the nurse who listened, the physician who stayed with him or her emotionally all the way, the family that felt welcome in the terminal care situation, the overall impression of a world one could depend upon when one could no longer depend upon one's own body.

This seldom happens when there is a relentless undercurrent of jockeying for control among the principals. The physician who hoards control throughout the terminal care process is virtually guaranteeing that the environment as a whole will have a depleted, impoverished aspect. Nurse, patient, and relative were not entrusted with significant control, and now can offer little comfort to each other. The physician packed all the control into his little black bag, and then walked away with it at the critical time.

The physician who exercises his control *through* others creates quite a different situation. Everybody has had the opportunity to acquire, maintain, share, and utilize all the reasonable control maneuvers available. The physician himself can let go of the reins here and there as certain responsibilities lose their significance, but this does not create a vacuum or emotional desert. Others in the situation pick up those reins of control that remain functional in their hands. The patient can still trust. The world he is dying through has been secure and comforting enough to provide him the freedom to let go.

BIBLIOGRAPHY

Buckingham, R.W., S.A. Lack, B.M. Mount, L.D. MacLean and J.T. Collins: "Living with the Dying: Use of the Technique of Participant Observation," *Canadian Medical Journal*, **115**:1211–1215, 1976.

Glaser, B.G. and A.L. Strauss: *Awareness of Dying*, Aldine, Chicago, 1965.

Kastenbaum, R.: "Beer, Wine and Mutual Gratification in the Gerontopolis," in D.P. Spence, R. Kastenbaum and S. Sherwood (eds.), *Research, Planning and Action for the Elderly*, Behavioral Publications, New York, 1972, pp. 365–394.

———: *Death, Society and Human Experience*, Mosby, St. Louis, 1977.

Seligman, M.: *Helplessness*, Freeman, San Francisco, 1975.

Weisman, A.D. and J.J. Worden: "Psychosocial Analysis of Cancer Deaths," *Omega*, **6**:61–75, 1975.

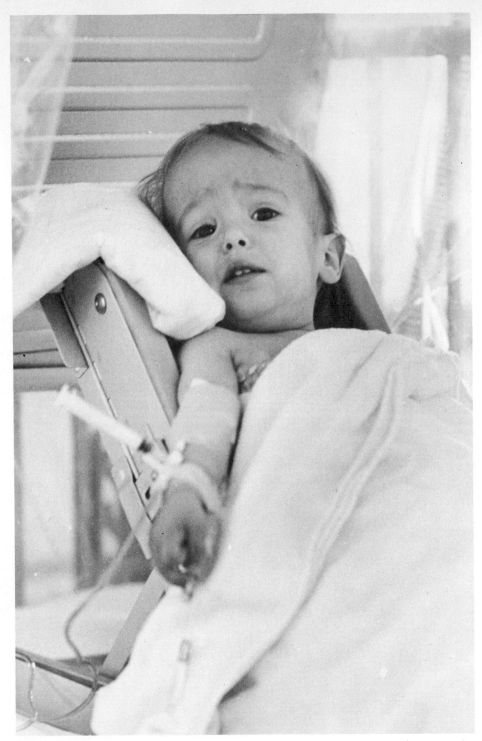

Courtesy of Arlene Bernstein

Part 6

Counseling the Patient's Family

Chapter 24

Family Mediation of Stress

David M. Kaplan
Aaron Smith
Rose Grobstein
Stanley E. Fischman

Serious and prolonged illness such as childhood leukemia is a common source of stress that poses major problems of adjustment, not only for the patient but also for family members. It is important to emphasize family as well as individual reactions in coping with stress since the family has a unique responsibility for mediating the reactions of its members.

When individuals belong to families, they do not resolve their own problems of stress independently, nor are they immune to effects of stress that may be concentrated in another member of the family. Vincent states that the family is uniquely organized to carry out its stress-mediating responsibility and is in a strategic position to do so.[1] No other social institution has demonstrated a comparable capability for mediation that affects as many people in the community.

Because the family has a commitment to protect its members under a wide range of stressful conditions and over long periods of time, physicians, social workers, and other professionals working with a severely ill child must extend their concern beyond the child, at least to members of the immediate family and perhaps to other close relatives. They must offer parents and other family members, as appropriate, help when

The study on which this article is based was conducted, 1969–1972, at the Stanford University Medical Center with grant support from the American Cancer Society.
Reprinted from *Social Work*, **18**:60–69, July 1973.

they need it to handle and resolve specific problems of stress. If stress is great enough and sufficiently prolonged, the role of a family as a buffer for its members can be permanently impaired or even destroyed. To prevent this, more must be learned about effective individual and family coping—and more help given to improve this coping.

A better understanding of the process of coping with severe stress would have substantial clinical and preventive value. Adaptive coping by the family and its individual members—that is, mastery of the sociopsychological problems associated with stress— offers the greatest protection for family members confronted by stressful situations and the best assurance that the family will continue as a viable unit, able to meet the changing needs of its members after they have gotten over the stress.

This article describes the effect of serious illness on the family, delineates the family's critical role in resolving problems related to stress, and provides data needed for organizing preventive and clinical programs that will protect the family's stress-mediating function and mitigate the impact of stress on individual family members. The article is based on the authors' clinical review of more than fifty families with a child diagnosed and treated for leukemia at the Stanford University Department of Pediatrics. Each family was studied from the date the parents were informed of the diagnosis until two months after the child died.

IDENTIFYING EARLY REACTIONS

The aim of the study was to identify adaptive and maladaptive coping responses by the family as early as possible after diagnosis—within three weeks or four at most. It was hoped that developing a method of early case-finding would make intervention feasible during this crucial period and reduce the incidence of families who failed to cope adequately.

Early identification was attempted because studies of the concept of crisis suggest that both individual and family reactions to such threats as prolonged illness are fashioned from one to four weeks after the diagnosis is confirmed.[2] Both adaptive and maladaptive coping responses become evident then. These responses tend to persist and to be reinforced throughout the course of the illness, which may run for years. Rapoport indicates that coping patterns are not as fixed and unyielding during these first weeks as they become in time.[3] Therefore, the ideal time to discover that families are coping inadequately is during this early phase.

Families with a leukemic child constitute a high-risk group. The severe stress precipitated by the diagnosis of the illness generates many problems in addition to those involved in caring for the leukemic child. Both clinical and research observations indicate that a disturbingly large number of families who face this situation fail to cope successfully with the problems it poses.[4] Binger et al. reported that following this diagnosis, at least one member in more than half the families in a 1969 study required psychiatric treatment.[5] Bozeman et al. noted that in families with a leukemic child, school difficulties with the healthy children, divorce, and illness occurred frequently.[6] In the study on which this article is based, 87 percent of the families in the sample failed to cope adequately with the consequences of childhood leukemia, and this failure created a variety of individual and interpersonal problems that were superimposed on the stresses posed by the illness itself. The success or failure of the family's coping behavior was assessed on the criterion that Friedman and his associates outlined:

> Coping mechanisms observed in parents should be viewed in terms of how such behavior contributes or interferes with meeting the needs of the ill child and other family members.

In addition to demonstrable risks associated with a fatal illness such as childhood leukemia, many critical problems of management that involve the family confront medical and social work personnel. Research has not yet provided data helpful for resolving these problems. The following are among the common unsolved questions of management:

1   What should the parents, the leukemic child, healthy siblings, and members of the extended family be told about leukemia—that is, about its course, treatment, and prognosis?

2   Who should give each family member the information deemed appropriate?

3   What advice should be given to parents who consider major family changes after they hear about the child's diagnosis—for example, having another child soon, separating from each other, remarrying, or moving to a new community?

4   What should be done to help parents who seriously disagree about the handling of fatal illness in the family?

5   What help can be offered to single-parent families faced with long-term illness?

6   During the period in which the parents are preoccupied with the leukemic child and tend to neglect the healthy siblings, how can the needs of these other children be protected?

7   What should be done to help parents who avoid visiting the leukemic child during hospitalization—and to help the child?

8   How can morbid preoccupation over the lost child be avoided?

COPING TASKS

The tasks of coping with stress occur in order and relate to the characteristic, sequential phases of the illness—that is, diagnosis, remission, exacerbation, and terminal state. These phase-related tasks must be resolved in proper sequence within the time limits set by the duration of the successive phases of the illness. Failure to resolve them in this manner is likely to jeopardize the total coping process of the entire family and the outcome of the stressful situation faced.[8]

Successfully resolving any crisis depends largely on each individual's ability to experience with minimum delay the immediately painful consequences of a stress-producing event and to comprehend and anticipate, even though dimly, the later consequences—that is, the pain, sorrow, and sacrifice that the trauma will cause. Comprehension in this context means learning to accept one's new life circumstances, however painful, and then acting in accordance with the new conditions that follow the original crisis-precipitating event. The family, primarily through its adult members, can either facilitate or obstruct individual efforts to master a situation of stress.

The development of preventive or clinical programs that are capable of reversing maladaptive coping responses to any illness is contingent on having detailed knowledge of the process of adaptation specific to each illness, including relevant coping tasks and methods of task accomplishment. Because coping tasks vary significantly from one illness to another, it is first necessary to identify the problems posed by each illness.

The birth of a premature infant, for example, requires the family to anticipate the infant's possible loss. If it survives, the family must face the possibility of its being defective. Even when the prognosis is favorable, the parents must prepare themselves to care for an infant who has special early needs that yield in time to normal patterns. Many families with premature babies manage these tasks well, but a large minority do not. This minority continues to think of and treat the premature baby as though it were permanently damaged, even after its development follows normal patterns.[9]

The family with a leukemic child is also suddenly confronted with major alterations in its circumstances that threaten cherished hopes and values for all its members and involve drastic alterations in their lifestyle. Each family member must comprehend these new circumstances and adapt to them by making suitable role changes, despite an understandable reluctance to face painful losses. While coping problems are unique for each illness, crises do fall into common groupings. Principles relevant for coping with leukemia apply with some modification to problems of family coping with other severe and fatal illnesses in children and adults.

FAMILY COPING

For any serious illness, coping demands and responses are not static, but change as the medical treatment of the illness changes. At any point in time, families confronted by childhood leukemia will have dissimilar experiences that reflect differences in the course of the illness as well as variations in medical treatment. Physicians and hospitals also have important differences in their philosophy of "managing" families who have a fatally ill member.

From the authors' observations, it is clear that certain methods of medical management facilitate family coping, while others hinder families struggling to master the consequences of leukemia in a child. For example, some physicians are vague and obscure when communicating with families concerning the diagnosis and prognosis. Others realistically describe the illness and its prognosis, but are eager to sustain hope by emphasizing possible breakthroughs in research. Still another group describes the illness realistically, but tries to focus the family's hopes on lengthy remissions during which the child may live comfortably and actively at home. The authors' experiences indicate that describing leukemia and its prognosis honestly and holding out hope of good remissions is the most helpful approach in dealing with patients and their families.

The marked differences in the medical management of families must be delineated before a demonstration program aimed at enhancing family coping with childhood leukemia can be established. However, it is possible and important at this point—without analyzing how this significant variable affects the coping process—to describe the essential factors in adaptive and maladaptive family coping with this fatal illness.

The typical experience with childhood leukemia today begins when a community physician who suspects a child of having leukemia refers that child to a medical center to confirm the diagnosis. The center usually makes this diagnostic evaluation with the child admitted as an inpatient. The family and the child (if old enough to understand the situation) await the news of the diagnosis with considerable apprehension; the parents may have received forewarning that serious illness is possible. However, the symptomatic behavior of the leukemic child prior to diagnosis rarely prepares the family adequately for the bad news to come, since the symptoms are rarely severe or frightening to the layman and may have been evident only for a short time.

ADAPTIVE COPING

Although what physicians tell parents about the diagnosis varies considerably, it is important for both parents to understand the essential nature of the illness as early as possible, preferably before the hospital that makes the initial diagnosis discharges the child.

According to the authors' observations, in families that achieve adaptive coping, parents understand that leukemia is a serious, ultimately fatal illness involving remissions and exacerbations but moving progressively toward a terminal state. These parents often reach this understanding within a few days after the diagnosis is confirmed. They do not spend an inordinate amount of time blaming themselves or others for the illness; instead, they accept the fact that the etiology of leukemia does not seem to be related to genetic characteristics or certain patterns of child care.

These parents do not arrive at this realistic understanding of the illness and what it holds for the future without considerable anguish. As a prelude to making the necessary changes in living that the child requires, they must accept the fact that they have a chronically and seriously ill child instead of a normal one. The realization that a child until recently considered healthy is seriously ill in itself provides reason for family mourning. Furthermore, the recognition that there is neither a cure nor a good prospect of long-term survival (over five years) adds to the shock and grief these parents experience initially as they anticipate the eventual loss of their child.

Early comprehension of the consequences of a stress-producing event does not mean having detailed knowledge of what the future holds. The parents cannot know at the outset how long the child will live or what symptoms he will experience at each stage of the illness—but they should understand that since leukemia is a chronic and fatal disease, the diagnosis constitutes bad news and will involve painful losses and sacrifices for the family. The course of the illness varies with the type of leukemia; some forms have a rapid development and are short-lived, while other types continue for many years with proper treatment. The average life expectancy after diagnosis is from two to three years.

It is important for both parents to inform the family about the true nature of the illness. At the outset it is sufficient to tell all family members that the child suffers from a serious illness which will require regular and continuous medical care. Medical care is aimed at bringing the child home from the hospital.

Communicating the nature of the illness within the family leads to a period of grief that involves many if not all members. The diagnosis ushers in a phase of shared family mourning and mutual consolation that includes the leukemic child.

Those in the fields of health and social services have long known that mourning is a healthy, natural response to the news of impending loss. They realize what patients and family survivors must experience to accept fatal illness and death.[10] In the instance of childhood leukemia, each family member should have the opportunity to experience grief for current and anticipated losses. This should include the leukemic child, who gathers from his hospital experience and the behavior of staff and family that he is seriously ill.

The family as a group offers its members the potential of mutual support and access to its collective coping experience. When a healthy child becomes seriously ill, all members of the family need to find comfort and solace in each other in their grief. With such support they can face losses and make the sacrifices required by severe trauma.

Mourning may extend over a long period and be an intermittent process in which family members participate. Many losses are associated with a child's serious illness—such as goals that must be postponed indefinitely or relinquished forever. Some families are able to face the inevitable outcome realistically and talk about it frankly.

John D was the eldest of seven children, an active 12-year-old boy involved in many activities. The family was close, and Mr. D's job provided them with a reasonably good financial situation. The parents were understandably shocked when told that John had leukemia. Their initial reactions were typical of those of other parents, but they expressed their shock and grief openly and together. They understood that leukemia is a fatal illness for which there is no cure, respected and trusted the physicians, and made no attempt to seek corroborative or contradictory diagnoses from other physicians. The parents did not try to hide their feelings from each other but found strength and encouragement in grieving together.

From the start, Mr. and Mrs. D knew they must talk to their son about the diagnosis. They told him he had a serious illness that most children did not survive and encouraged him to trust the physicians, who would do everything within their power to keep him as well as possible as long as they could. John and his parents were able to cry together over the implications of the illness. Mr. and Mrs. D also talked with John's 10-year-old sister about the situation, since the two children were especially close.

The parents clearly wanted to be as honest as possible with John. The limited time remaining was doubly precious and was not to be wasted playing games or jeopardizing relationships. The pain of accepting their child's impending death would be even more unbearable if he turned away from them and no longer trusted them. They had never lied to him and were sure their frankness allowed them to trust, respect, and love each other.

At times the family had to express feelings of sadness by crying and mourning and no one tried to inhibit this. Mr. and Mrs. D allowed John time to himself but he was always free to go back to one or both of them with questions that were bothering him. He was a remarkable child whom everyone enjoyed. He was a bright, sensitive boy wrote a science paper on leukemia for which he received an "A."

The D family's open discussion of survival with the child at an early stage attests to their unusual strength as a family. Not all families need to be as frank at the outset. Some may prefer merely to indicate to the child the seriousness of the diagnosis.

MALADAPTIVE COPING

Of the families studied, 87 percent failed to resolve successfully even the initial tasks of coping—that is, the tasks associated with confirmation of the diagnosis. Parents' reactions vary but fall into certain recognizable classes. Their most common reaction is to deny the reality of the diagnosis in as many ways as possible. Such parents avoid those who refer to the illness as leukemia. They themselves use euphemisms (for example, virus, anemia, blood disease) in speaking of the child's illness. They may even be fearful that the child will hear the news from someone outside the family.

> Mr. and Mrs. R refused to allow anyone to tell their 8-year-old daughter what her illness was or what implications it had. When the child asked her father what was wrong, he told her not to worry—there was nothing seriously wrong—she had the gout, just as he did. One evening he called his neighbors for a meeting at which he asked them not to tell their own children that his daughter had leukemia for fear they would reveal the secret.

Reality-denying parents seek convincing reasons for their actions.

> Mr. and Mrs. H said their 15-year-old son was not emotionally strong enough to be told about his diagnosis. When the child asked his parents what was wrong, they told him he had a long-term virus but would be O.K. After the child died several months later, his best friend informed the parents that their son knew he had leukemia but could not tell them he knew.

Parents who strongly reject facts cling to the possibility of a mistaken diagnosis and often seek other medical opinions to confirm their suspicions. Interestingly enough, parents who deny the existence of leukemia, who fight on many fronts to block out both thoughts and feelings associated with this illness, rarely deny their children the medical treatment offered for leukemia.

> Mrs. T, 24 years old, was devastated when told her 4-month-old son had leukemia. Her mother encouraged her not to accept one physician's opinion but to see others, hoping that the diagnosis was wrong. As a result, the family was almost overwhelmed by financial problems, with bills from seven physicians and two university medical centers.

In some cases these parents deny the obvious symptoms of the illness and the effects of treatment.

> The face of the once slender and attractive 4-year-old son of Mr. R became puffy and round soon after steroid treatment began. The physical change in the child was

obvious to everyone except his father. When his wife reminded him of these changes, he became angry and refused to talk to her for several days.

Often these parents take elaborate precautions to keep the child unaware of the diagnosis.

> Mr. and Mrs. B insisted that their 12-year-old son be protected from knowing the nature of his illness or how serious it was. They mounted a 24-hour watch over his hospital bed, never leaving the child alone. One parent or family member was always present. The child asked his parents to explain why they never left him as other parents did.

FEAR OF DISASTER

Such extreme precautions seem to stem from fear that the child's knowing about the illness will lead to disaster—for example, mental breakdown or suicide. Parents use this fear to justify concealing the diagnosis, but it often reflects their own inability to face the facts. One parent's open expression of fear or depression is perceived as confirming the other's worst fears and may lead to the other's repression of grief. One parent's emotion is frequently seen as "weakness," requiring the partner to inhibit expression of feeling because "someone has to be strong." The strong spouse who suppresses his own fears and grief is the one to be concerned about, not only for his sake but for the rest of the family, whose coping he jeopardizes.

> Mr. and Mrs. D, although quite close, seemed to have disparate ways of handling their grief. Mr. D was an open, sensitive person who cried whenever his son had a serious exacerbation of the illness. Mrs. D was secretive about her feelings, stating that both of them could not afford to break down because there were six other children to consider.

Some parents talk about postponing grief until the illness has reached advanced stages. These parents may have severe reactions in the later phases.

> Mrs. W, the mother of six children, resisted everyone's efforts to get her to express her feelings about the illness of her 4-year-old boy. Even when tears would have been appropriate, she refused to express any emotion. She rationalized the importance of remaining strong because she had to think of the other children. Because no one would promise her it would be better if she cried, Mrs. W insisted on waiting until later to cry and mourn. When her child's condition worsened, she was completely unprepared for the change. She became frantic and hysterical and required sedation. Even when her child called for her to be with him, she was so overwhelmed that she proved ineffective.

"Flights into activity" may accompany inability to grieve. Parents may try to escape from grief by becoming involved in new activities that keep them from thinking about the illness or the future—such as starting a new pregnancy, making other changes in family composition, or moving to a new home. Unfortunately, such activities increase the family's burdens and divert resources urgently needed to contend with the illness and its demands.

HOSTILE REACTIONS

Parents who refuse to accept the diagnosis occasionally display overt and massive hostility to members of the health center staff. If this lasts long, it usually evokes a counterhostility among the staff toward the family. The leukemic child is generally the chief victim of such family-staff warfare.

> Mr. and Mrs. A. seldom left their child during his hospitalization. They refused to allow anyone to talk with them about his illness. Mrs. A would run away if anyone mentioned the word "leukemia." Both parents expressed great hostility toward everyone. Mr. A would curse the nurses; he refused to share pertinent information concerning his son's prior illnesses and infections with the physicians. As a result, the staff questioned his sanity.

Some families accept the diagnosis, but refuse to believe that leukemia is incurable or fatal even when the course of the illness confirms both facts. Shopping for a cure, resorting to faith healing, and placing the child on a special diet in the belief that food restriction will cure or arrest the illness are not uncommon practices among these families.

> Mr. H, a dairy farmer, refused to believe there was no cure for leukemia. He was sure the disease was transmitted to his 14-year-old son by the farm animals and therefore refused to allow the boy to eat milk products, restricting him to vegetables and grains. Mr. H also believed that iron-rich foods such as liver would enrich his son's blood. His theory involved overcoming his son's "bad blood" with "good blood."

In a few families the parents can accept the diagnosis and also can anticipate the additional care the illness will require of them. However, they fail to cope by refusing from the start to take on the actual care of the leukemic child because it is "too much for them to handle." These parents claim that they cannot help the child and should not be expected to care for him. This early abdication of parental responsibility is not to be confused with the later abdication that occurs in families only after the parents have taken care of the leukemic child for months or years.

> Mr. and Mrs. K could admit to themselves and others that their 3-year-old son had leukemia, but they could not cope with or adjust to the illness. They refused to visit the child when he was hospitalized, explaining that it was too hard on him when they left. Mrs. K claimed she was too ill to drive from their home to the hospital. Furthermore, since they couldn't take care of him when he was really sick, they didn't see why they should bother to visit him. They also refused to allow their 17-year-old son to visit the ill boy, stating that his school work would suffer

and he would not be able to graduate with his class. The leukemic child was literally abandoned by his family, and no appeal from the staff changed their attitude. The child became withdrawn and frightened during each hospitalization.

DISCREPANT COPING

However capable one parent may be in facing and resolving the issues, the family's success in coping with childhood leukemia is in jeopardy if the parents take opposing positions at an early stage of the coping process. The family's ability to manage the illness depends on successful coping by both parents in the tasks that follow diagnosis. When the parents have different emotional reactions to leukemia and when they disagree on how to define the illness, whom to discuss it with, and what to tell others about it—then the essential ingredients for failure in individual and family coping are present.

> From the time the diagnosis was confirmed, Mr. and Mrs. D had difficulty communicating with each other. Mrs. D wanted to talk with her husband about their child's illness. He insisted that nothing could be accomplished by talking or crying over the situation. He offered no support to his wife, who constantly needed and expected him to comfort her. This gap in communication and mutual support continued for over two years. Mrs. D's anger toward her husband finally became quite apparent. She was on one occasion able to receive comfort from her father, with whom she did not usually feel close, but never from her husband.

Discrepant parental reactions to the coping tasks that follow diagnosis may be responsible for (1) producing garbled and dishonest communication about the illness or preventing communication about it, (2) prohibiting and interrupting individual and collective grieving within the family, and (3) weakening family relationships precisely when they most need to be strengthened. Relationships between parents are undermined by dissatisfaction with the amount of support one gives to the other. Dishonest communication about the illness creates distrust and undermines relationships between parents and children. When parents fail to accomplish coping tasks that follow diagnosis, the net result is to compromise the family's ability to address itself to the next coping tasks, that is, preparing for and making the adaptations necessary in the siege phase of serious illness. Successful early resolution of the tasks following diagnosis is considered a most critical coping assignment because achieving further coping tasks depends on the effectiveness of this initial effort.

In the family system of reciprocal relationships, in which one function is to provide mutual assistance to members under stress, members expect others in the family to help them meet their needs—whether these needs are for emotional support or assistance with family functions and labors. When one family member fails to respond to what another considers legitimate expectations under stress, the inevitable resentment and dissatisfaction that follow decrease the effectiveness of the joint effort essential for successful family coping. The parents' failure to cope successfully with the initial tasks after diagnosis largely precludes sound coping by the rest of the family.

A family must have the closest possible cooperative relations to attain the discipline it requires for living through the siege imposed by a child's serious illness. Such close relations are based on trust, honesty, and mutual support and are virtually impossible to maintain if the family fails to handle the initial coping tasks adequately.

One purpose of the authors' study was to provide the groundwork for effectively assisting at an early stage those families who experienced difficulty in coping with severe illness—specifically, childhood leukemia. Preliminary attempts have been made to correct maladaptive family responses to the diagnosis of leukemia. The following case summary is an example of early efforts to develop appropriate techniques of intervention:

> The reaction of Mr. and Mrs. S to the diagnosis of leukemia was typical of many parents. The mother recognized the seriousness of the illness and felt frightened and depressed. When she cried and sought consolation from her husband, he became angry. "What in hell are you crying about?" he asked. He refused to believe or accept the diagnosis. Mrs. S became angry with his failure to support her and they fought frequently.
>
> Peter, their 13-year-old leukemic boy, resisted treatment procedures during his first hospitalization and an early rehospitalization, loudly proclaiming that the medication did not help and he knew he was "going to die." His parents had steadfastly refused to talk to Peter about the seriousness of his illness. When the project worker insisted, they finally consented to let the physician discuss Peter's illness with him because staff had continuing difficulty in managing him. The physician told the boy, while his mother was present, that he had a serious illness requiring continuous hospital and clinic care. Peter became upset and cried, but soon was less agitated. Just before his mother left the ward, he asked her to lean over so he could whisper to her. He threw his arms around her and they both sobbed bitterly. Then Peter said, "I'm all right now. You can go home." His mother, after a day or two, expressed pleasure that she and Peter were close once again. She was relieved that she no longer had to evade his questions or lie to him about his illness. He told her he now understood why she and his father were worried about him and why she cried. She had thought she had successfully concealed her worry and tears from him.

This case illustrates one method of reopening and clarifying communication in families whose members refuse to talk honestly with one another about leukemia. It is also clear that since coping is a family problem, coping tasks cannot be successfully resolved if key family figures are not included. In this instance, the reopening of family communication did not involve the father and an adolescent sister. After the boy died, the sister refused to go near his room. The family had to sell the house and move to a new home. These omissions limited the success of this interventive effort.

GUIDELINES

Certain guidelines for clinical management can be outlined at this point on the basis of the limited research data available. The following principles were derived from the authors' study findings, plus consultation with a physician who had broad clinical experience.[11]

1. The successful management of the seriously ill child and his family is based on a trusting relationship with the physician treating the child. The psychiatrist is not a practical alternate for the physician, although he may serve as a consultant. Social workers, nurses, technicians, and other health and social service personnel who may be available can help deal with these problems, but they cannot take over for the physician.

2. Perhaps the most important function the physician or social worker can fulfill is to share the anguish, the grief, and the fears of these families without "turning them off." Listening without offering false hope is essential. Giving them long, intellectual descriptions of disease processes and chemotherapy alone is of small value.

3. The parents' denial of the significance of the illness is natural at the outset; however, persistent denial lasting for weeks and months should be probed gently but persistently. Sources of denial such as guilt may be mentioned to them as natural feelings. That the physician and the social worker can face the bad news with them offers the parents the hope that they can somehow survive the child's death.

4. Since families often must endure years of siege with a leukemic child, it is important to help them conserve their energies and resources for the long haul. Physicians and social workers should anticipate and discourage common family reactions that lead to such flights into activity as early pregnancy, divorce, remarriage, and changing jobs or residence. The most useful advice to families contemplating these activities is "Don't just do something, stand there." Each additional major change adds stress to an already overloaded circuit.

Appointments with the parents after the child's death are extremely valuable in assessing whether the family is managing adequately or needs additional help. All members of the family should be considered at that time since all are vulnerable as a result of the leukemic experience. Unresolved problems of grief are not uncommon long after the death of the child. The physician or social worker can help resolve problems of grief by indicating that such reactions are normal and that mourning often takes months to complete.

NOTES AND REFERENCES

1   Clark E. Vincent, "Mental Health and the Family," *Journal of Marriage and the Family* (February 1967), pp. 22–28.

2   See, for example, Gerald Caplan, *Principles of Preventive Psychiatry* (New York: Basic Books, 1964), pp. 39–54.

3   Lydia Rapoport, "The Concept of Prevention in Social Work," *Social Work,* 6 (January 1961), pp. 3–12.

4   See for example, Mary F. Bozeman et al., "Psychological Impact of Cancer and Its Treatment, III: The Adaptation of Mothers to the Threatened Loss of Their Children Through Leukemia, Part I," *Cancer,* 8 (January–February 1955), pp. 1–20; and Maurice B. Hamovitch, *The Parent and the Fatally Ill Child* (Duarte, Calif.: City of Hope Medical Center, 1964).

5 C.M. Binger et al., "Childhood Leukemia: Emotional Impact on Patient and Family," *New England Journal of Medicine* (February 20, 1969), pp. 414–417.
6 Bozeman et al., op. cit., p. 12.
7 S.B. Friedman et al., "Behavioral Observations on Parents Anticipating the Death of a Child," in Robert I. Noland, ed., *Counseling Parents of the Ill and the Handicapped* (Springfield, Ill.: Charles C. Thomas, 1971), p. 453.
8 David M. Kaplan, "Observations on Crisis Theory and Practice," *Social Casework,* 49 (March 1968), pp. 151–155.
9 Paul Glasser and Lois Glasser, eds., *Families in Crisis* (New York: Harper & Row, 1969), pp. 273–290.
10 See Erich Lindemann, "Symptomatology and Management of Acute Grief," *American Journal of Psychiatry,* 101 (September 1944), pp. 1–11.
11 The authors discussed clinical management of the leukemic child and his family with Dr. Dane Prugh, Professor, Department of Pediatrics, University of Colorado Medical Center.

Chapter 25

The Physician
and the Dying Patient
and His Family

Robert E. Taubman

Enormous demands fall on the physician when illness threatens life itself: demands for technical knowledge and competence; demands for interpersonal relationship skills; demands for internal wisdom and strength in coping with loss (death).

The physician must first formulate a strategy of intervention on which to base his or her treatment of seriously ill patients and their families. Discussed here is the concept that the appropriate unit of study and care for the physician is the configuration of significant persons in a family; and that this behavioral system has its own field of forces beyond the vectors directing the behavior of individuals, including that of the identified patient. Working with the family unit enables the physician to reduce the potential for his or her overinvolvement with the identified patient; to deal with the process of family adjustment to great disequilibrium; to promote useful defense mechanisms; and to assist with appropriate grief and mourning.

Primary care physicians and particularly family physicians have a remarkable opportunity to provide continuity of care and health counselorship based on an intimate knowledge of and concern for the patient and his or her family. Skillful and sensitive integration of health care by the primary physician enables the patient and his or her relatives to look to this doctor for expert medical knowledge, care, and treatment, including the involvement and coordination of diagnostic studies and treatment programs instituted by other competent specialists.

The primary physician is in a unique position to assess the strengths and assets of the patient and his or her family; he knows their history over a relatively long period of personal acquaintance. He knows whom to tell and what to tell about sickness and its implications. He tells the truth. But he is judicious in determining how much knowledge to convey to patient and family. He knows that patients hear selectively and partially. He knows how regularly patients misinterpret the data they are given.

The physician needs to individualize his approach to the emotional content of illness. He does so partly because of his own feelings toward illness and death and he does so partly because of his respect for and understanding of the patient's needs.

There is, however, an important question for the physician to decide: when should he pursue aggressively the emotional aspects of illness in a given person? How should he offer the patient a choice of expressing or not expressing feelings about his or her illness?

Initially, our patient, Linda, appreciated the doctor's intellectualized approach to her monocytic leukemia. But then the internal pressures arising out of concern with her imminent death overwhelmed her. The following transcript presents part of an interview between the author and the patient.

R.E.T.*: You know there are some things that I'm puzzled by and perhaps you could share some of your thoughts and feelings with me. You have tried to maintain a very stoical outward appearance, even in front of Dr. P., your first physician here at the medical school. I don't understand it. I wonder if you could tell me why it was so important for you not to cry when he told you such important news?

Linda: I don't know if I can answer that.

R.E.T.: Try.

Linda: It's kind of a problem I have worked on for a long time, not only with the leukemia. I guess I don't want to be a weak person. I have discovered a couple of things just recently. I think that my image of myself is to be the perfect counselor, the perfect student, the perfect daughter, the perfect whatever, and now I am being the perfect patient—the one who holds up under stress, the one who does not cry and feel sorry for herself. Even when you're in pain, you ask for something for the pain but you don't whine. It is pretty important to me to be the perfect patient, I guess, and I must say I think I'm doing a very good job, although I'm not necessarily pleased with that.

R.E.T.: How do you mean?

Linda: I don't think it's all that honest. It doesn't really reveal what I am feeling all the time but it puts up a good front. And evidently it is an effective way for me to deal with my situation.

R.E.T.: But you have second thoughts sometimes?

*Robert E. Taubman

Linda: Well, yes, because it's been hard for me to get my feelings out and discuss them with other people, and that has limited the things I could deal with. Lately I have been more able to, I guess, and have been sort of pushing myself in the direction of, if I feel like crying, crying. If I want to say, I'm scared to death, then I can say it.

R.E.T.:   And how easy is it for you at this moment to say those things about your feelings, to say, "I'm scared, I'm frightened?"

Linda: I'm sorry?

R.E.T.:   How easy is it for you at this moment to say those things about yourself?

Linda: Well, I don't like to hear it out loud. That makes it much more realistic.

R.E.T.:   So the sound of your own voice saying, "I'm frightened," makes it more real for you and you suffer twice.

Linda: .   Well, I admit it. If I don't admit it I guess I think that it is not there, but I've realized that I can't keep it inside very much longer—I have to deal with it. And so I have been saying it and Dr. G. and I have spent quite a few sessions talking about it.

R.E.T.:   Without your betraying any personal data, would it be possible for you to share with us the content of some of the things you've discussed with him?

Linda: Well, we have talked about death and my feelings about that. I came out of the hospital this last time feeling very down because it seemed much more . . . it seemed like death was a lot closer. I feel like I'm running out of things and I said this to him and so he said, "What you are really afraid of is dying, isn't it?" and I said, "Yeah." So we talked about that and what it means, what just saying the word *death* implies, the shock value of the word, and I have done some reading on the subject. I can say it now. It doesn't shake me up quite so much now to say, "Look, Linda, you have leukemia and you will probably die from it and your death may not be too far away." I went through a period of a couple of weeks when it was right there all the time and I knew that I had to get that out of the way or I wouldn't do very well. I think one of the things that helped me was just to say it and to visualize it, you know. We talked about funerals and what our society says about death and how we pretty much try to keep it hidden from people and how it is something that is a taboo sort of subject, and we talked about dignity in dying. How do you help someone die?

R.E.T.:   What are your thoughts?

Linda: I haven't any really. . . . Well, I think I sort of feel that the people who are close to you should be included. The book that I have been reading is *On Death and Denying*. I think the author's name is Avery Weisman. He says some really good things that I think that I . . . he says that the dying need the support of their relatives or people who are close to them. So I have decided for myself that I am going to tell my family where I am now, the things I am thinking about and the way I am dealing with them, so that when I am ready to die it won't be a surprise and everybody won't be shocked.

R.E.T.:   At this point you haven't shared your diagnosis with them?

Linda: Yes, they know.

R.E.T.:   When did you tell them?

Linda: I told them about 2 months after I found out but I haven't mentioned dying. I think we all sort of go along with the idea that I will be the one exception. I don't know because they have never brought the subject up to me either.

R.E.T.:   You know, I would like to return to the topic of your family because I know very little about them other than there are four girls. But right now I want to get back to what you were saying about how you dealt with your feelings with your physician and I also want to tell you that I respect what you are saying because I really believe in what you are doing. Can you tell me, then, is it still so difficult for you to express your feelings of sorrow and grief, and do you feel you have to keep face even with me?

Linda: Yeah.

R.E.T.:   For what purpose?

Linda: For my own personal satisfaction, I guess.

R.E.T.:   But how do you figure out in advance that you must not show despair or sorrow or frustration, even with me? You really don't know me very well.

Linda: I don't think it matters who the other people are or what the subject is, as long as I must "maintain." I will talk about something when I can deal with the problem without getting uptight. That's not always true but it is most of the time.

R.E.T.:   It's a tough problem for me to deal with because you've given me conflicting signals—it's O.K. intellectually, in your brain, but not in your heart. And there have been times, when we have spoken, when I have wondered why we have had to protect your feelings so much. So from time to time I have not known in my brief relationship with you whether to say, "Look, you can cerebrate all you want to, I know you have a fine mind, but there are other things you allude to that I think also need to be paid attention to"; or whether to say, go ahead. I know you are having feelings and a number of times you have expressed with your face and your eyes something much more than your cerebral activity.

Linda: Like right now. (She begins to cry.)

R.E.T.:   Yeah. It's O.K.

Linda: Thank you. I feel like I want something to happen now. I don't know what.

R.E.T.:   It's hard to deal with your feelings?

Linda: Well, yes it is, here. I . . . lately have been more able to deal with them but I have been forced into it, I think, because there are too many of them. I'm not, I have given up just trying to control them.

R.E.T.:   Well, you know up to a point, that's fine. But you do have dignity and you do need to maintain that. And that's O.K., but you expend a hell of a lot of energy trying to keep those feelings that are so powerful from even showing themselves a little bit and that is all I was trying to point out to you. So I have a lot of respect for what you are doing, but I like you so much better when I know that sometimes you do have these feelings that can't be controlled. So as much as you have such a lovely smile—if that's valid, that smile—certainly this is valid too, in my opinion. Have I made myself clear? (Linda nods her head.) So I see you as dignified when you cry, just as I also see you as dignified when you are smiling and thinking carefully.

We can see the doctor's dilemma in dealing with a person such as this bright, highly trained, sensitive, and attractive young woman. On the one hand, we could have continued to discuss with Linda the medical history, the course, and the treatment of her disease and its probable outcome—all from the ideational-cognitive standpoint. After all, this young woman is easy to talk to—she approximates the doctor's educational background, his social-cultural milieu, his vocabulary. She has a serious and interesting organic disease. Her obsessional and compulsive character make it possible for her to order her thinking in ideational terms and to deny the emotional components of her illness. She maintains her dignity by denying the implications of early death. It is easy for the physician to relate to such a patient; and he can do so without assuming the burden of *caring* for the person (2, 3).

On the other hand, Linda tells us that she can no longer internalize and deny her feelings. Hence, we decide to share with Linda our awareness that her defenses are no longer adequate to deal with the tremendous feelings within her. We tell her that we can respect the expression of her emotional life. We give her the opportunity to reveal her concern about dying, while, at the same time, maintaining her dignity. She can cry without losing face.

The family needs the knowing, seasoned, total approach of the physician whose *mental set* or attitude orients him or her toward dealing with the person identified as the patient, as well as with the significant others in the patient's support system. It is this special set that enables the doctor to understand the basic notion that sickness is a family thing, that sickness produces family disequilibrium that must be resolved (4).

For example, consider the following family situation. Gary and Barbara are 41-year-old parents of five children ranging in age from 8 to 20 years. Gary was a power company lineman and is now employed by the same company in another capacity. Barbara is a housewife. Five years prior to our consultation, Gary came into contact with 12,000 volts, 40 feet above ground. He was seriously disabled both mentally and physically. His burns destroyed his left arm and hand, which were replaced with a prosthetic device. Barbara assumed nearly complete control of the family. For nearly 2 years she functioned as head of the family while Gary achieved a slow but remarkably successful recovery. Gary eventually became, he said, "a better man than I ever was." He was happy that he had refused medical retirement. His company placed him in charge of testing the very equipment that had saved his own life.

Three months prior to our meeting, Gary had his first myocardial infarction. "It was a dilly," he said. "I am one scared dude."

The family had gone through its earlier adjustment to Gary's obvious, severe injury. Now, he had suffered a severe, internal injury, one to his heart. There followed still another period of adjustment to Gary's condition and personality changes—he became so autocratic, demanding, and rigid that it was difficult for the family to live in harmony. Barbara found the transition extremely difficult partly because, as she put it:

> Before, for months, I was the boss. [during Gary's first period of rehabilitation] He could hardly talk or walk; these kids took him walking every day . . . to help him. We were involved a little bit more. Maybe for once I was the boss. Maybe it went to my head because I made all the decisions. I still make an awful lot of them. But he has come back into the role of the father. Maybe I don't like this. Maybe. I don't know, but the heart attack seemed to bust it all up. After 20 years, I don't know— I don't know whether I care.

The shift in authority and power within the family was confusing to parents and children alike. Barbara's new roles were upsetting to her; she underwent enormous changes from collaborating with a dominant husband to assuming sole leadership of the family. The interview gave Gary an opportunity to express for the first time how frightened he was for his life, in spite of his seeming strength, drive, authority, and competitiveness. A technical problem arose for us in this sense: it was clear that Gary's mental ability had been significantly affected by his electrical burn. We felt that we should not focus on this issue of central nervous system impairment because we believed that such an emphasis would further undermine Gary in his role of father.

The physician must support the patient and his or her family. He must support the spouse or the parents or the children. He must be humble in predicting outcome and he must offer hope. He must convey even to young children that although the family member is sick, they themselves will be all right and safe. He must give the patient and family a chance to talk about the illness and its implications, and he must give them repeated opportunities to talk (5, 6). He must use language appropriate to the patient and the family. He must use other allied health workers to provide the best care.

In managing patient and family effectively, the physician must be knowledgeable in the following areas of patient care:

1   The detection, analysis, clarification, synthesis, and perhaps modification of the vectors that support the adaptive, homeostatic mechanisms of the family.
2   The family's assignment of various roles to its members, including the *sick* and *healthy* roles.
3   The disclosure of and maintenance of secrecy around sensitive information. Such maneuvers may themselves be overt or covert.
4   Therapeutic and antitherapeutic alliances formed ostensibly to protect the person who is identified as sick.
5   The dynamic changes in family subgroup affiliations that tend to reinforce behaviors valued by family members or to extinguish those behaviors intolerable to the family.
6   Mechanisms of defense such as denial (e.g., in the face of the imminent death of a loved one).
7   Affective reactions, such as reactive depressions, anger, and the grief associated with the consequences of serious and terminal illness.

Presented below is the partial transcript of an interview between the author and a family that has serious health problems and whose intelligence and capability require sophistication and skill on the part of the treating physician.

Bill and Ethel are 50-year-old parents of three children who are present during the interview (they range from 15 to 20 years of age). Father, an agricultural investigator, makes frequent and extended business trips out of state. Mother, a housewife, is also very involved in church activities and community projects.

Our identified patient is Ethel. We know she has been treated for breast cancer. Bill leads the family in open criticism of Ethel's (1) failure to disclose extension of her illness; (2) delay in initiating medical treatment.

Our interview discloses Ethel's concealment of salient personal data and further reveals that her secrecy is based partly on her fear of causing Bill a cardiovascular accident or another myocardial infarction.

For the first time we now learn that Bill has a significant medical history that he minimizes and denies to himself, his family, and his physician (who is present during the interview).

Bill: I remember something else I think that she—but this is more to the point, this lump. I think that you had that lump 3 weeks or so before you called Dr. P.

Ethel: No, it was, I forgot . . . what I . . . I think it was a month.

Bill: Before you called Dr. P?

Ethel: Uh Huh.

Bill: I don't think that you've brought that out before, I think that is a pertinent observation.

R.E.T.: What's pertinent about it, can you tell us?

Bill: Why any woman or man would let something unusual go and think that maybe it's going to go away all by itself.

Ethel: Well, I thought I would wait until my next period and check it again.

Bill: And it was still there?

Ethel: Uh Huh.

R.E.T.: It sounds like you still have some resentment about the way Ethel handled it.

Bill: No, not resentment really, I don't think that it would have . . .

Ethel: He was gone most of the time.

Bill: I don't think it would have changed the course of the whole thing; once the lump is there, it's there, it's either malignant or it isn't.

R.E.T.: Just like that.

Bill: I'm not a doctor and I don't know whether 1 month will make that much difference. But I have done a little reading and the medical profession tells us, don't wait, go right away, and Dr. P. didn't wait when he heard about this lump—"Get yourself in here," he said.

R.E.T.: But Mama says that you weren't even there.

Bill: I don't remember. I would have to check my vouchers.

R.E.T.: He has to check his vouchers?

Ethel: You got back just in time for us to take that spring vacation.

Bill: Oh . . . well, anyway I heard about the lump whether I was home or not 1 month after I should have heard about it.

Ethel: Well, then I . . .

R.E.T.: Well, you didn't tell him either.

Ethel: No, I have a habit of not telling my family lots of things.

Bill: She was going to let me go to Idaho before the second operation and then at the last minute told me, "Oh, by the way I'm going in, I've got another lump under the left arm. I'm going to have it examined."

R.E.T.: What did you make of that?

Bill: I didn't think very much of it. Boy, if you had let me go out of town . . . I mean that's serious.

Ethel: I wasn't about to let you go out of town.

Bill: You were going into the hospital Tuesday morning.

Ethel: I just didn't want you to have another heart attack! I waited until the last minute to tell you.

R.E.T.: So you were not telling him out of concern for his health?

Ethel: Right.

Chris: Why didn't you tell me?

R.E.T.: Wait a minute, Chris says she didn't know either.

Chris: Nobody knew. All I knew was when you were getting in the car and leaving and you said, "Bye, I'm going to the hospital."

Ethel: Oh no.

Chris: Oh yes.

Ethel: Let's not argue about it here.

R.E.T.: Well, now let's find out about Kathy and Larry. Were you aware of Mom's going into the hospital that Monday or Tuesday morning, or the night before?

Chris: I knew the night before.

Ethel: Was this the second time or the first time?

Chris: This was the second time.

Larry: I heard from Kathy or my father that she was going into the hospital the night before.

R.E.T.: So somehow the family didn't know about it until it was very close to the time and you were . . .

Ethel: My main concern was my husband. I didn't want to worry him or give him too long a time to worry or think about it. So I waited until the last minute to tell him and the family also—because, speaking of impact of illness, I guess I thought that, you know, tempers might flare again and automobiles might get banged up again and there might be more arguments, so I just wanted to keep it at a minimum.

R.E.T.: How would you folks have preferred your Mom to have dealt with you about this?

Bill: Openly and frankly.

R.E.T.: How so?

Bill: How so? As soon as she felt that second lump, she should have said, "Bill, I had better call Dr. P. This morning I discovered another lump." I had a trip scheduled, but I could have put it off or I could have adjusted my schedule.

Ethel: Well, again, you weren't even there. I was sitting at my desk at work when I discovered the second lump under my arm.

Bill: Wasn't I home all that time?

Ethel: No, you were gone all that month again.

Bill: When did you go into the hospital the second time . . . oh, just 2 months ago.

R.E.T.:   You need your vouchers again?

Bill: Not quite. I got back from Arizona and then I was around Portland for weeks and I think the next trip was . . .

Ethel: No you weren't here. It was September.

R.E.T.:   O.K., now listen. I think we are missing the point that Papa is making. What's the point?

Ethel: That I didn't tell him when I first discovered it, or tell him first.

R.E.T.:   Yeah, or tell him very soon thereafter. So he would have been able to make some kind of adjustments and deal with the fact that you were heading for the hospital again and so on. What do you think of that now?

Ethel: Well, he has high blood pressure and he has a tendency to fly off the handle and lose his temper. And when he is concerned about me, and I've seen him do this in the past, he's apt to take it out on the kids, and I wanted to keep that down to a minimum.

R.E.T.:   Hey, we have some secrets here between father and son. Can you tell us?

Bill: What do you think about that Larry, after a little prodding from your father?

R.E.T.:   Yeah, you are taking my job away from me.

Bill: Yeah, boy, all of these people are looking at me and thinking, Wow, what a cad he is. His wife gets a lump and she has to go to the hospital and he beats his kids.

Ethel: No, I didn't mean that!

Bill: This is what I observed.

Ethel: I'm sorry. (Laughing)

R.E.T.:   Larry, Papa wants you to tell us something.

Bill: Be honest, Larry.

Larry: Well, he just leaned over to me and said, "That's not true." So . . .

R.E.T.:   Wait, what's not true?

Larry: About what my mom said, that sometimes he really loses his temper and takes it out on us kids.

R.E.T.:   He's reassuring you, in case you don't know. O.K., but you are really worried about him and we haven't heard that he has some really big things going on with him. You know what—what's this business about your high blood pressure?

Bill: I wish my doctor weren't here now.

R.E.T.:   You want to tell him?

Bill: Well, I really don't think I had much of a heart attack; he assures me that I did have. I haven't followed his instructions too closely on diet, and smoking and whatnot, which is apparent.

R.E.T.:   Which is apparent?

Bill: That I don't take him too seriously about this heart attack, and I won't, not until I really have one of *those*, you know, when the pain shoots up your arm and you wake up in the intensive care unit.

R.E.T.:   If you wake up.

Bill: If you wake up—then I'll believe I have heart trouble.

R.E.T.:   You like to gamble for big stakes.

Bill: No, let's not put it that way, let's just say that I am a skeptic when it comes to the pains that I had.

R.E.T.:   You're a skeptic?

Bill: But let's talk more about Ethel's cancer.

R.E.T.:   What do you think of that? He says, Get off of my back. Let's get back to Ethel. You mean you don't think you have anything to worry about?

Bill: I don't think so.

R.E.T.:   No? With high blood pressure, heart attack, a hell of a temper, and what else?

Aggressive interviewing of the family thus elicits crucial information about significant family health matters. Secrets about family illness may be uncovered and important issues centering upon sickness may be clarified. Often, this very process may break down the elaborate wall of fantasy and myth that the patient has constructed to protect himself. Exposure of defenses (such as denial) that are used by family members to cope with the impact of life-threatening illness enables the physician to confront the family in regard to its typical ways of managing stress, and he or she can help the family choose more constructive ways of adapting to illness.

Betty and Jim were extremely difficult to interview. The following transcript reveals classical examples of the use of coping behaviors such as denial, anger, depression, and rigidity in an attempt to come to grips with devastating life problems.

Kelly, a boy of 8, has acute monocytic leukemia. This diagnosis was made 2 months prior to our interview with Kelly's parents, Betty and Jim. Both parents had prior marriages that terminated in divorce. Betty's three teen-age daughters by her first marriage were adopted by Jim. But Kelly is the only child born to the second marriage. Jim, 35, is a craftsman for a large electronics company. Betty, 32, is a housewife.

Betty: Our house is pretty disrupted with our 13-year-old. She is a real handful for Jim and now even myself . . .

Jim: It's not that. We have a personality clash.

Betty: He just can't get along with her and when she isn't around there isn't nearly as much trouble at home. Her counselor said that she would love to have a fatal disease so that she could get the attention that Kelly has been getting.

R.E.T.:   How do you feel about that?

Betty: I have thought a lot about that. I've wondered if it were her instead of Kelly, how I would feel . . . I try not to answer that.

R.E.T.:   So you are proud that you are a father and that's great. But you are still a young man and you are still a young woman. Now what?

Jim:	If you are asking if there will be any more children, there won't be. That was taken care of.
Betty:	When I had the miscarriage, the doctor . . . We didn't want any more to begin with. We felt that four was plenty. And when I had the miscarriage, the doctor recommended that I not have any more, which was fine with me.
R.E.T.:	O.K., were there any other alternatives for you?
Betty:	You mean adoption?
R.E.T.:	Yeah!
Betty:	No.
R.E.T.:	What's the matter with that?
Jim:	That would be, in my mind, like trying to replace him if something did happen . . . and I don't want to do that.
R.E.T.:	I understand what you are saying but I don't understand the feeling behind it.
Jim:	Well, it should be pretty obvious. I just don't want any more.
Betty:	I couldn't raise another child. Not a boy.
R.E.T.:	But now listen. What do you expect is going to happen with Kelly? What are you betting on? We hope for the best, but really what are you betting on?
Betty:	I am shooting for a star I guess, I just . . . I won't believe it . . . I can't . . . Well, I can't look at him and say that one day he will be gone. Somebody is going to come up with something. Even maybe my carrot juice will work. I don't know. I don't look at it like he is going to be gone. I just don't look at it that way and I don't know whether that is good or bad.
Jim:	We both do pretty good when he is home with us but when he is in the hospital she can't stand to come home. She spends most of her time here at the hospital and most of the nights too. As long as . . . as long as he is with us it doesn't seem too bad. It's a lot easier to have him with us than it is to have him in the hospital. I am real grateful that he has been able to be home most of the time.
R.E.T.:	But you have an ultimate faith that won't let you even consider that, maybe even with all of your faith, sometimes bad things happen.
Betty:	That's what I have been told. I won't believe it unless it happens.
R.E.T.:	But what then?
Betty:	Fall apart.
R.E.T.:	How could we help you then?
Betty:	Then? Well, I hope you won't have to.
R.E.T.:	I hope so too.
Betty:	I don't know but I . . . I'm scared to even think what will happen to me or to him [Jim]. Am I supposed to think about that?
R.E.T.:	I don't know. I want you to have hope and faith but what *if?*
Jim:	(Unintelligible)
R.E.T.:	I'm sorry, I didn't hear you, Jim.
Jim:	We haven't thought about it and I don't want to have to be pushed into thinking about it either.

R.E.T.:   Yeah, I don't want to do that to you either. We all agree on that. But I think Betty wonders whether she should have an alternative plan . . . just in case. She doesn't like it either.

Jim: Well, for the time being I think we are just going to go right on thinking that it's not going to happen.

Jim was already depressed and Betty chose to play the role of the "tough woman" who would support her husband. Both parents resisted considering how to compensate for Kelly's loss. Betty's steadfast denial prevented her from preparing herself for Kelly's demise. Jim used anger to prevent himself from contemplating alternatives and this anger came on top of his rather profound depressions; yet additional work with him might have made it possible for Jim to bridge the anticipated loss of his son by establishing better relationships with his three stepdaughters, or eventually by adopting another child. We offered Betty and Jim additional sessions through the oncologist who had initially presented the family, but the parents rejected any such offer of help. Medical attempts to work through the bitterness associated with Kelly's tragedy were frustrated by them in every way.

In caring for patients, the physician is positively reinforced when his patients become well. Conversely, when his patients fail to improve or when they die the doctor is negatively reinforced. His self-image suffers (8). He may become frustrated, angry, anxious, depressed, and withdrawn (1). He may indeed manifest those defensive maneuvers designed to protect his own vulnerability but that distance him from those who need him most. At such particularly difficult moments, both personally and professionally, the physician needs the support of his or her colleagues. Often enough, physicians who are closely involved with the care and treatment of seriously ill patients require and benefit from personal consultation with a psychiatrist because of the inordinate strain these physicians themselves experience when some of their patients die (7).

REFERENCES

1 Artiss, K.L. and A.S. Levine: "Doctor-Patient Relation in Severe Illness," *New England Journal of Medicine*, **288**:1210–1214, 1973.

2 Crane, D.: "Decisions to Treat Critically Ill Patients: A Comparison of Social Versus Medical Considerations," *Milbank Memorial Fund Quarterly*, **1**:1–33, Winter 1975.

3 Lipkin, M.: *The Care of Patients—Concepts and Tactics*, Oxford, New York, 1974.

4 Olsen, E.H.: "The Impact of Serious Illness on the Family System," *Postgraduate Medicine*,   :169–174, February 1970.

5 Rosenbaum, E.H.: *Living with Cancer*, Praeger, New York, 1975.

6 Taubman, R.E.: "Family Counselling," address given to the American Academy of Family Physicians, New York, September 27, 1972.

7 Taubman, R.E.: "The Emotional Components of Life-Threatening Illness," a videotape program presented at the annual meeting of the American Psychiatric Association, Miami Beach, Florida, May 9–14, 1976.

8 White, L.P.: "The Self-Image of the Physician and the Care of the Dying Patient," in L.P. White (ed.), *Care of Patients with Fatal Illness, Annals of the New York Academy of Science*, **164**:822–837, December 19, 1969.

Chapter 26

Psychological Aspects of Sudden Unexpected Death in Infants and Children

Abraham B. Bergman

By virtue of our training, and possibly our temperament, few of us modern physicians tend to be very good at dealing with death. We learn about the pathophysiologic mechanisms leading to death, but little about what to do when the event occurs. Even the practice of clinicians attending autopsies on their patients is going out of style—in favor of reviewing the pathologist's typewritten summary. Our ethos is cure rather than care, and death, after all, represents failure. We quickly turn back to tasks where the tools we possess can be applied.

I never remember being prepared during my training about what to say to a family whose child has died. I do have a vivid memory of my instruction as an intern on how to obtain permission for an autopsy on my first patient who died. My resident told me, "Go in and get the autopsy permission signed."

Seldom do students get the opportunity to watch a senior physician serving as a model in some of the tough, human jobs in medicine, such as comforting a dying patient, telling a mother her baby is deformed, or managing a case of sudden infant death syndrome. The American system of clinical training called "giving the house officer maximum responsibility" sometimes passes for "trial by ordeal."

Many of the ideas expressed in this paper have come from my friend and colleague, Dr. J. Bruce Beckwith, a brilliant pathologist who has provided solace to hundreds of families who have lost children to sudden infant death syndrome.
Reprinted from *Pediatric Clinics of North America*, **21**:115--121, February 1974.

Last year, a 14-year-old boy who suddenly collapsed on the street was rushed to our hospital emergency room. Even though there were no clinical signs of life, at least six physicians frantically attempted resuscitative measures. In the hallway outside the emergency room, I came upon two stunned parents who were standing absolutely alone. None of the physicians wanted to leave the dramatic scene to obtain a history, let alone provide any solace. I did not want to either, the boy was dead (possibly from a cardiac conduction defect—even the autopsy later was unrevealing); but I forced myself to sit down in an adjoining room and listen while they talked of their hopes and their son's aspirations. I am used to talking with parents whose children die of sudden infant death syndrome; this was different and I was overwhelmed. Afterward, I went to my office and cried. I later thought that I should have let my interns and residents witness me cry to learn that professionalism does not preclude expression of human feeling.

A notable exception during my training, who served as a model on how to communicate with grief-stricken parents, was Dr. Rudolph Toch who formerly headed the clinical oncology service at Boston Children's Hospital. He personally spoke with the parents of newly diagnosed leukemia patients and encouraged house officers to sit in on what we called the "Toch talk." The basic theme with many variations was simple: the cause of the disease remains unknown and the parents did not cause, nor could they have prevented, its onset. Some vivid impressions emerged from watching this master physician in action which later aided me immeasurably in facing similar situations.

Friedman lucidly outlines the dynamics involved when families experience sudden, unexpected death in their children.[3] Several of his points need underlining. A predictable grieving *process* must be experienced when loved ones die. This process is related more to the manner of death than to the specific disease entity. Thus, when death is preceded by an illness, some of the separation process can take place beforehand, which allows a degree of comfort to the family. I used to decry the practice of placing children with obviously mortal head injuries on respirators for one or two days. I have now come to feel that even a respite of 12 hours before death is pronounced gives the parents some opportunity to prepare for the dread event, a time which seems to assist their later adjustment. Sudden, unexpected death, whether due to trauma, overwhelming infection, sudden infant death syndrome, or other catastrophes, allows no preparation and, as Friedman states, "The grief reaction is intense, disruptive and almost intolerable." An understanding of the *normal* grief reaction is imperative if the physician is to fulfill his obligation to comfort as well as to cure.

In the course of dealing with over a thousand families who have lost children to sudden infant death syndrome, either through personal conversation or correspondence, I have developed an appreciation of the family's point of view regarding the physician's management of sudden, unexpected death. Overall, our profession does not come off with high marks.

What follows are some of the more common complaints that I hear, accompanied by some editorial comments:

"I couldn't reach my doctor." There is debate whether a personal physician is necessary for routine pediatric care. There can be no question, however, about the benefit of having one's own doctor present during times of serious illness. Invariably, the families who come through the crib death experience in the best shape are those who have

been supported throughout by a personal physician. Doctors should not have to be constantly "on call" but alternative coverage in the form of another physician, instead of a faceless hospital emergency room, is a necessity for those desirous of practicing quality medicine.

Because of the inverse relationship between sudden infant death syndrome and socioeconomic class, a disproportionate number of families lack any personal physician and thus tend to suffer the worst consequences. In other words, the less educated families who have the least information about sudden infant death syndrome and are least likely to get sympathetic treatment from "the system" are the very ones who would benefit most from a supportive physician at their side. Alas, the world does not work that way. An appropriate alternative, however, is utilization of specially trained public health nurses to provide information and counseling to all families who lose babies to sudden infant death syndrome. The training required is not elaborate; it involves learning some basic facts about sudden infant death syndrome and the attendant grief reactions. Pediatricians should take the lead in insisting that cooperative programs exist in each and every community between the coroner or medical examiner's office and the health department to provide this urgently needed service for all families.

"I reached my doctor but he said there was nothing he could do and wouldn't come." To my mind, such inaction on the part of a physician is blatant malpractice. The explanation is that the physician is frightened at his own inadequacy in dealing with death and has to "run away." Physicians, of course, must also cope with their own guilt feelings. Whenever I talk about sudden infant death syndrome at a medical meeting, invariably one or two members of the audience wander up afterward to relive a case in which they were involved far in the past. "I had just examined that baby 2 days before and couldn't find anything." is an oft repeated phrase. I spend a good deal of time explaining to angry parents that physicians who are not knowledgeable about sudden infant death syndrome often carry a great deal of guilt on themselves, wondering "What did I miss?" I do not feel that aggrieved parents must feel sorry for their physicians when they display callous behavior, but at least it is helpful to them to understand the reason for the behavior.

I always knew that Dr. Charles McClelland of Cleveland was one of the best pediatricians in the country, but my respect for him became even greater on hearing the following story last year: An anxious mother in his practice made several calls to the office about her infant who had a cold. Dr. McClelland made a house call and confirmed that the baby had only a minor upper respiratory illness. At the time, the mother pleaded with him to hospitalize the child, which Dr. McClelland advised against, stating that therapy in the hospital would be no more beneficial than therapy at home. That night the baby died. I suspect that most ordinary pediatricians would have wanted to go and hide after that shaking episode. Instead, Charlie McClelland spent considerable time with both parents to help them through their grief. He explained, rightfully, that the episode probably would not have been averted even if the child had been in the hospital. He is a doctor with both guts and sensitivity.

"The doctor told us an autopsy wasn't necessary—it wouldn't show anything." If at all possible, autopsies should be performed on all cases of sudden, unexpected infant. death. Certainty, however harsh, is better than lingering doubt. It is well to remember that in from 10 to 15 percent of infants dying suddenly and unexpectedly,

a cause such as overwhelming infection or intracranial hemorrhage will be found. The concept that "nothing will be found at autopsy" stems from the lack of agreement among pathologists until recent years on criteria for the diagnosis of sudden infant death syndrome. The most important product of research in the last decade has been the establishment that sudden infant death syndrome is a definite disease entity with defined clinical and pathologic criteria for diagnosis.[2] I have spoken with numerous families who regret terribly that an autopsy was not performed on their child. I have never talked with a family who regretted the procedure.

Because of the shortage of trained pathologists, there are some areas in the country where it is simply impossible to obtain a competent postmortem examination. It is possible for the clinician to make a diagnosis of sudden infant death syndrome with a high degree of probability if the clinical picture is typical (previously well infant between the ages of 2 weeks and 10 months discovered lifeless during apparent sleep); postmortem x-ray, blood culture, and lumbar puncture, which are negative, serve as additional confirmatory evidence of sudden infant death syndrome. In such situations, one should be as certain as possible in providing a diagnosis to the family, not leaving them to agonize that some "will-o'-the-wisp" killed their baby.

"The doctor told me my baby died of crib death but something else was written on the death certificate." An incredible variety of diagnoses are listed on death certificates for so-called crib death. Some physicians use sudden infant death syndrome or an analogous term such as crib death not to mean the specific disease entity but rather to mean a death that occurred in a crib according to their own pet theory of cause. Some think that sudden infant death syndrome is caused by another disease and will prefer to use that disease as a cause on the death certificate (e.g., pneumonia, upper respiratory infection) either because they feel it is more scientifically correct or because they feel the parents need to be told something "more definite" than sudden infant death syndrome. We feel it is extremely important that parents know that their child died of a disease entity and advocate general use of the term "sudden infant death syndrome."[1]

My pathologist colleague, Dr. J. Bruce Beckwith, uses the following philosophy: "The diagnosis of sudden infant death syndrome at autopsy involves two issues— scientific and humanistic. It is necessary that one be willing to render a reasonably positive diagnosis immediately if effective counseling is to be accomplished. We, therefore, make a diagnosis of sudden infant death syndrome for *counseling purposes* on the basis of gross autopsies alone in the vast majority of instances. If subsequent work-up reveals additional information and we deem this important for the family to know, we so notify them. Usually our approach is to tell them that the infant did in fact die of sudden infant death syndrome, but in working up the case in detail, something was found which we feel they should know about. Usually this pertains if an unsuspected genetically determined condition is found."

"I didn't understand all that scientific stuff he was explaining to me." Many of us tend to talk to relieve our own anxiety when faced with oppressive gloom. "Therapeutic listening" is a difficult art to master. When families are in the shock state of grief, one should not attempt to impart much information. "Being there," physically and spiritually, is more important than what is said. The most vividly remembered event in the minds of Seattle area parents whose children died of sudden infant death

syndrome is the telephone call they receive from Dr. Beckwith after he performs the autopsy on their baby. Though the conversation may go on for 30 or 40 minutes, the highlights from the family's point of view are: (1) The pathologist actually called, (2) he said it was a real disease, and (3) he said we were not responsible. When parents ask, "Why did my baby die?" they are not talking about pathophysiologic mechanisms. Thus, a discussion of research theories is not appropriate during the initial grief period. The unsaid question is invariably, "What could I have done to prevent my child's death?" Reassurance must be repeatedly directed to this point.

A Seattle pediatrician lost her baby to sudden infant death syndrome in the past year and had an unusually severe grief-guilt reaction. This was alleviated only after she was treated as a grieving mother rather than as a fellow pediatrician. At one point she told me, "I know all about your research work but I can't get it out of my head that the baby suffocated."

I rarely discuss our scientific work with these parents. I say that "there are many theories, some of which seem to be more promising than others, but much more scientific research must be done; the cause of sudden infant death syndrome remains unknown." I classify theories about sudden infant death syndrome into those that are wicked and those that are benign. The wicked ones imply that the death could have been prevented by some action of the parent, such as diet, close observation during colds (whatever that means), whiplash injury, or, worst of all, child abuse. A special place in hell should be reserved for those who feel impelled to impose pet theories that aggravate guilt on newly bereaved parents.

"He kept wanting to tell us about his experiences with crib death rather than listen to ours." While physicians tend to lump patients into disease categories, parents see their children as individuals and often resent close comparisons. It is important to impart to parents that one is familiar with the disease entity and has in fact seen it before, but it is not necessary to go into details of other cases.

"He told me to get pregnant again right away." Dead children cannot be replaced. The physician's attempt to discuss future pregnancy during the initial grief period is usually bitterly resented. Genetic counseling is appropriate at a later stage but should be provided on the parents' rather than physician's initiative. When the subject does arise, I state the following: "Though sudden infant death syndrome is not an inherited disease, the risk in a subsequent child is *slightly* higher than in the normal population. The overall odds are 349 chances out of 350 that a baby will *not* die of sudden infant death syndrome. If the event has occurred already in a family, the odds are on the order of 345 chances out of 350 that a subsequent child will *not* succumb to sudden infant death syndrome."

Written information about sudden infant death syndrome is extremely helpful. Families can review the information at their leisure and also can give it to relatives and friends in lieu of answering the invariable questions. Initially, we give parents the blue brochure of the National Foundation for Sudden Infant Death, "Facts About SIDS." Later, when questions about future children arise, we recommend the pamphlet, "The Subsequent Child," by Carolyn Szybist.*

*Both pamphlets are available from the National Foundation for Sudden Infant Death, 1501 Broadway, New York, New York 10036.

"When I took my other child in to be checked, the doctor didn't even mention the child who died of crib death." Again, parents expect physicians to be infallible. They do not understand (why should they?) that the physician's reluctance to discuss painful material is because of his own discomfort. In our nationwide study of sudden infant death syndrome management, parents tended to be more grateful to nonprofessionals, such as policemen and firemen, for their sympathetic efforts, than to professionals such as physicians and nurses who maintained professional cool (distance). Also, many women received more support from their obstetricians than from their pediatricians. A reason that an obstetrician might be more comfortable talking about sudden infant death syndrome is that he might know the parents better and not feel any personal responsibility for "missing anything."

"We didn't get any help with what to say to the other children." The reactions to sudden infant death syndrome can be particularly devastating to siblings, as outlined by Friedman. Painful as it is, families must be encouraged to allay the invariable guilt feelings of siblings. When discussing a dead sibling with children, I employ the "third person option play" as recommended by Gould and Rothenberg.[4] This technique is an indirect way to explore sensitive subjects. For example, one says, "When a baby brother or sister like yours dies, some kids I know worry that they might have done something to cause it even if they don't talk about it. Does that make sense?" The child then has three options: (1) "No!" (2) "Yes, I imagine some kids might worry about that but I don't." (3) "Yes, and I'm glad you mentioned it." In either option, the frightening subject is exhumed in a nonthreatening manner.

SUMMARY

No greater opportunity for preventive psychiatry exists than in the management of sudden infant death syndrome. Proper management depends upon understanding of the basic grief-guilt reactions experienced by families. These reactions occur not only in sudden infant death syndrome but in other diseases characterized by overwhelming tragedy for which there is no time to prepare. Of paramount importance is the necessity for the physician to feel comfortable with his own feelings about death and willingness to function as one who comforts as well as heals.

REFERENCES

1 American Academy of Pediatrics, Committee on Infant and Preschool Child: A statement on the sudden infant death syndrome. Pediatrics, **50**:964–965, 1972.
2 Beckwith, J.B.: The sudden infant death syndrome. Current Problems in Pediatrics, III–8. Chicago, Illinois, Yearbook Medical Publishers, Inc., June, 1973.
3 Friedman, S.: Psychological aspects of sudden and unexpected deaths in infants and children," *Pediatric Clinics of North America,* **21**(1):103–111, February, 1974.
4 Gould, R.K., and Rothenberg, M.B.: The chronically ill child facing death—how can the pediatrician help? Clin. Pediat., **12**:447–449, 1973.

Chapter 27

After the Child Dies

J. Fischoff
N. O'Brien

Today the death of a child from an illness or accident is a relatively uncommon event in America, and yet in the not too distant past, adults, including parents whose child had died, were quite familiar with the fact of a child's death. This is not so today. Parents of a child who died tend to go through the psychic events of shock, mourning, confusion, and seeking an answer for the absolute or mystery after the child dies, in relative isolation with relatively little support from the family or community though they have each other.

Parents experience the death of their child in a way that is different from the death of their parents, brother, or sister. Becoming a parent is a unique event. The parents feel the loss of their child as if they have lost a part of themselves, which, indeed, they have. Although mourning is all pervasive and colors all other activities and thoughts, it may not be apparent to others after a period of several months. The mourning process will last for months or years with some parents, whereas some parents mourn for a lifetime if appropriate intervention is not forthcoming. The events surrounding the child's death are usually remembered with extreme clarity, as if permanently recorded on a photograph, and recalled over and over as is any overwhelming traumatic experience. The mental process of giving up the child who was recently alive proceeds very

Reprinted from *The Journal of Pediatrics*, 88(1):140–146, January 1976.

slowly. Parents often "hear" and "see" the child at fleeting intervals for months after the child dies.

The search for a "reason" why the child died and a search for the meaning of life and death, the absolute and the mystery, is present during the mourning process. Parents seek consolation, meaning, and faith from any source that is available. However, many parents mourn the loss of their child in isolation and solitude. We did not find, in a review of the literature, a description of the following type of intervention.

Since February, 1974, a group of couples from the metropolitan Detroit area have been meeting bi-monthly to share their individual experiences of losing a child. One couple started the group. They had lost their daughter in June, 1973. Six months later they were still searching for answers and meaning in their child's death. They called the chaplain at the hospital where their daughter had died and he gave them the names of other couples who had lost children. Within four weeks, four couples began meeting as a group. A few weeks later a hospital chaplain began meeting with them regularly.

The couples are self-selected and participate in open-ended discussions where nothing said is out of place. Through communications via newspapers, radio, chaplains, and couples themselves, approximately 35 couples have joined the group. Some attend regularly while others attend on an irregular basis. Some come with their spouses and some without. They feel free to discuss any aspect of their feelings toward their child's death and their ways of coping with it. They speak about the impending death, the death itself, the health professionals and their attitudes and involvements with them, the funerals, and the reactions of the siblings, friends, and relatives.

Some couples speak freely while others sit quietly and cry silently. Some speak about what occurred while the child was ill and dying while others speak about the events that occurred after the death. They talk about the mourning process, the trial of continuing to live, the feelings of isolation and depression, attempts at restitution, and the search to find the meaning of life and death.

When a new couple comes in, they, as a rule, take over the conversation immediately. Those couples who have attended before listen attentively, being aware that the new couple needs to have someone listen to them and needs to know someone else has also gone through this.

The following excerpts will illustrate what occurs in the group meetings.

WHILE THE CHILD IS DYING

That was a big shock to see my daughter on all the tubes and a respirator and a heart machine and whatever else she was on.

They kept him in an incubator and he was sweating. Oh, it was just a nightmare. He was very unique though. He was my son and I knew him, but I could not hold him nor tell him. . . . It was awful seeing him all hooked up. He was naked. It was like seeing your child crucified!

The doctor then told me, "We may save him for a few years, he may live to be five." I told him I have already gone through his death. If you give me five more years, I will be very grateful.

I prayed, Take her now! I never believed such a prayer could be uttered and I said it.

The thought that he may die anytime, it was terrible. I was walking this baby up and down in a room thinking, My God, this baby is going to die!

I remember asking the doctor, If the baby dies, what will he feel? Will there be pain? Will he suffocate?

He said, "This baby is fighting a battle, if it was just a little hole it could be patched up." It hit me like a bomb!

Then they told me the little one was gone. . . . God hates me!

. . . a tumor . . . , an unknown virus . . . , fibrosis . . . I wanted to hammer that tumor out.

Comments

Parents experience a wide variety of emotions and thoughts when they are told their child has a fatal illness and while he is dying. Though some thoughts and feelings such as shock and disbelief are somewhat predictable, many other responses occur within the context of the personality structure and past life experience of the parent. The pediatrician should expect individual differences—verbal, emotional, and physical—to manifest themselves. A parent may appear depressed, enraged, or deny the truth of what the physician has said. The pediatrician should not express surprise or pass judgment on the parents' utterances or behavior. The reality of the child's impending death cannot be denied and parents are bereft of hope. The pediatrician's role is to be supportive and this can be done with or without words, as the situation indicates.

REACTIONS AFTER THE CHILD'S DEATH

We were kind of on a fast track for maybe four or five months. It is kind of hard to slow down.

We go to the cemetery all the time. I think about all the changes I'm going through and I just can't get myself together for nothing.

I feel like screaming a lot of times. I feel like getting into my car and just going, where I don't know, just to go and get away.

We have an angel in heaven, now that feels good. But, it doesn't feel as good as seeing, touching, having him here.

I'd rather have a devil on earth than an angel in heaven.

I tell you one thing, you'll be scared, like she was saying, letting your children go out.

You forget so many things—like putting the wash away and making dinner.

I have wanted to die, I have really wanted to die, because so much of me has been buried.

There were times when I felt anger and disbelief and then one day I thought to myself, all I have are some clothes and a crib. Maybe God has something better, I don't know.

The times it hits me I just go off by myself and fight with it.

I had been so used to buying four items, and for a while I would actually forget, you know, and get four things, and I would just keep the other for myself.

I've been numb from my toes to my head and I can hardly breathe at night . . . . I have weird reactions, fantasies . . . . I'm scared. I have been a person I don't know.

Maybe the anger will last for a day, or two days. Maybe the depression will last for a month or two, maybe three or four. And then the denial, maybe it will last for an hour. But everybody goes through those different stages at a different pace.

Should we have another child? Would it be the same? . . . We had another child. Named the same . . . the other children want a replacement. Adopt!

I just don't want to go on. There are times when I'm suspended . . . . I think that the normal reaction after six months is that so many little things come up. There is such a gap between just knowing and really feeling all this.

There's this hopeful mother right up until a quarter to twelve and at 1:25, boom! Her child is dead! So really for months I felt like I was shot out of a cannon . . . there is no such thing as forgetting.

Comments

The length of time that parents are in shock and mourning can be and often is much longer than a few months. It is helpful, as a form of anticipatory guidance, for parents to be told by their pediatrician that they may feel dazed and depressed continuously or intermittently for quite some time and that they will think about the absent child and cry. It is helpful for the parents to hear from the pediatrician that they will feel numb, angry, guilty, think "unusual or strange" thoughts, wish they were dead, and experience waves of emotion or thoughts that seem intolerable and interminable. It is reassuring for parents to hear that they are not losing control of themselves when these events occur. It is helpful to know that their reactions are not unique, that they are not decompensating, and that with the passage of time these feelings will diminish.

MEMORIES

We just can't return to the hospital or to the scene of the accident.

I've overcome that. I volunteer in pediatrics several hours each week.

No way could I do that. . . . I can't drive by the high school, but I follow his class and graduation preparations.

The birthday of the child is traumatic. . . . If only I could fix his breakfast once more.

I supported that child. I took that child to school the first day. I took that child to the doctor. And now what the hell do I do?

Comments

The memories parents have of their child prior to his death and while he is dying are very poignant, vivid, and enduring. To give up the memories is to give up the child. The physician must be aware that at times the parents may seem to ruminate about the past. Certainly during the first year after the death, recalling the memories is not unusual and should be expected. It appears that the cycle of having lost a child for an entire year and then returning to the anniversary of the child's death has some significance. Facing the first year of birthdays, holidays, and vacations is extremely difficult for the parents. It seems, however, that once the parents have lived through the four seasons with all the memories, they will experience a sense of finality and acceptance when the anniversary of the child's death comes again and the child is not there. However, only with the passage of time will the parents be able to remember without pain.

SPOUSES

You can help her. If she wants to cry you have got to cry with her.

My wife had immediate acceptance. But me! I said to God, Why such a hurt? Why such a pain? Why did you call?

My husband is unable to come to this meeting—he has to get through this experience in silence.

Comment

Each parent can be expected to react to the child's death in his own way. To some degree they may be able to share their feelings, cry together, or sit silently together. On the other hand, it is important that the parents understand that their spouses will feel and express in a manner characteristic to himself in addition to having the same feelings. The more the parents share their bereavement the better it is for both. However, if parents are told that each will respond in an individual way, each will feel less distraught and isolated when the other does not react as expected.

GOD AND CLERGY

Then I told God to take the baby quickly so that he would not suffer.

After I lost my son, sometimes I would get up and walk out of church. I think it was resentment of God, really.

We called our pastor and explained our troubles. He said that it had already been four whole months and that we had better get to a psychiatrist fast.

Comment

Faith and belief in religion are sufficient to sustain some parents. At times the religious advisor is helpful, but when parents are told, "You had better go to a psychiatrist fast," or, "You didn't pray hard enough," they are not helpful. Many parents continue to feel frightened, depressed, and confused and find in the group what they did not find elsewhere. This by no means indicates that they lost faith in religion, but that the group serves as an additional source of support not available previously.

SIBLINGS

I've got three teen-agers and when they are down I have to go to them and tell them to go ahead and cry because I cry too. The teen-agers had a need to affirm that everything would return to normal. The teens always prayed . . . and then were the most turned off.

And my little one was in the car with me and said to me, "Mom, if I die can they make a head transplant so my sister will be better?"

And my older son was admitted to the hospital because of his nerves. Right now he is in and out of bed all night long, he can't sleep.

He's not coming home this time. "O.K." Anything else? "No." Then his brother took flight to the tree house. Solitude.

Comment

Many parents are aware that their surviving children require special attention and are sensitive to their needs. Children of various ages have specific needs. If these needs are not recognized and met, the children can decompensate in a variety of ways. They may regress, experience somatic symptoms, develop fears of impending death, isolate their feelings, or express anxiety in various forms of behavior. The pediatrician should alert parents that their children might respond in a number of ways to the death of a sibling. Verbal communication between the child and his parents should be encouraged. When parents and children share their feelings about the child's death, the task of mourning, painful at best, is shared and has the best opportunity for normal resolution.

HOSPITALS

You know, hospitals are very cold. They don't realize that parents panic, even more than the child.

My son was at the hospital an hour before he died. A nurse came out, and abruptly said, "He's gone," and I was totally shocked. I'm sitting in the waiting room thinking he probably broke a leg, wondering how long he's going to be out of school and, well, they come out and just dump it on you and go home.

If the doctors would ask the parents to stay at the hospital with their child to see if anything develops, would be better than sending the parents home.

Maybe because they see death every day, the doctors and nurses don't put the two together, but a parent and a child is another thing and they must realize this.

I think these doctors need the education, even if they have to go back to school to learn how, to talk to parents that have lost children, or to parents that are going to lose children.

My doctor stammered, foot to foot, sweating, deeply, personally involved. "The struggle is over for your daughter."

I talked to the older doctor first and he said, "This doctor is great but he's losing too many little ones and it's getting to him." The doctor of the terminally ill child hates to see them suffer, I think that's one of the hardest things for him to go through.

Your child has died but all this intense communication ends. We knew we would see the doctor about the autopsy and thank goodness there was that because I needed to talk to him again.

The pediatrician told me I would probably visualize the child, and talk back to the child. It happens at home, at the cemetery. I feel his presence. You gotta be prepared. Being informed was a help. I anticipated those reactions. We need the pediatrician and the clergy.

The doctor came out and told us that our son never came out of the coma. He was so cold-hearted, just like saying to me, "Well, your son is a vegetable."

What the doctor was trying to do was soften the blow which I appreciated.

He said, "Daddy, just tell them to leave me alone, I want to go to sleep," and the doctor pushed me out the door and pushed me out of the room and that was it.

I saw how afraid the nurses were of the dying patient.

The nurse let me go in and stay with her. She was in a coma, and I knew she was dying, and I didn't want them to keep telling me she was dying. I guess one nurse thought I was trying to avoid reality and felt she had to get through to me. She said, "Why don't you face up to it, your daughter is dying, she's almost dead, she's like, did you ever see a chicken with its head cut off, moving around sort of wild, that's how your daughter is, she's really dead."

And the nurse said, "The staff and I feel you have not come to accept the death of your child," and he had not died yet.

Comment

The parents had a wide variety of experiences with doctors, nurses, and the other hospital personnel. In acute situations parents feel helpless, ignorant, and frightened, and when the child dies after an acute or chronic illness or accident, the parents feel abandoned, lost, and confused. In either circumstance they are in need of appropriate emotional support, not random reactions by the doctors, nurses, and others. The great need appears to be for continuous education of the staff. The child with a terminal illness arouses a visceral response in staff which may be tempered by education, support, and advice by experienced, wise clinicians. When all is said and done, the ultimate crisis in human experience is one's own death or the death of a loved one. Children and parents deserve the best emotional support we can give and it is incumbent on staff to provide the support. It is our belief that the staff can be taught how to provide this care.

MOTHER AND CHILD

I think the first impression I got was that my daughter felt that she was being neglected. In other words, she felt we were too tied up with the loss of our son.

She wanted to talk Wednesday night but she didn't know how to say, "Mom, stay home, I need to talk," so she talked on Thursday and her conversation was, "Is there a God and will I go to heaven?" . . . and these kids have to have answers.

They want to know if you feel the same way they do, if you feel bad. They don't want to see a rock sitting there.

Comment

It is apparent that the dying child not only is willing but he has a need to talk to an adult, usually the mother, about death. The child needs to get close to someone and feel he is not alone. The child does not fear death as much as the threat of being abandoned. Pediatricians can tell parents that although they may not be able to answer all their children's questions, answers are not what the children need as much as talking to someone and realizing they are not alone.

When a child unburdens himself by sharing his worries, he may quickly terminate the discussion and turn to topics of everyday living and the realities of the everyday world. At the same time his mood may change very radically for the better because he has felt a close relationship with someone.

GROUP

We found it helps a lot to share our experiences, that's why we keep coming back to the meetings.

Sharing here together is so important. But even more important is giving support to each other at home.

Well, I certainly learned we've all experienced the same agony.

After six months our relatives had their own lives again.

But to the parent it just doesn't go away, it keeps popping right back in there, you need someone to talk to sometimes.

Even if we go to a meeting and we don't open our mouths, it's just nice being in the room with people who have gone through a fantastic trauma.

I was desperate. I went through the whole thing for months. You get to the point where you feel guilty letting your friends know this, because you don't want them to say to you, "Maybe you should go and see somebody."

Comment

The group provides a setting for sharing any and all experiences and feelings. Support of the group comes from knowing that all the members have undergone a similar and profound emotional experience and to some degree understand the others' feelings. The need to share, if only in silence, is self-evident. Parents speak about the isolation they feel several months after their child's death. Relatives and the community at large are not involved with how the parents feel and it is at this point, if not before, that their sense of isolation may be the greatest. The group, with its support, serves as a vehicle for sharing and attenuating the sense of isolation. The parents feel they are not alone even though there are no immediate answers to the loss of their child. However, as they share a common experience the blow is softened, the pain diminishes, and they gradually integrate the event into their life experience.

DISCUSSION

The parents of a child who dies may have inner resources to console and support themselves and one another during the mourning process. Some, in addition to having each other, have an extended family or relatives who are helpful. Parents may turn to pastors or counselors in the community for help, but as we have indicated a number of changes have occurred in our society so that the traditional sources of support are not readily available. Children die infrequently today in the United States in contrast to 40 years ago. In our very mobile society where 20 percent of the population move every year, very often the nuclear family must support itself without benefit of the extended family nearby. Owing to the factors of high mobility and relative infrequency of children's deaths, the parents, of a child who dies, often mourn in solitude and isolation.

This group of parents arose out of a spontaneous need for outside support. From its inception, other couples have taken the initiative to inquire and to eventually join. The needs of the parents are self-evident, indicating that such a group does help couples in mourning. The ready availability of the group allows parents to attend when they feel it is necessary. Some parents come regularly while others come irregularly. Some attend for prolonged periods of time while others attend intermittently. The group creates an atmosphere in which the parents feel that they are not abnormal and that they are entitled to their individual feelings. Nothing said is out of place. They become aware that other couples have gone through or are going through a similar mourning period while other couples may have mourned differently. Some couples listen quietly while others lend advice as to how they have coped with their loss. Any member is free to accept or reject any advice offered.

From its beginning, the group has grown via word of mouth, other couples, various media, and hospital communications. There have been inquiries from various parts of the United States and Canada regarding the group's formation, function, and operation and the possibility for one to begin elsewhere. From the inquiries, it is apparent that others see the group as being helpful to parents whose child has died.

The purpose of the paper is to inform pediatricians that the need for such a group may arise in their own practice or in their community and that from our experience this type of group is beneficial to parents.

In the words of the noted pioneer chest physician, Dr. Edward Livingston Trudeau: "The physician's duty is to heal sometimes, to relieve often, to comfort always."

APPENDIX

The following are the unedited transcripts of two mothers' experiences.

Mother I

The child is a real person and I felt that so much with my child, he was a baby three months old but I knew him so well. He could not talk to me but I knew who he was. You see this child and you shouldn't identify this child with the sickness he has. I will tell a story that has impressed me a great deal. I watched a movie in which a doctor, taking care of a girl dying of leukemia, got extremely involved with her and loved her very much. When the end came he couldn't take it any more and he just couldn't go into the room and face her. Another doctor came by and said, "You must learn to say good-bye," and so he got hold of himself and went in and the girl looked at him and she understood what was going through the doctor's mind and said to him, "I am not cancer, I am not leukemia, I am a person," and it made a tremendous point to me. I think it even helped me through this ordeal. When the doctors and nurses came to me saying, "He's going to die, he's very sick, he's a very sick child," I kept looking at him and all I could see was my son, a person whole, not defected, not dying, whole. What I mean by not dying is that I just saw the spirit of this child and to this day I'm with the assurance and hope that he's not dead. And, maybe his body is still gone apparently to us but there is more to human beings than the body and I think that's what sorrow is, it puts us all in awe of life. I saw doctors at the end that didn't even know my son was dying, they'd say, "Go home and don't worry about him." Although the doctors study many, many years about the functions of the body, the spirit is something you cannot capture. I guess that is what I wanted to share with you, to think of a child with love and compassion and never identify him with the sickness. You know, I feel badly and I wanted to join this group. I think you mentioned in your paper that a parent goes through a transformation when a child dies. There's something that happens to you that wouldn't happen otherwise. He was such a beautiful child. And really that is maybe the most creative moment in anybody's life.

To make it easy for the parents, I think a lot of clarification would be helpful, when you do something don't say, "Something has to be done, the doctors ordered it." If you would explain just a little bit about it, the parents wouldn't be so nervous about it. And don't chase the parents away, although it is very painful for them. I don't think you can make the pain any less, but to chase the parents away when the child is suffering, when the parent wants to be there and be with the child, I think it's unfair. There's a tremendous bond that shouldn't be cut, that shouldn't even be taken for granted.

Mother II

So I'll tell you my experience, it's very personal, it's a mother's feelings and it was kind of stupid, of how filled with hope we were. Our daughter was diagnosed eighteen months before she died as having myocardiopathy. Our doctor was a man of great hope, and of course you don't have to give a parent much hope. They just take the first straw of hope that's there and they just run off with it and with me I could really build a straw of hope into an oak tree. I was very optimistic. You just never think it's going to happen to you. In fact you don't even think of a child dying. She was in the hospital and on the second night I was at home with my husband and I remember saying, You don't think she could die do you? He answered me with, "You don't think she could do you?" and really that was the first time we had approached it and really that wasn't much of an approach because we both just dropped it. I really don't think that my husband and I lack in communication, that just goes to show that we really were filled with hope. Well, when our daughter did die she was never termed a terminal patient. She didn't have leukemia, she didn't have a brain tumor. Really no medical person could say "Your daughter is terminal" because she could go on. And of course I just took that aspect of it. I stayed the first night with her. I was there about 24 hours. I came back that Friday morning. There were some delays early in the morning so I guess I wasn't there as early as I wanted. It was really late. She was always very considerate of me. She never really reproached me. She never really reproached any-one even when she was in pain. And she had a lot of suffering for that last month. So that morning I came in with my usual rah rah attitude, you know, "what can I do to make you happy today" and entertain the mind. She was a child, and I was aware that I had to keep her mind busy. She did very well in school. In April or May, she had taken an IQ test, the computer just ran out of paper it was so high. But she was just a regular kid, so I was always thinking of things to keep her up, because I knew she was down. I turned on the TV and she said, "Mom, I want you to hold me," and I did. She was in my arms and she wasn't interested in the TV so we turned it off. Then she said, "I have to get back in bed to find a place to breathe better." She had been in an oxygen tent and it frustrated her so much. I think that day she was allowed a few minutes out of it and I started reading aloud, and I said let's read *Winnie the Pooh*, one of her favorite books. I started out and she said she wanted me to hold her again. Of course what we were going through were her stages of congestive heart failure. I had heard that the child starts going into a fetal position to make himself more com-fortable to breathe. She started calling for more oxygen. Then I realized she was going through the oppression that one might feel when they are going to die, and of course she wanted the only thing in the world that counted, her mother to hold her and be close to her. But I wasn't picking this up and I just wasn't picking up the signals until I saw her moving around and calling for the oxygen. Then the nurse came and turned up the oxygen. My daughter called for more and the nurse came back and said, "It doesn't go up any further," and she heard this and she looked up at me and said, "I'm going to die. Am I going to die?" She asked me the question and answered it herself so really she kind of prepared me. And of course I figured out times afterward what I wasn't aware of. So then I started talking to her. I made up a story of long lost words and perhaps since she had asked the question and she had answered it, I figured that was it, and we were both in the same boat of knowledge. I told her she was God's child, that He had just given her to us as a loan to take care of as best we could, that He wanted her back and that He was really the one who made her and loved her and He was going to take care of her, and I talked to her about this for quite a while. This is a child, remember, who was not in a coma, who died with the brain going right to the last minute, and absorbed everything, and when the audio was going I knew she could still hear me so I had until 1:25 to say something that would go with her into eternity. I really felt that she prayed. She listened to everything I said. She said three sentences that have comforted me and will comfort me until the day I die and I hope I will say the same three sentences when I die. This was a beautiful thing for a mother. She said, "I love you God, I'm sorry for my sins, and please don't let me die." I didn't realize she had any concept of sin but this is all part of training, but the fact she said I love you, God, first, and she was really short of breath. I held her for about an hour and I held her a long time after she died and nobody made me budge. I stayed in that room with her about 40 or 50 minutes after she died and it was really neat. But my little girl did have a message. She has a message for me, she has a message for everybody here: the only thing when the chips are down that really matters is kindness. That's the only thing that matters. You can spell it anyway you want. Some people say love, some say compassion but when you act it out what is it, it's kindness. and that's the only thing you can give to this person that's dying. She didn't need anymore needles, anymore tests, or anymore anything. What she did ask, was for me just to be with her and hold her, and that's the message. When the chips are down what else have you got—it's one human being communicating with another and it's time to get that person ready for the absolute. It depends on your faith. I guess, I'm not sure. That's all I have to say, just be kind. And to you who are professionals, to you who have been in this hospital all day long with sick kids and dying kids, I know you have to go home at night and live with yourself and your own family and it's hard. I know you have to turn it off but please, in educating yourself to turn it off, so you can carry on your normal life and carry on functions that you have to do, please don't stifle your compassions, or your kindness.

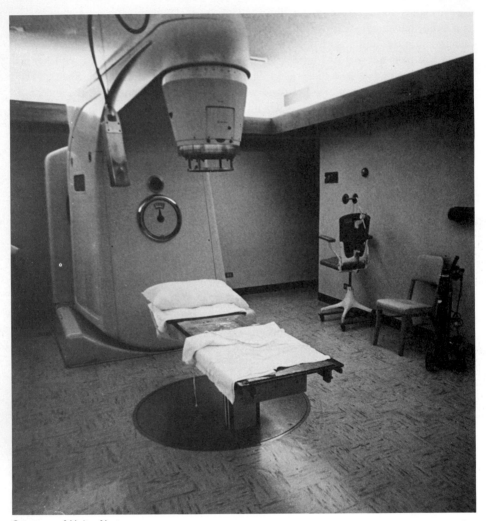

Courtesy of Helen Nestor

Part 7

Specific Issues

Chapter 28

Notes of a Biology Watcher: The Long Habit

Lewis Thomas

We continue to share with our remotest ancestors the most tangled and evasive attitudes about death, despite the great distance we have come in understanding some of the profound aspects of biology. We have as much distaste for talking about personal death as for thinking about it; it is an indelicacy, like talking in mixed company about venereal disease or abortion in the old days. Death on a grand scale does not bother us in the same special way: we can sit around a dinner table and discuss war, involving 60 million volatilized human deaths, as though we were talking about bad weather; we can watch abrupt bloody death every day, in color, on films and television, without blinking back a tear. It is when the numbers of dead are very small, and very close, that we begin to think in scurrying circles. At the very center of the problem is the naked cold deadness of one's own self, the only reality in nature of which we can have absolute certainty, and it is unmentionable, unthinkable. We may be even less willing to face the issue at first hand than our predecessors because of a secret new hope that maybe it will go away. We like to think, hiding the thought, that with all the marvelous ways in which we seem now to lead nature around by the nose, perhaps we can avoid the central problem if we just become, next year, say, a bit smarter.

"The long habit of living," said Thomas Browne, "indisposeth us to dying." These days, the habit has become an addiction: we are hooked on living; the tenacity of its

Reprinted from *The New England Journal of Medicine*, **286**(15):825–826, April 13, 1972.

grip on us, and ours on it, grows in intensity. We cannot think of giving it up, even when living loses its zest—even when we have lost the zest for zest.

We have come a long way in our technologic capacity to put death off, and it is imaginable that we might learn to stall it for even longer periods, perhaps matching the life-spans of the Abkhasian Russians, who are said to go on, springily, for a century and a half. If we can rid ourselves of some of our chronic, degenerative diseases, and cancer, strokes and coronaries, we might go on and on. It sounds attractive and reasonable, but it is no certainty. If we became free of disease, we would make a much better run of it for the last decade or so, but might still terminate on about the same schedule as now. We may be like the genetically different lines of mice, or like Hayflick's different tissue-culture lines, programmed to die after a predetermined number of days, clocked by their genomes. If this is the way it is, some of us will continue to wear out and come unhinged in the sixth decade, and some much later, depending on genetic timetables.

If we ever do achieve freedom from most of today's diseases, or even complete freedom from disease, we will perhaps terminate by drying out and blowing away on a light breeze, but we will still die.

Most of my friends do not like this way of looking at it. They prefer to take it for granted that we only die because we get sick, with one lethal ailment or another, and if we did not have our diseases we might go on indefinitely. Even biologists choose to think this about themselves, despite the evidences of the absolute inevitability of death that surround their professional lives. Everything dies, all around, trees, planktons, lichens, mice, whales, flies, mitochondria. In the simplest creatures it is sometimes difficult to see it as death, since the strands of replicating DNA they leave behind are more conspicuously the living parts of themselves than with us (not that it is fundamentally any different, but it seems so). Flies do not develop a ward round of diseases that carry them off, one by one. They simply age, and die, like flies.

We hanker to go on, even in the face of plain evidence that long, long lives are not necessarily pleasurable in the kind of society we have arranged thus far. We will be lucky if we can postpone the search for new technologies for a while, until we have discovered some satisfactory things to do with the extra time. Something will surely have to be found to take the place of sitting on the porch reexamining one's watch.

Perhaps we would not be so anxious to prolong life if we did not detest so much the sickness of withdrawal. It is astonishing how little information we have about this universal process, with all the other dazzling advances in biology. It is almost as though we wanted not to know about it. Even if we could imagine the act of death in isolation, without any preliminary stage of being struck down by disease, we would be fearful of it.

There are signs that medicine may be taking a new interest in the process, partly from interest, partly from an embarrassed realization that we have not been handling this aspect of disease with as much skill as physicians once displayed, back in the days before they became convinced that disease was their solitary and sometimes defeatable enemy. It used to be the hardest and most important of all the services of a good doctor to be on hand at the time of death, and to provide comfort, usually in the home. Now it is done in hospitals, in secrecy (one of the reasons for the increased fear of death these days may be that so many people are totally unfamiliar with it; they never actually see it happen in real life). Some of our technology permits us to deny its existence, and we maintain flickers of life for long stretches in one community of cells or another, as though we were keeping a flag flying. Death is not a sudden-all-at-once affair; cells go down in sequence, one by one. You can, if you like, recover great numbers of them many hours after the lights have gone out, and grow them out in cultures. It takes hours, even days, before the irreversible word finally gets around to all the provinces.

We may be about to rediscover that dying is not such a bad thing to do after all. Sir William Osler took this view; he disapproved of people who spoke of the agony of death, maintaining that there was no such thing.

In a 19th-century memoir about an expedition in Africa, there is a story about an explorer who was caught by a lion, crushed across the chest in the animal's great jaws, and saved in the instant by a lucky shot from a friend. Later, he remembered the episode in clear detail. He was so amazed by the extraordinary sense of peace and calm, and total painlessness, associated with his partial experience of being killed, that he constructed a theory that all creatures are provided with a protective physiologic mechanism, switched on at the verge of death, carrying them through in a haze of tranquility.

I have seen agony in death only once, in a patient with rabies, who remained acutely aware of every stage in the process of his own disintegration over a 24-hour period, right up to his final moment. It was as though, in the special neuropathology of rabies, the switch had been prevented from turning.

We will be having new opportunities to learn more about the physiology of death at first hand, from the increasing numbers of cardiac patients who have been through the whole process and then back again. Judging from what has been found out thus far, from the first generation of people resuscitated from cardiac standstill (already termed the Lazarus syndrome), Osler seems to have been right. Those who remember parts or all of their episodes do not recall any fear, or anguish. Several people who remained conscious throughout, while appearing to have been quite dead, could only describe a remarkable sensation of detachment. One man underwent coronary occlusion with cessation of the heart and dropped for all practical purposes dead, in front of a hospital, and within a few minutes his heart had been restarted by electrodes and he breathed his way back into life. According to his account, the strangest thing was that there were so many people around him, moving so urgently, handling his body with such excitement, while all his awareness was of quietude.

In a recent study of the reaction to dying in patients with obstructive disease of the lungs, it was concluded that the process was considerably more shattering for the professional observers than the observed. Most of the patients appeared to be preparing themselves with equanimity for death, as though intuitively familiar with the business. One elderly woman reported that the only painful and distressing part of the process was in being interrupted; on several occasions she was provided with conventional therapeutic measures to maintain oxygenation or restore fluids and electrolytes, and each time she found the experience of coming back harrowing; she deeply resented the interference with her dying.

I find myself surprised by the thought that dying is an all-right thing to do, but perhaps it should not surprise. It is, after all, the most ancient and fundamental of biologic functions, with its mechanisms worked out with the same attention to detail, the same provision for the advantage of the organism, the same abundance of genetic information for guidance through the stages, that we have long since become accustomed to finding in all the crucial acts of living.

Very well. But even so, if the transformation is a co-ordinated, integrated physiologic process in its initial, local stages, there is still that permanent vanishing of consciousness to be accounted for. Are we to be stuck forever with this problem? Where on earth does it go? Is it simply stopped dead in its tracks, lost in humus, wasted? Considering the tendency of nature to find uses for complex and intricate mechanisms, this seems to me unnatural. I prefer to think of it as somehow separated off at the filaments of its attachment, and then drawn like an easy breath back into the membrane of its origin, a fresh memory for a biospherical nervous system, but I have no data on the matter.

This is for another science, another day. It may turn out, as some scientists suggest, that we are forever precluded from investigating consciousness, by a sort of indeterminacy principle that stipulates that the very act of looking will make it twitch and blur out of sight. If this is true, we will never learn. I envy some of my friends who are convinced about telepathy; oddly enough, it is my European scientist acquaintances who believe it most freely and take it most lightly. All their aunts have received Communications, and there they sit, with proof of the motility of consciousness at their fingertips, and the making of a new science. It is discouraging to have had the wrong aunts, and never the ghost of a message.

Chapter 29

Reflections on Life and Death

Ernlé W. D. Young

I will suggest there is a difference between extending life and prolonging death. Yet, it must be recognized there are physicians who (in practice, at least) seem not to be aware of this distinction. For them, life may be represented diagrammatically (Figure 1) as a continuum between birth (X) and death (Y) without any intervening point (Z) at which the process of dying may be said to have begun. Since no point Z is discerned, any discrimination between extending life (the X-Z line) and prolonging death (the Z-Y line) is excluded de facto.

For those who see life only in terms of the X-Y continuum, medical care inevitably takes the form of the unrelenting attempt to cure—irrespective of the fact that the treatment may be more detrimental to the patient's total well-being than the disease itself. This appears to be the present policy of some physicians. It was the explicit philosophy of the late Dr. David A. Karnofsky (Class '40) of the Sloan-Kettering Institute for Cancer Research, to adduce a concrete example. Karnofsky enthusiastically advocated continuous "aggressive or extraordinary means of treatment," in the

Reprinted from *Stanford M.D.*, **15**(1):20–24, Winter 1976.

Figure 1

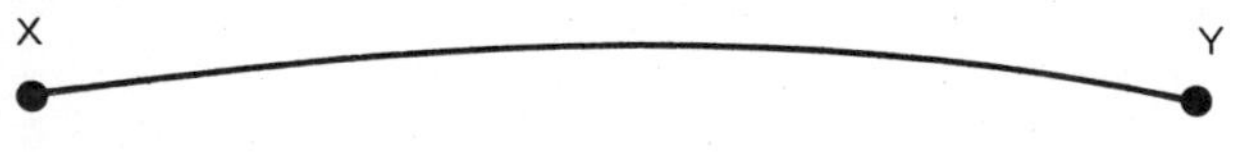

X   Y

belief that "the medical imperative . . . is to apply one temporary relief after another, stretching the life of a patient with cancer of the large bowel to ten months who would have died within weeks if any one massive remedy had not been used."[1] As Karnofsky himself wrote:

> The sense of mission . . . is diminished (by) the view that the fight against cancer should not be continuously waged on all sectors.
> The achievements and triumphs that may occur in the fight against cancer will come from doctors who do too much—who continue to treat the patient when the odds may appear overwhelming—and not from those who do too little.
> The physicians . . . can learn a great deal from the study of these patients. . . . In facing every challenge, even if doctors usually fail, they are kept in training to handle the remediable situations more effectively.[2]

We shall offer a critique of this view of medical care later. However, it may be of interest to note that the physician's "duty" always to seek to preserve life is being called into question by many doctors for whom this obligation once represented the cornerstone of their professional ethic.[3]

Now let us turn to those who do intuit that there is a distinction between extending life and prolonging death—however difficult it may be to define empirically and thus locate precisely. For such physicians there is, discernibly, a point Z along the curve X-Y (Figure 2) where the dying process may be regarded as having begun. Let it be frankly acknowledged that only an experienced clinician can fix a point Z along the line X-Y—and then only in a highly imprecise way, by means of "educated guesswork." From a medical perspective, point Z may be said to have arrived when irreversible damage is observed in any one of the human life-support systems.[4] From a theological standpoint, if a central constituent of the *humanum* be the capacity for autonomous self-determination and responsiveness to others in faith, hope, and love (to offer a rough definition), then point Z could be said to have occurred once that capacity were irrevocably lost.

Difficult though it may be to locate point Z exactly, once the possibility of there being such a decisive turning point is admitted, it does make sense to differentiate between extending life and prolonging death. Then options in terms of the care of the dying patient other than the unyielding determination to cure become apparent— and these lead us to the heart of the "euthanasia debate." From X-Z, the obligation to care will require that the physician do everything humanly possible to cure the

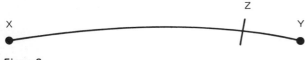

Figure 2

patient's disease. Not to do so would be negligence. However, from Z-Y at least four other alternatives to "cure" may be delineated:

1 Allowing the disease to take its course while providing only palliative drug therapy for pain (benemortasia);[5]
2 Withdrawing a regimen of treatment already begun so that the patient may die peacefully (euthanasia);
3 Doing something to the patient to end her or his life ("mercy" killing); and
4 Allowing the patient to take her or his own life (suicide).

Before we explore these four options I would insist, with Paul Ramsey, that, whichever we choose, it is our additional obligation, from Z-Y, to "company with" the dying person as an expression of care. It is regrettable that we, the living, are often so threatened by death that—psychologically as well as physically—we isolate or abandon the dying. Persons journeying from Z-Y are frequently wheeled into the most remote rooms on our units and left to do their dying in more or less lonely segregation from friends, family members, nurses, doctors, and even ministers, who devote progressively less attention to them as persons. Part of what it means to *care* for those between points Z and Y is to surround them with love, and life, and even laughter, so that their final passage may be an experience, not of loneliness and loss, but of the warmth and strength of the companionship of their fellows. That is the enlightened modus operandum of the St. Christopher's Hospice in London, and of similar institutions coming into being in this country. Paul Ramsey has long been an advocate of "companying with" the dying as a form of care, and his sentiments are therefore worth quoting:

> It can certainly be said that our duties to the dying differ radically from our duties to the living. Just as it would be negligence to the sick to treat them as if they were about to die, so it is another sort of "negligence" to treat the dying as if they were going to get well. The right medical practice will provide those who may get well with the assistance they need, and it will provide those who are dying with the care and assistance they need in their final passage.[6]

1. *Benemortasia* signifies a good death resulting from a disease or disability simply being allowed to take its course or have its effect, while providing the patient with palliative drug treatment for pain, without any therapeutic intent. Pneumonia is often called "the old man's friend." Benemortasia would be practiced when, instead of treating the pneumonia in a patient also suffering from terminal metastatic melanoma of the brain in a comatose condition, the pneumonia were simply allowed to take the patient's life. To attempt to cure a 9-year-old victim of leukemia is both justifiable and laudable. But it might not be so if the patient were 90 years of age, whose life-span could only be extended by a few months through treatments that are far more deleterious than the leukemia itself.

2. *Euthanasia.* Advances in medical technology are in large part responsible for the emergent possibility of euthanasia. Prior to our being able to treat incurable diseases, the real alternatives were benemortasia (that which used to be called euthanasia),

"mercy" killing, or suicide. But now, increasingly, we have the power to extend life (as well as prolong death) by treating once-fatal illnesses. Euthanasia thus becomes an option for someone who, from X-Z, is being treated for an incurable disease, but who, once point Z has arrived and the journey from Z-Y has been started, wishes no longer to be treated but presses the right to die in peace. I, for one, am glad and grateful that more and more physicians are willing to agree to this type of euthanasia—where the patient clearly desires this alternative form of care to be adopted.

For example, Mr. R. S. was a 68-year-old man with leukemia. Had he been 88, to have attempted to treat his disease would have made little sense. Being 65 when the disease was first diagnosed, vigorous chemotherapy was offered him and this extended his life three years, with a "quality of life" of an acceptably high level. But then, three weeks before his death, he announced that the side effects of the treatment were more burdensome than the disease itself, and he wished to be allowed to die peacefully. He and his wife and family had completed all their "unfinished business"; furthermore, they concurred with him in his wanting the treatment to be discontinued. The attending physicians, with enlightened understanding of what was in the patient's best interests, agreed to stop treating him. They prescribed a good scotch whiskey, three times a day, for his pain. Surrounded by Mozart's music— which he had grown to love since the onset of his leukemia—Mr. R. S. died as he had wished just three weeks after making his feelings known. Technically, this was euthanasia—for life-sustaining measures were withdrawn in order that he might have a good death.

The decision to practice euthanasia—as an expression of care—is infinitely more difficult where the patient is too tiny or too sick to participate in the decision. Then the parents (in the case of an infant) or family (in the case of an adult), together with the physician, have a far more onerous role. Then, understandably, physicians will tend to be more than usually defensive in their practice of medicine. The so-called "living will,"[7] though not yet a legal document, may be of considerable help to physicians in arriving at a decision with which they can be comfortable—especially if it is regularly updated, so that the intentions of a patient over a span of years is clearly evidenced. But this presupposes a continuing physician-patient relationship. Regrettably, such continuing relationships are rare almost to the point of being nonexistent, at least so far as our major medical centers (which have the most sophisticated technology) are concerned.

3. *"Mercy" killing.* As the name implies, this means doing something to kill the patient. The presumption is that this is done for reasons of mercy—though this presumption will have to be called into question later. Dr. Vincent A. Montemarano was accused of killing Eugene Bauer, a terminally ill cancer patient, on December 17, 1972, at the Nassau County Medical Center by injecting potassium chloride into his arm.[8] Lester Zygmaniak was similarly accused of killing his brother, George (paralyzed in a motorcycle accident):

> Lester testified he told his brother: "I am here to end your pain." I walked over to the room, looked in and saw my brother. I asked him if he was in pain, a lot of pain. He nodded: "Yes." Then, according to Lester's testimony he shot his brother

with a sawed-off shotgun once in the head, and, after he had put his hand on his brother's heart said: "God bless you, George, I'm sorry it had to happen like this." George died 27 hours later.[9]

Mercy killing is clearly illegal, but no one prosecuted for mercy killing in this country has ever been convicted. In all cases those charged have been acquitted.

Although there is a legal difference between killing and letting die, there are those who argue there is no moral difference between these two options. Writing recently in the *New England Journal of Medicine*, James Rachels concludes:

> I have argued that killing is not in itself any worse than letting die; if my contention is right, it follows that active (mercy killing) is not any worse than passive euthanasia.[10]

Other writers, such as Karl Barth, take a very different view:

> It can hardly be said of this form of deliberate killing that it can ever seem to be really commanded by any emergency, and therefore to be anything but murder.[11]

These conflicting views will have to weighed in the critical part of this paper.

4. *Suicide.* The fourth possible way of expressing care for the patient journeying between points Z-Y on the diagram (Figure 2) is that of allowing the individual to take her or his own life. There is a difference between allowing and enabling suicide. For a physician or nurse to enable a patient to commit suicide would, strictly speaking, be a form of "mercy" killing. To allow a patient that "right" is simply to recognize the inviolable autonomy of the individual—a principle which has acquired semi-religious sanctions and stature in our "emancipated" era.

How are we to decide between these four alternatives—benemortasia, euthanasia, "mercy" killing, and allowing the patient to commit suicide—and the view which urges that care should take the form of the attempt to cure from X-Y? What are we to make of all five practices from an ethical standpoint? To these questions, and to the necessary work of ethical criticism which they entail, we must now turn.

The belief that care should take the form of a determined and stubborn attempt to cure has much, on the surface, to commend it. It is arguable, for example, that cancer is one of the principal scourges of humankind, that breakthroughs in the fight against disease are constantly occurring, and that for advances to be made in medicine, experimental data must be accumulated. That the accumulation of data may cause the patient more suffering than the disease itself is offset by the prospect of alleviating the suffering of great numbers of future patients.

Underlying this argument are certain values. From my own point of view, any ethic which reduces persons from ends in themselves to mere means, or which argues that the end justifies the means, is highly suspect.

The difference between benemortasia and euthanasia is that of doing or not doing—in the first place--what medical technology has made it possible for us to do. Until fairly recently, technology was so highly valued that there was a widespread assumption that what could be done should be done. If a patient was brought into the emergency room with cardiac arrest, that heart could—and therefore automatically would—be started again; only later when irreversible brain damage was seen to have occurred, would the questions be asked, "Why didn't we simply allow the patient to die?" and, "Can we now take this patient off the machines (i.e., perform euthanasia)?" The advocates of benemortasia question whether the stopped heart ought always and inevitably be made to beat again. That this view is gaining acceptance, that we are no longer automatically doing what it is within our power to do, is a welcome indication that the technological imperative—always to do what can be done—is, at least by many, being called seriously into question.

The difference between benemortasia (where the patient is in a position to request that no treatment be begun) and suicide is in one's point of view. For those who accept the technological imperative, there will be no difference: to refuse treatment is a form of suicide. But for those who cannot accept the technological imperative, the difference between benemortasia and suicide is perceived at the level of intention: the primary intention in refusing treatment is the avoidance of something possibly more burdensome than the disease itself (a life of enormously diminished quality), with the second consequence being the patient's death; the primary intention in suicide (in a situation of terminal illness) is death as a release from suffering (either that of the patient or his family).

What about euthanasia? Where the patient is sufficiently conscious to request that a regimen of treatment be now discontinued, or where, though unconscious, the patient has, by an instrument such as the so-called euthanasia will, made his wishes clear over a number of years, then deciding to comply with this wish is very much easier for both family and physician. For them, all that will be required will be a recognition that:

> Our first responsibility is not to save a physical life and then only later to worry about the whole person. Our first responsibility is to take into consideration the person's wholeness—involving emotions and significant relationships—at each step of the way. Our first responsibility is to care. This is even more basic than curing, and acts of care will center principally upon the person rather than principally upon the disease.[12]

However, if the patient is comatose, and has left no long-term indication of how she or he would want to be cared for in these circumstances, the physician's responsibility is far more onerous. Most physicians take the position—and I tend to concur with them—that until irreversible damage has occurred to one or other of the body's life support systems treatment cannot under any circumstances be discontinued. Once point Z has clearly (and empirically) arrived, euthanasia—where this accords with the family's wishes as well as their understanding of what the patient would want—is a moral option.

The distinction between "letting die," in this sense, and negligence is twofold. On the one hand, the question is, "Has point Z discernibly arrived or not?" If it has not, to discontinue treatment would be negligence; if it has, then Nelson's principle (quoted above) clearly applies. And on the other hand, the difference again lies at the level of intention. In a case of negligence, intention (negatively stated) is not to care. In euthanasia, the intention is to care, not by continuing a now useless regimen of treatment, but by respecting the integrity of the whole person.

Is there a moral difference between euthanasia and "mercy" killing, between "letting die" and actively doing something to end the patient's life? I take issue with Rachels in asserting that there is.[13] Any action includes at least three components: the intention, the means used to accomplish it, and the consequences which result. Ethics takes account of all three components together. Intention and consequences cannot be excluded from the discussion (as Rachels excludes them) in order to arrive at the conclusion that one means of ending the life of a suffering patient (letting the patient die) is the same as another (killing the patient). The intention may well be one of mercy in a case of "mercy" killing. But the intention could well be quite different.

> Originally, in the trial that began January 14, 1974, Cahn, the prosecuting district attorney, had characterized the death of Eugene Bauer as "a mercy killing." Later, however, he described the death as a "murder of convenience" so that Montemarano would not have to return that night to pronounce the death of the man.[14]

Equally, the intention in a so-called mercy killing could be to collect on an insurance policy, to avoid one's own pain, or to reduce mounting medical costs. Killing cuts short the possibility of testing intentionality; letting die allows time for assessing the motivation of all parties involved.

The means used to end life have uneven moral calibrations. Generally speaking, ethics is happier with means having a so-called double effect than with means that have a single effect: the death of the patient. Morphine would be a "double effect" means: the primary effect is the amelioration of pain; the secondary effect is that of shortening the patient's life. Such a "double effect" means recognizes that life itself has not an *absolute* value; that the expression of compassion (administering the drug to relieve suffering) justifies the concomitant reduction of the patient's lifespan. This is morally more acceptable than a means with only one effect: a revolver, a dose of cyanide, a stick of dynamite under the bed. The closer a means comes to expressing care, the more acceptable it is to the Judaeo-Christian ethic; the nearer a means comes to expressing what could be interpreted as a violent or murderous intention, the less acceptable.

The consequences for the patient might well be the same, whether we allowed the patient to die or killed him. But the consequences for society could be vastly different. In a recent article, John Fletcher mentions three. One is the "potential brutalization of those who participate in (mercy killing)." A second is a straining (if not a tearing) of the delicate fabric of trust which binds physicians and patients together. And a third would be the depletion of the reservoir of compassion so slowly and painstakingly accumulated in our Western culture. If those deserving of our compassion and succor were simply killed, then the reservoir of concern for others would dry up, and society as a whole would be immeasurably poorer. Fletcher concludes that:

The crucial difference between "mercy" killing and allowing to die is that the self-restraint imposed by the latter choice is more consistent with ethical and legal norms that physicians . . . do no harm.[15]

The present legal posture of this country towards "mercy" killing seems to me to be eminently sound: unambiguous sanctions against "mercy" killing (because of the difficulty of knowing precisely the intentions behind and the consequences of the act), coupled with as compassionate and lenient treatment as possible of those who—genuinely for mercy's sake—have killed another human being to end her or his suffering.[16]

The fourth, and final, option in terms of caring for those travelling between points Z and Y on our diagram is that of allowing them the right to commit suicide. While suicide has, in the West, traditionally been thought of as a "cop out"—an act of cowardice—or as a final, defiant expression of absolute autonomy, it is capable of other interpretations. It can result from the loss of any sense of meaning in what is happening (faith), any sense of there being potentially creative future options left (hope), and any sense that others care (love). Or it can be an act of heroic self-sacrifice, taking one's own life so that others may be spared agonizing emotional suffering or crippling financial burdens.

Speaking as a theologian, I am compelled to say that it is not our business to be moralistic or judgmental about those for whom the only recourse left them seems to be that of taking their own lives. It is our duty to strive to prevent the loss of others' faith, hope, and love—by caring for them continuously and conscientiously as *whole* persons—not as "one-dimensional" beings. It is also incumbent upon us to recognize that some things are more precious than life itself: the desire to set another's well-being above one's own, among them.[17] However, I agree with John Bennett when he asserts:

Without seeing it as my duty to pass judgment on others, I do not favor suicide as anything but a last resort in the gravest of situations.[18]

Certainly, to involve the physician, the nurse, or even a member of the family in the patient's suicide would be unthinkable. Almost by definition, the decision to commit suicide and to carry through with that decision is profoundly personal. To involve another human being either in the decision or in carrying it out represents the abdication of the very autonomy which the act itself finally claims. Those who take this desperate step deserve our compassion, our understanding, and our nonjudgmental love. But they may not demand—so far as the act itself is concerned—our help.

NOTES

[1] To quote the paraphrase of Karnofsky's position presented by Paul Ramsey in *The Patient as Person*, Yale University Press, New Haven and London, p. 147.

[2] Karnofsky, David A., Why Prolong the Life of a Patient with Advanced Cancer? *Cancer Journal for Clinicians*, No. 10, January-February 1960, p. 10.

[3] Reich, Walter, The Physician's 'Duty' to Preserve Life, *The Hastings Center Report*, Vol. 5, No. 2, April 1975, p. 15.

[4] Such physical "life-support systems" would be, for example, the body's cerebral, renal, or respiratory functions.

[5] The word "benemortasia" was coined, so far as I am aware, by Arthur J. Dyck in An Alternative to the Ethic of Euthanasia, *To Live and To Die: When, Why, and How*, ed. by Robert H. Williams, Springer-Verlag, New York, 1973. Since the term "euthanasia" (from the Greek words "eu," good, and "thanatos," death) has come to mean good death caused by someone stopping a treatment once started, Dyck goes back to the Latin equivalents ("bene," good and "mort," death) for a word that designates a good death resulting, not from the cessation of therapeutic efforts, but simply from the disease itself.

[6] Ramsey, op. cit., p. 133.

[7] The best known "living will" is that prepared by the Euthanasia Educational Council, 250 West 57th Street, New York, N.Y. 10019. Draft legislation on euthanasia is, to my knowledge, before the house in three states: West Virginia, Florida, and Idaho. None of these three drafts have yet become law.

[8] Reported in the *Palo Alto Times*, June 28, 1973, p. 2.

[9] Reported in the *Palo Alto Times*, November 6, 1973.

[10] Rachels, James, Active and Passive Euthanasia, *The New England Journal of Medicine*, Vol. 292, No. 2, January 9, 1975, pp. 78–80.

[11] Barth, Karl, *Church Dogmatics III. 4*, T & T Clark, Edinburgh, 1961, p. 427.

[12] Nelson, James B., *Human Medicine*, Augsburg Publishing House, Minneapolis, Minnesota, 1973, p. 133.

[13] See my letter in *The New England Journal of Medicine*, Vol. 292, No. 16, April 17, 1975.

[14] Reported in the *Palo Alto Times,* February 6, 1974.

[15] Fletcher, John, Abortion, Euthanasia, and Care of Defective Newborns, *The New England Journal of Medicine*, Vol. 292, No. 2, January 9, 1975, p. 77.

[16] It is significant that no one, to my knowledge, has yet been convicted of murder in a "mercy" killing trial in this country.

[17] It seems to me that the church has always implicitly recognized this in the honor it has accorded martyrs, those who have counted integrity, truth, or loyalty to another as more valuable than their own continued physical existence.

[18] Bennett, John C., Viewpoint: The Van Dusens' Suicide Pact, *Christianity and Crisis*, March 31, 1975, p. 67.

Chapter 30

Ethics in Human Biology

Milton D. Heifetz

Physicians have always made decisions affecting the life and death of patients. These decisions are supported by a body of knowledge and skills unique to the physician. But the rapid development of new medical life support systems that can prolong dying without dignity, or even hide the fact that death has already taken place, has resulted in difficult ethical and sometimes tragic dilemmas. These problems need discussion and solution.

Although the topic of ethics as it applies to human biology is a broad one and any discussion of it would include consideration of such areas as genetic engineering, abortion, human experimentation, problems of informed consent, and so on, I would like to restrict this study primarily to a discussion of the right of the individual to refuse life-saving treatment, the question of to treat or not to treat the hopelessly ill, euthanasia, suicide, the management of the severely deformed newborn, and the definition of death.

The fundamental principles underlying these dilemmas should apply equally to all other areas of bioethics.

What must be the ethical basis of decision making in medicine?

Ethics is a contrivance of man. Its base, its direction will depend upon the attitudes of the specific society. It is therefore only as absolute as we wish to make it. The essence of our (Western society's) ethics is the realization that freedom, i.e., the right to privacy, the right to independence, the right of self-determination, is most fundamental to our concept of ourselves, and that, ideally, the absolute freedom of the individual should be inviolable. But we also realize the danger and the impracticality of absolute freedom. We therefore counter and temper this freedom with the doctrine of *parens patria*—state paternalism—in order to prevent the misuse of that freedom.

The result of this social formula is an ethical base that states that we are free to speak, to act, to live as we wish as long as in the exercise of that freedom no one else is harmed, e.g., as in the case of a person who refuses vaccination when there is danger of an epidemic; of the mother who refuses to be treated for illness and would, should she die, abandon an infant; or of the person who shouts "Fire!" in a theatre. In order for society to continue functioning, freedom of the individual must be balanced by consideration of other people and the good of society as a whole.

This ethical doctrine is implicit in every major religion and every humanistic society and may be expressed by the dictum: "Do not to others as you would not have others do to you."

This fundamental axiom embodies our ethic. It expresses the understanding that the absolute freedom of every individual would conflict with the desire of every individual to be free from harm.

In 1928, Supreme Court Justice Louis Brandeis stated:

> The makers of our Constitution . . . sought to protect Americans in their beliefs, their thoughts, emotions, and their sensations . . . they conferred . . . the right to be left alone . . . the most comprehensive of rights and the right most valued by civilized man.[1]

This fundamental concept not only implies the right of the individual to do wise things, but also the right to be foolish.

In complex medical situations we sometimes cannot see, or do not wish to see, how this basic principle applies, and therefore we attempt to solve bioethical problems by means of the application of secondary ethical concepts such as the sanctity of life, economic considerations, the meaningfulness of suffering, or the thought that only God can determine the course of life. There is undoubtedly a certain validity to all such ethical factors, but never, in a secular, free society, should any of these secondary concepts be given the same weight as the right of self-determination, which is the basis of individual dignity and the hallmark of a free man.

The difficulty we may have in understanding the ethical basis of a given situation should not lead us to seek new ethical values.

Ethical values do not change just because of the ongoing increase in medical technology and expertise. Value judgments of what is right or good are not relative to changing circumstances. Changing circumstances may demand a greater flexibility in the law but not the invention of a new or less morally stringent ethical code.

How does this apply to the right to refuse therapy—the right to die?

The most important factor in this issue is not what the physician would or would not wish to do, but the will of the patient, i.e., the patient's rights. The physician has no rights in such circumstances. He has only a role to play. That role is to inform, to advise, to recommend, to persuade. It is the patient who has full power. The patient has the right to know the most important details of the illness, the right to refuse treatment, and the right to be informed of that right, the right to direct, manage, live, and die as he or she wishes, as long as no one else is harmed in the process.

This fundamental right of the patient who is competent to say "No" to a doctor and thereby refuse treatment must be preserved. This right reflects the individual's freedom. If the refusal of treatment results in death, that is the individual's prerogative. The physician may try to persuade the individual to do what is medically wise, but to persuade does not imply the right to coerce, as long as the individual is an adult and competent.

In order to properly evaluate this basic right, we may have to rethink our thoughts concerning the meaning of life and our fear of death.

The platitude that as long as there is life there is hope and that therefore we must prolong life regardless of its quality can be inhumane and its implementation, if contrary to the individual's desire, can be a violation of that individual's fundamental rights. There are humane qualities in death. Life is precious and awesome. To hold it lightly dehumanizes it, but to divorce it from the dignity of personal freedom debases it.

Those who would aggressively treat a dying brain-damaged patient with no hope of recovery, contrary to the patient's request, when they would not wish to be treated if they themselves were in that condition, act hypocritically. They hide behind a mask of morality. The doctor who believes that his function is to preserve life as long as he has the ability to do so, in spite of his patient's wishes, is, unless adhering to a religious precept, in moral error. His safety lies in the fact that doctors can rarely be blamed by society for prolonging life. These doctors are secure in the knowledge that when the patient dies, the family can say that everything was done to keep the patient alive, even if the patient has lived as a vegetable.

Many physicians accept this approach. It helps them medically. It helps them legally. It helps them psychologically. We must condemn it.

How many men or women would want to live if recovery of their human qualities was impossible? Many, if not most, would beg to be allowed to die. If this is true, how moral is that man or woman or society that would prevent an individual's right to make that decision? Those who would deny that right of self-determination to others fall into the trap of doing to others what they would not have others do to them.

We must understand that when physicians permit a patient to die who wishes to do so, there is no breach of moral faith. On the contrary, there is a facing of responsibility; there is adherence to the individual's right of self-determination.

The right of the individual to refuse medical treatment has been upheld repeatedly in our courts. In 1962 Judge Bernard S. Meyer Jr. refused to force a competent adult member of the Jehovah's Witness faith to accept a blood transfusion under the doctrine of self-determination. He said:

> It is the individual . . . who has the final say, and this must be necessarily so in a system of government which gives the greatest possible protection to the individual in the furtherance of his own desires.

In another ruling this right of self-determination was overruled. Again it involved a member of the Jehovah's Witness faith. In 1964 a 25-year-old mother of a 7-month-old child was seriously ill and in need of blood. She refused a blood transfusion. A court order sought by the doctor and hospital was approved by Circuit Court Judge J. Skelly Wright, who overruled a lower court decision.[3] He rightfully invoked the doctrine of *parens patriae*—the right and obligation of the State to protect those unable to care for themselves—on the basis that the death of the mother would have been tantamount to the abandonment of her child and therefore contrary to the child's welfare. This doctrine of state paternalism reflects the concern a civilized society must have for the welfare of all its members and that we should all have for each other. But such concern must not become distorted into self-righteousness and interfere with the individual's right of self-determination when others are not harmed.

The right of self-determination as it applies to the incompetent patient has also been tested in the courts.

In 1972 in Allentown, Pennsylvania, Mrs. Maida Yetter refused to undergo surgery for the removal of a breast cancer. At the time of this refusal Mrs. Yetter was alert, oriented, and totally competent. Approximately 1 year later Mrs. Yetter became delusional because of her fear of possible surgery. At the time of her delusional state, when she was obviously incompetent, her brother asked the court to appoint him guardian so that he could authorize the surgery. The court rejected the brother's request, noting that "the Constitutional right of privacy includes the right of a mature, competent, adult to refuse to accept medical recommendation that may prolong one's life." The court ruled that she was competent at the time of the initial decision, and added that:

> Balancing the risks involved in our refusal to act in favor of compulsory treatment against giving the greatest possible protection to the individual in furtherance of his own desires, we are unwilling now to overrule Mrs. Yetter's original . . . competent decision.[4]

The court upheld the important principle of Mrs. Yetter's right of privacy and self-determination, her right to refuse treatment even though it meant her death.

This case gives legal support to the concept that the wish of an individual expressed while competent must be respected even if that individual subsequently becomes incompetent. This principle was further supported at the federal level in a 1971 decision by the Second Circuit Court of Appeal that refused to authorize a blood transfusion for an unconscious patient who, while conscious, had specifically refused a blood transfusion. This refusal was based on the understanding that the administration of blood under such circumstances would violate that individual's civil rights.

Since a patient has the right to refuse any treatment—and thereby to choose death—the individual already has the right to die. This right to die has existed throughout our nation's history.

Why is this right so frequently ignored? Why do physicians hesitate to inform patients of their right to say no? Why do we so often treat patients when only to prolong their dying without dignity? I am inclined to reject the often-stated opinion that physicians cannot accept the death of their patients because of their own fear of death or their inability to accept what they perceive as defeat.

The probable explanation of the situation lies in the physician as healer's tradition to continue to treat the patient combined with the physician's fear of criticism or legal action by the patient's survivors if the treatment is stopped.

This attitude must be understood if we are to protect the right of the individual to refuse treatment, especially during a possible future state of the individual's incompetency.

In order to protect the individual's wishes it is necessary to protect the physician for obeying those wishes as well. This demands a properly written statement to the physician. It must be precise and it must make the physician legally liable for disobeying it. A sample of such a directive may be as follows:

DIRECTIVE TO MY PHYSICIAN

This directive is written while I am of sound mind and fully competent.

I insist that I have the complete right to refuse any medical and surgical treatment unless a court order affirms that my decision would bring undue or unexpected hardship on my family or on society.

Therefore:

If I become incompetent, in consideration of my legal rights to refuse medical or surgical treatment regardless of the consequences to my health and life, I hereby direct and order my physician or any physician in charge of my care to cease and refrain from any medical or surgical treatment that would prolong my life if I am in a condition of:

1 Unconsciousness from which I cannot recover
2 Unconsciousness over a period of 6 months
3 Irreversible mental incompetency

However, although mentally incompetent, if conscious, I must be informed of the situation, and if I wish to be treated I am to be treated in spite of my original request made while competent.*

If there is any reasonable doubt of the diagnosis of my illness and the prognosis, then consultation with available specialists should be obtained.

This directive to my physician also applies to any hospital or sanitarium at which I may be at the time of my illness, and relieves them of any and all responsibility in the action or lack of action of any physician acting according to my demands.

If any action is taken contrary to these express demands I hereby request my next of kin or my legal representatives to consider—and if necessary, to take—legal action against those involved.

I hereby absolve my physician or any physician taking care of me from any legal liability pertaining to the fulfillment of any of my demands.

Signed _____

---

*This paradox must be understood. It is the only time a request or demand made while incompetent can override one made while competent. It is conceivable, although rare, that next of kin may attempt to take advantage of such a state of incompetency and to too readily take advantage of a prior directive ordering cessation of therapy.

EUTHANASIA

What is the relationship between this right of self-determination—the right to die—and euthanasia?

Euthanasia literally translated from the Greek means "well" or "easy death," but since 1869[5] it has commonly been accepted to mean the act of inducing an easy death. Therefore the word euthanasia should only be used to connote the willful putting to death of an individual with the intent to prevent suffering; in other words— mercy killing.

The act of removing a respirator from a patient who no longer can recover from a state of coma that subsequently results in that patient's death is not euthanasia. On the other hand, the injection of a massive dose of morphine into the same patient that produces death would be euthanasia. The difference is twofold. Euthanasia is an act of commission as opposed to an act of omission. But more more important, and most crucial, euthanasia induces death by interfering with life's natural course. The act itself is the cause of death. Actions that militate against treatment, that either fail to initiate treatment or that discontinue treatment, allow nature to take its course. In this case, the disease process itself is the cause of death.

There are those who would legalize euthanasia. This I believe is dangerous.

Euthanasia for the seriously deformed and retarded newborn, or for that matter, in the rare case of the adult, can at times be humane and correct, moral and right. The doctor or parent who overdoses an anencephalic monster is committing infanticide, a variant of euthanasia that may be considered as euthanasia. To end the life of such an organism is valid and correct, but to kill, regardless of the circumstances, must remain subject to the scrutiny of our courts. Never should the taking of a life be free of the court's judgment.

In the United States motivation is not a defense in cases of homicide. Consent to or request for euthanasia is not legally acceptable. Our law considers the deliberate and premeditated taking of life as murder in the first degree; however, the *attitude* of our courts has been more reasonable. Altruistic motivation has been considered as an extenuating circumstance in judging homicides. Other countries in the world have accepted motivation as a legitimate defense in court; it behooves us to do the same. Therefore we should pass laws that grant our courts the right to consider and honor motivation and intent in cases of euthanasia, and the right to declare no penalty.

SUICIDE

The same principle that underlies the right of a competent adult to die by refusal of medical care underlies the ethical and legal right of the individual to suicide.

Three groups of people attempt suicide; those suffering from transient or chronic emotional disorders; those emotionally sound but aged, alone, and without a sense of purpose in life; and those near death who do not deem their remaining days or weeks worth living.

The first and second groups are in need of psychological and sociological support.

We must encourage the development of suicide prevention centers and increase the availability of psychological help for these two groups of people.

The third category—those physically devastated and near death—is another matter. The members of this group, although under emotional stress, are frequently still capable of reasoned judgments. I believe that if they desire to leave life through suicide we should not only give them the courtesy of respecting their wish, but also offer them medical assistance to commit suicide if they wish to have it.

At times death-dealing medication left by the bedside of a dying person can be the answer to that person's prayers for relief from pain and suffering, and thus a most humane solution. It is illegal to do this in the United States. Maybe it is time to change this law. But this concept of assisting suicide must be kept within tightly controlled circumstances; it must be allowed only for those alert and competent humans, unequivocally near death, who do not wish to continue their dying state in spite of psychiatric help, and who specifically ask for this type of assistance.

We must cease forcing decisions upon others because of our own personal beliefs and preferences. At times we should look at death as a welcome release from an untenable life. Death is part of life's pattern. At times it should be sought, not avoided. I do not mean to imply that we should hold life less dear, but that we should consider death less terrifying.

Nature frequently removes the fear of death from the elderly, infirm, or hopelessly ill, and, in fact, often allows these people to welcome death.

If living becomes a hopeless state of anguish for a coherent and sentient adult, does anyone have the right to insist that someone live in that state against his or her will? Where is a person's free choice? Who is the transgressed if even the agonized is not? Certainly psychiatric help should be utilized to assist such people to adapt to their tragic lot, but to insist that life must be lived when all efforts to help have failed is a presumptuous imposition on a fellow human's right of self-determination.

Death is a natural process that in the proper scheme of things ought neither to be feared nor resented. What should be feared more is the inability to feel the joy and serenity of life.

THE TRAGIC NEWBORN

How does this ethical base apply to the management of the severely deformed newborn—that newborn who does not have the potential of achieving even near normal human mental or physical qualities?

We speak of the right of self-determination. But the newborn cannot speak for itself and therefore any action or lack of action that may ensue may not necessarily be in accordance with that newborn's wish. But this holds true even for the child and adolescent who can, but cannot legally, speak for themselves. Their right to decide, their authority, is relegated to their parents. Therefore, parents have been granted the right to decide whether their newborn should or should not be treated. But this does not mean that parents have absolute control over their offspring. Their right to decide is tempered by that same doctrine of *parens patriae* that reflects society's desire to protect the weak and incompetent.

How do we balance this equation of parents' right of decision and society's obligation to protect the weak?

Let us apply this equation to the tragic newborn. These infants fall into three categories:

1 Those who are so damaged that nothing can keep them alive
2 Those damaged infants who could live without medical care
3 Those newborns who could not live without medical care and, even with medical care, could live only a subhuman existence

I am discussing only children in this *last* category. Should these hopelessly damaged newborns receive the full benefit of medical science if that science can enable them to live only on a subhuman level? Should medical aid ever be withheld?

What are the factors that must enter into this decision process?

First and foremost, parents must be *fully* informed as to the degree and significance of the damage, as well as to the prognosis for the child.

Second, they must be informed as to their legal right to give or withhold consent for treatment.

What should society, as reflected in the recommendations and actions of the physician, consider as pertinent factors in order to exercise its obligation of concern for the weak in case parents refuse to authorize life-saving medical or surgical treatment for their newborn? In general, we must evaluate what can be coldly termed the *salvage value*. This factor is vital in our decision making and includes consideration of the following questions. What kind of child will result? Can the child be relatively self-sustaining in the future? Will life be one continuous form of agony for the child? Will life be meaningful to any degree? What is meaningful, and to whom?

When evaluating what action to take in the case of the tragic newborn it is necessary to balance the present and future condition of the child against its effect on parents and siblings. In order to do this we must better understand at the time of birth what effects its continued existence would have on all those involved. We must ask whether pregnancy and birth are so sanctified that all other factors become irrelevant in spite of the fact that for a healthy, normal woman impregnation is a relatively easy thing to achieve.

We must weigh the value of that *future, subhuman* existence, and the right to maintain such a life, against the sadness and cruelty that living with such a child would impose on parents and siblings. In other words, what happens to the child and the family after all the doctors and the other experts have gone away and those concerned with the problem are left alone to live with it?

Our society makes life itself an absolute and places it before all else and makes no provision for the effect of what is essentially a living death on the family of the afflicted child. Certainly some families are drawn closer together as its members cooperate with each other to shield the child and to find aid for him or her, if such aid is possible. Yet, regardless of how well family members work together to help the mentally retarded and deformed child, the parents inevitably ask: What will happen to the child when we are dead? Many families disintegrate under this kind of pressure.

The anguish that is experienced by a family of a newborn who is drastically deformed and/or mentally damaged, without hope of recovery to even a near-normal state, and who is nevertheless alive in the physiological sense of the word, is one of the most heartbreaking emotional states I have ever witnessed.

It is not uncommon for physicians to recommend and for parents to authorize that every effort be made to save the child although they intend to put the child into an institution—never to be seen again by the parents. Is this humaneness?

People should visit state and private institutions flooded with mentally retarded children and adults and see for themselves the quality of their lives, the horror of their existence, and the effect of such tragic states on families so they might better understand this problem.

A baby was born hopelessly paralyzed from the waist down with a severe myelomeningocele. But there was no evidence of mental retardation. The parents had two normal children, ages 3 and 5. They asked me not to operate to prevent the possible occurrence of meningitis. I agreed. The child contracted meningitis and died.

Even though they may have a normal brain and therefore normal intelligence, I do not believe that newborns afflicted with such hopeless and devastating deformities should be treated.

The late Donald D. Matson, M.D., a respected pediatric neurosurgeon of the Children's Hospital Medical Center and Harvard Medical School, has stated:

> In our clinic, it is not customary to operate upon newborn infants or those in the first few months of life . . . who exhibit complete sphincter paralysis and total paraplegia . . . . This is true whether or not there is significant hydrocephalus at the time. When examination on the first day of life therefore confirms total absence of neurological function below the upper lumbar levels, custodial care only is recommended . . . . It is the doctor's and the community's responsibility to provide this care and to minimize suffering; but, at the same time, it is also their responsibility not to prolong individual, familiar, and community suffering unnecessarily . . . in an infant whose chance for acceptable growth and development is negligible.[6]

> "How many doctors familiar with the condition would willingly accept the lifelong commitment [to] a severely affected offspring with myelomeningocele if such a misfortune occurred in their own family?" asks Dr. John Lorber of Sheffield, England, . . . "To minimize the suffering caused by this condition, [an] operation at birth should not be recommended for those cases for whom severe disability can be predicted."[7]

Yale University pediatrician Raymond S. Duff and pediatrician A. G. M. Campbell of the University of Aberdeen, Scotland reported in 1973 that forty-three infants were permitted to die during a 30-month period at Yale-New Haven Hospital, New Haven, Connecticut, because parents and staff members there felt those children had "little or no hope of achieving (what theologian and ethicist Dr. Joseph Fletcher terms) meaningful *humanhood*." The children, all of whom had profound and irreversible mental and/or physical defects, died because essential medical treatment was withheld from them.[8]

In each case, the child was hopelessly ill and had multiple handicaps, but could have lived, at least for some period of time. Not all were newborn. One of the infants, the victim of an incurable lung disease, was kept alive for 5 months in spite of an inadequate respiratory system and a weak heart. He lived only because of special oxygen treatment. The hopelessness of the situation and the continuous distress of the infant compounded by the severe emotional trauma to the parents and the other children in the family forced the decision to shut off the oxygen. The child died in 3 hours.

"When maximum treatment was viewed as unacceptable by families and physicians in our units," writes Drs. Duff and Campbell, "there was a growing tendency to seek early death.

"In lengthy, frank discussions, the anguish of the parents was shared and attempts were made to support fully the reasoned choices, whether for active treatment and rehabilitation or for an early death."

In all forty-three cases parents and physicians concurred.

Drs. Duff and Campbell acknowledge "the awesome finality" of their decisions and the "potential for error," but they insist these life-or-death matters must be dealt with candidly. Both men charge that medicine has been "hiding" from this issue:

Since major research, teaching and patient care efforts were being made, professionals expected to discover, transmit and apply knowledge and skill; patients and families were supposed to cooperate fully [even] if they were not always grateful. Some physicians recognized that the wishes of families went against their own, but they were resolute. They [the doctors] *commonly agreed* that if they were the parents of very defective children, withholding treatment would be most desirable for them [italics added]. However, they argued that aggressive treatment should be done for the children of others.

Such an arrogant, autocratic approach perpetuated under the guise of research must be condemned.

Dr. Anthony Shaw, pediatric surgeon at the University of Virginia Medical Center, Charlottesville, Virginia, who also believes that the quality of life must be considered in addition to the idea of life for its own sake, comments on the identical point:[9]

I was called to the newborn nursery to see baby C whose father was a busy surgeon with three teen-age children. The diagnosis of imperforate anus and microcephalus were obvious. [The father] called me after being informed of the situation by the pediatrician. "I'm not going to sign the op [operation] permit" he said. When I didn't reply, he said, "what would you do doctor, if he were your baby?" "I wouldn't let him be operated on either," I replied.[9]

The infant was kept comfortable and died 48 hours later.

This pointed question—"What would you do?"—put to the physician by parents of tragic newborns should be asked more often. It would prevent extraordinary and life-long heartache.

For years some physicians have accepted and supported parental decisions that death is the kindest response to the tragically deformed newborn. "The treatment of severely deformed children is a common denominator at every nursery in the country," says Dr. Lawrence K. Pickett, chief of staff at Yale–New Haven Hospital.[10] "Other hospitals follow similar practices but are afraid to report them."

This fear is understandable. The world press in 1971 condemned the 'inhumanity" of a husband and wife and the staff of a major American medical center. A child with Down's syndrome was born with an intestinal obstruction at Johns Hopkins Hospital in Baltimore. The parents, who had two normal children, refused to give consent to correct the obstruction. The infant could not be fed and died within 15 days.

The parents agonized over the problem. They decided that the impact of a mongoloid infant on the lives of their other children, as well as on their own, could not be endured.

The child's death caused a furor in medical and lay circles. It was a major topic at an international symposium concerning medical ethics.[11] Panelists disagreed with the parents. They suggested the child's right to life, to the limit of happiness possible, was more important than the years of anguish and burden the child would bring upon the family.

Thus, the right to live, they argued, must be the basis of any such decision. The effect of that life on others is secondary.

If this is true, and if we are reasonable people, then it follows that we must affirm that the sanctity of life overrides all else. At that point, however, we reach a precipice.

We are faced with a question asked by the social critic and writer Michael Harrington: "What if the defect had been much greater?"[12] To answer his question and to remain consistent, we must also preserve the life of the anencephalic child, the newborn without a brain. That life is equally sanctified. But our society comfortably says, "No, that would be going too far."

But if we do not operate to preserve an anencephalic child and thus fail to affirm that child's right to live, we are making a comparative judgment. Comparative judgments deny the sanctity of life over all else. The two are in conflict. We cannot go both ways.

We must draw the line somewhere. But that line cannot use as its base the sanctity of life. That is too narrow. We must ask that basic question: What would you or I want if such a child were our infant?

The technical advances that have been made in medicine and surgery are superb. But the question is: Does treatment always permit a liveable life? We must not only ask, Can it be done?, but also, Should it be done?

David Patrick Houle was born on February 9, 1974, in the Maine Medical Center. He had multiple deformities. He did not have a left eye or a left ear. He was physically and mentally defective. His esophagus was not connected properly to his stomach; he was therefore unable to eat.[13]

His parents, Air Force Sergeant and Mrs. Robert B. T. Houle of Westbrook, Maine, asked that life-sustaining measures be stopped, that surgery to prolong David's life not be performed. But the hospital sought and obtained a court order to allow surgery.

The baby's physician told the court, "We have passed the point where the correction will be of any benefit to the infant. The infant would be physically and mentally retarded and probable brain damage has rendered life not worth preserving."

In spite of his testimony and the parents' wishes, Justice David G. Roberts of the Cumberland County Superior Court authorized consent for surgery. Justice Roberts's ruling: "The parents have no right to withhold such treatment and that to do so constitutes neglect in a legal sense. The basic right enjoyed by every human being is the right to life itself." The issue, he said, "is not the prospective quality of the life to be preserved."

The court order was obeyed.

For Justice Roberts to be consistent, he would have to order surgery to be performed to preserve the life of a brainless, armless, legless infant, even if it were his own grandchild.

Or would he?

If we accept the concept that certain tragic newborns should not receive medical support, can we devise safeguards to prevent its misuse?

There is an implicit danger in trying to establish specific guidelines to evaluate physical or mental deficits accurately. The degree of the tragedy varies. There is certainly no sharp line of demarcation.

It is one thing to say that the child who is armless, legless, and without a brain of significant size should be allowed to die. But what of the newborn who will be mildly retarded, who, with proper training, will be totally self-sufficient, able to work at specified jobs, and able to enjoy life; and what of those children who fall in between these categories?

I cannot draw that line, and neither can that amorphous thing we call society.

If specific guidelines cannot be established, are there reasonable safeguards to prevent unwise actions? I believe there are—the *parents*.

We should not underestimate the ability of parents to make wise decisions affecting themselves and the welfare of their children.

Parents will go to extremes to protect their newborn children. It is the exceedingly rare parent who will allow a newborn to die without an exceptionally good reason. In some isolated cases, parents would rather see their newborn die if the child is not perfectly normal. The physician may actually find himself in the position of fighting the parents to save a child with a minor defect that can be corrected, although not completely, through surgery. In these unusual cases, the physician can easily countermand any distorted requests by parents by simply seeking and obtaining a court order to authorize treatment.

The total thrust of medicine is to preserve life. This is the second safeguard. Physicians *will not allow* emotionally distraught parents to prevent treatment when treatment is indicated.

Therefore, in spite of a remote possibility for error, I believe that the protectiveness of parents toward their children and the drive of physicians to preserve their lives are all the safeguards that are necessary in these tragic circumstances.

I would like to suggest what I believe should be the postulates underlying the relationship between the parents of a severely deformed newborn and their physician:

Parents have the right to understand the medical problems facing their child. Only then can they make decisions.

It is the obligation of the physician to explain the problems to parents adequately.

If an infant is so damaged that treatment will result in prolongation of the life of a severely mentally or physically defective child, the parents must be informed of their authority to withhold consent for treatment and their authority to demand their physician to stop treatment if it has been started.

If a physician believes that a child may be able to lead a relatively normal life after treatment—and the parents refuse to authorize treatment—it is his or her obligation to seek a court order to enable treatment to take place.

If the physician's religion demands preservation of life, regardless of its quality and contrary to parental demand, he or she should transfer the child's care to another physician and, if necessary, to another institution.

If parents request treatment after full information has been given to them, treatment must be given.

We are dealing with principles that may apply in individual cases. We cannot be absolute, but I do not believe the inability to be absolute should deter us.

NOTES

[1] *Olmstead v. United States*, 277 U.S. 438,478,48 Superior Court 564,572,72 L.Ed 944(1928).

[2] *Erickson v. Dilgard*, vol. 252 NYS 2d 705,706, Superior Court, Nassau County (1962).

[3] Application of the President and Directors of the Georgetown College 331 F.2d 1000 (D.C.-cir) 377 U.S. 978(1964).

[4] Dockett #1973–533, Pennsylvania Court of Common Pleas, Northhampton County Orphans Court(1973).

[5] William E. Lecky, *History of European Morals from Augustus to Charlemagne*, 1869.

[6] Donald D. Matson, "Surgical Treatment of Myelomeningocele," *Pediatrics*, **42**(2): 225–227, August 1968.

[7] J. Lorber, "Results of Treatment of Myelomeningocele," *Developmental Medicine and Child Neurology*, **13**:279–303, June 1971.

[8] R. S. Duff and A. G. M. Campbell, "Moral and Ethical Dilemmas in the Special-Care Nursery," *The New England Journal of Medicine*, **289**:890–894, October 25, 1973.

[9] A. Shaw, "Dilemmas of 'Informed Consent' in Children," *The New England Journal of Medicine*, **289**:885–890, October 25, 1973.

[10] *Associated Press*, October 30, 1973.

[11] International Symposium on Human Rights, Retardation and Research, Washington, D.C., October 16, 1971.

[12] Ibid.

[13] *New York Times*, February 16, 24, 1974.

Chapter 31

Human Sexuality and Serious Illness

Mona Wasow

THE PROBLEM

Most of the significant research on human sexuality has been conducted only within the last 30 years, following the pioneering work of Kinsey (1948, 1953). Masters and Johnson have written extensively on sexuality and healthy individuals, and other doctors and health care professionals have reported how chronic illnesses affect the sexuality of the patient. However, our review of the literature focusing on the correlation between disease and sexual behavior has revealed no studies by professionals of the relation between human sexuality and terminal illness. By contrast, in our work we have found that many fatally ill patients are vitally concerned with their changing sexuality.

In March 1975, the Council on Social Work Education presented a panel discussion about sexually oppressed groups in American society. The presentation concentrated on issues related to the sexuality of certain minority groups, such as the mentally retarded, the physically handicapped, the aged, and homosexuals.

After the discussion, Lois Jaffe, a social worker, approached the author participating in the panel to ask for information about literature pertaining to the sexuality of a minority group that had not been mentioned that day—the terminally ill. Ms. Jaffe then told her own story, that of a 49-year-old woman terminally ill with leukemia, who is concerned about her changing sexuality as a result of her illness; she

Susan Dean, Rodney Judd, Sue Mayer, June Maynard, and Dagmar Wyatt contributed to the development of this paper.

has spent much time in chemotherapy treatment, and has passed that time by informally interviewing other waiting cancer patients about the effects of their illnesses on their sexuality.

Even though Ms. Jaffe did not relate specific details about the information she had thus gathered, she reported that chemotherapy, the illness itself, and depression about the illness and impending death combined powerfully to adversely affect the sexuality of the patients she interviewed. Based on this information, as well as on her own experience as a terminally ill person, Ms. Jaffe felt strongly that there is a compelling need for a systematic study of the sexuality of terminally ill people, including interviews of both the patient's sexual partner and health care personnel. It was through Ms. Jaffe's encouragement that this research project was conceived.[1]

The lack of literature on the sexuality of the terminally ill indirectly documents a predominant cultural belief about this minority group, namely, that people who have been diagnosed as fatally ill are asexual. The medical and allied health professions have done little to challenge this assumption.

Our hypothesis is that patients who have a fatal illness, but are still in good enough health to enjoy some form of sexual activity, do have sexual concerns, thoughts, and feelings, and may very well desire some information and professional counseling about their sexuality. In a lecture at the University of Wisconsin Medical School, Dr. Ed Tyler stated that:

> A concept of permanent or irreversible sexual incapacity seems an appropriate description *only* of those patients whose total interest, energy, and attention has become occupied with their painful, debilitating terminal illness.[2]

In assessing medical problems, most physicians do not assume that no complications exist just because a patient does not initiate questioning. However, most health professionals do assume that a patient's sex life is satisfactory if he or she does not bring up the subject. We believe that patients often need encouragement from their physician to discuss sexual matters, and that they sometimes even require medical permission to experiment with new or modified patterns of sexual behavior.

Whereas the physical aspects of a terminal illness are easy to observe and describe, the psychological concomitants that might affect sexuality are less apparent and therefore harder to analyze. The professional literature includes very little about the psychological aspects of terminal illness, even though we can assume that many health care professionals have encountered situations in which a terminally ill person has asked for help with a sexual problem. With cancer of the reproductive organs and the breasts, it is easy to imagine that the disease and its treatment will profoundly affect the patient's sexuality. Nevertheless a physician is, understandably, more likely to be concerned with controlling the disease and prolonging the patient's life, than with the

---

[1] For the complete research proposal and literature review, write Mona Wasow, School of Social Work, 425 Henry Mall, University of Wisconsin, Madison, Wisconsin 53706.
[2] Dr. Ed Tyler, lecture at University of Wisconsin Medical School, March 3, 1974.

quality of the life he or she is working to prolong. The oncologist who has treated a malignancy may well consider his or her mission successfully accomplished if the patient develops no recurrence or complications. The value of the mode of therapy is measured solely in terms of its ability to assure a 5-year survival rate, and, indeed, what happens to sexual functioning may appear trivial to both patient and doctor at the time of treatment. The helping professionals, like the rest of the population, suffer from embarrassment about sexual matters; they often believe many of the prevailing myths about human sexuality and are often ignorant about sexual functioning. It is probably a combination of these priorities, attitudes, and shortcomings that causes health care professionals to deny or ignore the sexuality of terminally ill patients.

PATIENT'S VIEWPOINT

Although health personnel have not provided us with much information about the effects of terminal illness on sexuality, terminally ill patients have. One recently published book describes the changing sexuality of the terminally ill author (Smith, 1975), who talks about the loss of her sexuality and how it signifies the loss of life.

> My problems are deeply rooted in who I am as a sexual being. I feel that sexuality has been taken from me. [After the removal of my breast] I needed help in learning to accept myself (p. 18). . . .
> Before my illness, we often showed our love in a variety of physical ways. But my response gradually waned, and I often wanted no part of a physical relationship with him. I feel I have to forfeit any intimacy. . . . I just can't be responsive (p. 76).

Sex was always important to the author and her spouse; the decline of their physical intimacy deeply depressed her.

> But our sexual relationship has always been an important part of our marriage, and because its mutual enjoyment is gone, I now realize death has come to another area of human existence (p. 79). . . .

Ms. Smith also talks about problems concerning hospitalization.

> One of my strongest feelings about the hospital environment is that there should be two or three rooms equipped with double beds for conjugal visits. . . . I believe it should be possible for a husband or wife to stay with his or her mate, even if it is just overnight and if the patient doesn't need a lot of nursing care, particularly if it's a terminal disease (p. 18) . . . .

The literature covering the physical aspects of the relation between serious illness and sexuality describes how a variety of diseases and their related surgical interventions and methods of treatment affect a patient's sexual functioning. Various authors place very different emphasis on the importance of physical variables in determining an individual's sexual behavior. Only one of seventeen sources published between 1967 and 1975[3] considered the individual's physical condition to be the sole variable in predicting the nature of his or her sexual behavior. This single source (Belt, 1973) indicated that lesions of the central nervous system do devastate potency.

Other relevant findings about the effects of illness on the patient's sexual functioning include the following. There is a lack of correlation between occurrence of impotence and the control or severity of diabetes mellitus (Ellenberg, 1973). Similarly, sexual functioning need not end after urologic surgery (Amelar and Dubin, 1971). Impotence is more prevalent after rectal resection if surgery was due to carcinoma rather than colitis. The reasons for this difference are not clear. Psychological variables seem to be one possibility (Lyons, 1972). Sexual and psychological adjustment prior to diagnosis or surgery is a critical determinant of sexual behaviors after diagnosis and treatment (Kass et al., 1972; Drellich, 1967; Olin, 1972).

The psychological impact of surgery combined with the quality of the patient's preoperative sex life seem to be the major influences on a person's response to fatal illness (Drellich, 1967 and Amelar and Dubin, 1971). In a study of 500 patients who had undergone ileostomy or colostomy because of a life-threatening illness, Dlin and Perlman (1972) found that surgery did not influence masturbation, petting, or premarital sex. Although presurgery patient/physician discussions focused on survival, after surgery patient sexual interest was present and generally in working order. A 15 percent loss of potency found in male ostomates was lower than previous estimates. The study revealed a definite relationship between the nature of the patient's postoperative sex life and an active sex life earlier. Cooperative, understanding partners were found to be helpful in assisting with the coping process. Surgery altered patients' self-image and caused concern over odors and body image.

PHYSICIAN'S VIEWPOINT

Sick or well, people use sexual behavior in a variety of ways as a coping mechanism (Coley, 1973), ascribing a variety of meanings to it. Patients generally consider physicians to be the experts on the physical processes of the disease disabling the patient's body; nevertheless, many physicians pay little attention to how illness affects an individual's sexual activities.

In studying the effects of various chronic illnesses on the sexual functioning of the individual, Ford and Orfirer (1967) observed three patterns of adjustment: (1) appropriate adjustment, (2) overcompensation, and (3) withdrawal; they concluded that physical disability in the chronically ill patient is apparently less than has generally been assumed. Their article provides guidelines for sexual rehabilitation through the use of (1) the team approach, (2) family preparation, and (3) the physician's role.

Other professionals cite the need for frank discussion and counseling in treating

[3]Drellich, 1967; Epstein, 1969; Blumer, 1970; Amelar and Dubin, 1971; Kass, Updegraff, and Muffley, 1972; Malin, 1972; Olin, 1972; Bernstein, 1972; Lyons, 1972; Hellerstein and Friedman, 1969; Belt, 1973; Ellenberg, 1973; Greenberg, 1975; Siddiqui and Kerr, 1971.

patients with heart disease (Bakker et al., 1971; Proger et al., 1968; Griffith, 1973), and indicate the importance of recognizing that physical, economic, and social losses in chronic illness threaten the patient's emotional health. In our opinion, sexuality should also be considered an important part of emotional health.

Physician empathy and willingness to advise play a key role in helping patients adjust during the approximately 1-year transitional period following major surgery such as ileostomy and colostomy (Dlin and Perlman, 1972). Psychologic intervention may become necessary if the patient and physician cannot resolve the patient's concerns during this 1-year period. We would like to add that other members of the health care team, including social workers, could also help patients cope with their losses and find alternative sexual behaviors if necessary.

A survey of 307 inpatients (between the ages of 21 and 80) and 76 physicians, undertaken to determine the interrelationship between medical conditions and sexual functioning (Pinderhughes, Grace, Reyna, and Anderson, 1972), revealed a 15 percent discrepancy between the frequency with which *patients* reported physician-initiated discussion of sexual matters (25 percent) and the frequency with which *physicians* reported physician-initiated discussion of sexual matters (40 percent). Thirty-three to 50 percent of the patients surveyed felt that discussion of sex with a physician was helpful, and 54 percent of the patients felt that it was appropriate. Another interesting finding was that residents (18 percent) and staff physicians and consultants (24 percent) differ in their report of how frequently patients initiate discussion of sexual matters.

Some professionals do consider it important to counsel patients on sexual matters (Klagsburn, 1971; Castelnuovo-Tedesco, 1968; Ervin, 1973, Schon, 1968). However, Klagsburn reports that only infrequently do staff discuss the consequences of a biopsy with the patient and/or mate in terms of their lifestyle, sexuality, body image, and the overall effect of treatment. Such discussions should be an essential component of treatment. Writing on the mastectomy patient, Ervin records his step-by-step involvement from the first preoperative visit to the last postoperative visit. Sensitive to the "double whammy" of the threat of cancer and the potential loss of sexuality resulting from a mastectomy, Ervin stresses the importance of the social worker's role, the involvement of the patient's husband in the counseling process, and the use of community resources for the patient's benefit. The surgeon-author's basic principles in dealing with the psychological adjustment to mastectomy are: scrupulous honesty, the communication of hope, acknowledgment of anxiety and depression, and early discussion of the possibility of deformity and methods of dress. Castelnuovo-Tedesco feels that a physician should bring up the topic of sexuality when proper management of the patient's disease requires that some consideration be given to his or her sexual practices. He further maintains that it is the patient, not the doctor, who should determine whether a problem exists.

Considering the high incidence of sex-related problems afflicting the general population (e.g., see Calderone, 1970 and Tyler, 1974), it is essential that health professionals obtain a better understanding of the impact of fatal illness on sexual behavior if they are to develop the skills to help patients with their sexual problems. With the new drugs and treatments now available, patients are being kept alive for longer periods of time than in the past. They may therefore desire aid in working out sexual problems so that they can enjoy as active a sex life as possible. The fact of a fatal illness does not have to end a person's sexual life.

PHYSICAL AND PSYCHOLOGICAL SEXUAL PROBLEMS OF CHRONICALLY ILL PATIENTS

Chronically ill patients are no different than the rest of the population in their experience of a wide range of sexual problems. Patients reporting a hesitance to engage in coitus often express a sense of boredom, a fear of frustrating themselves or their sexual partner, and a concern with performance (Comarr, 1970). In sum, fatigue and actual physical discomfort during intercourse are the two most frequently reported physiological problems hindering the sexual functioning of patients. The reported psychological problems include the desire to have sexual activity more often than the spouse, problems of erection for males, feelings of being less sexually attractive since illness, inactivity of the partner, premature ejaculation, and feelings that the sexual partner is less sexually attractive (Woodburne, 1973).

Differences exist between patients and their spouses. Patients have reported feeling tired more often than their spouses; they also tend to feel less sexually attractive than their spouses. As a result, spouses often desire to have sexual activity more frequently than patients. Finally, more male patients and female spouses have reported sexual difficulties than have female patients and their male spouses.

AMOUNT OF SEXUAL ACTIVITY OF CHRONICALLY ILL PATIENTS

Although 70 percent of the subjects in the 1973 Woodburne study reported having intercourse at least some of the time, the majority of the patients interviewed reported a decrease in the frequency of intercourse following the onset of kidney failure. The responses of patients differed from those of their spouses in this questionnaire study, with the patients reporting a decrease in the frequency of intercourse more often than their spouses.

A similar decline in sexual activity was found among chronically ill or physically disabled patients (Sadoughi, Leshner, and Fine, 1972). Seventh-eight percent of a group of subjects who were chronically ill or physically disabled reported a decline in the frequency of sexual activity. Comarr (1970) confirmed these findings among spinal cord injury patients; more than 33 percent of the patients studied would not attempt sexual relations with their partners.

Fear of injury often inhibits the sexual functioning of chronically ill patients. For example, the fear of damaging their shunts is an overriding concern of terminal renal patients.

GUIDELINES FOR PHYSICIANS AND HEALTH CARE PROFESSIONALS

Physicians and other health care professionals are in a unique position with regard to death in that it becomes a part of their everyday reality (Peretz, 1970). Their accessibility to patients also places them in a unique position with respect to the sexual problems of the terminally ill. Yet studies indicate that physicians frequently avoid the issue of sexuality when treating terminally ill patients and their families. This avoidance is in some ways understandable: health care personnel are rarely taught to consider a patient's sexuality as integral to treatment. Their attitudes are also colored by the prevalent myths about sexuality, and finally, many suffer from the same anxieties that plague us all (Barton, 1972).

The aforementioned factors do not, however, diminish the obligation of health care personnel to treat the sexual problems of the seriously ill. One study on the sexual problems of the chronically ill and disabled found that over 50 percent of the patients would have liked to discuss their sexual concerns with a hospital staff member of the same sex if one had been available (Sadoughi, Leshner, and Fine, 1971).

The frequency with which patients bring their sexual problems to the attention of a physician depends upon (1) the physician's specialty; (2) whether the physician routinely asks about sex problems; and (3) the ease with which the physician discusses sexual questions with the patient. In general, patients are more likely to express their sexual concerns if their physician routinely discusses sexuality and appears to be comfortable in doing so (Beeson and McDermott, 1975).

To give adequate attention to the sexual problems of seriously ill patients, physicians will need to: (1) make an appraisal of their own sexual attitudes; (2) have a knowledge of human sexual development; (3) be respectful and sympathetic to the patient's needs; (4) assess to what degree the problems are based on misconceptions and misinformation; and (5) initiate discussion of the patient's sexual adjustment. The physician will also need to include the patient's spouse and other family in the treatment process.

Curriculum Changes

The inclusion of a course on sexuality in medical school curricula would help overcome physician avoidance of addressing the sexual concerns of patients. A combined didactic-experiential approach would give medical students the opportunity to work through their own biases, resistances, and discomfort (Jaffe, 1977). "A combined course on sexuality and terminality could synthesize these phenomena as integral parts of the natural life cycle rather than as subjects ridden with pathology and taboos."

Changes in the Hospital Environment

A quiet room furnished with couch, carpet, soft lights, *and an opportunity for privacy* would go a long way in counteracting the usual cold atmosphere of hospital rooms. The quiet room could replicate the home ambiance, which patients miss so badly, and might be used for family and conjugal visits as well as for counseling sessions.

Sexual Counseling

Hospital staff could offer individual and group sexual counseling to those patients who request it, using a treatment approach to counsel both the seriously ill patient and his or her family. The patient's medical work-up should include an evaluation of the patient's and his or her spouse's sexual functioning (Leviton, 1973). The physician or counselor might start by taking a sexual history. Wahl (1967) has offered some general principles to follow in recording a patient's sexual history:

> The history progresses from those topics which are easier to discuss to those more difficult; and the patient is asked first about how he acquired sexual information, before he is asked about sexual experience (p. 15).

Sexual counseling can also be preventive. A physician should inform the patient and his or her family of any anticipated changes in sexual drive and performance that might result from the treatment or illness. If the patient is able to return home, the physician should include sexuality in the home care treatment plan (if the couple so desires).

In addition, a physician or counselor may choose to utilize group counseling techniques. An ongoing group composed of patients and their spouses would allow couples to share information and express their feelings. Group counseling might be especially advantageous because most people have had some type of experience discussing sexuality within a group of peers. A group also allows for the modeling of coping behavior and provides a nonthreatening atmosphere in which group members can share emotional support (Romano, 1973).

CONCLUSION

It is time for us to change our cultural attitudes toward the sexuality of the seriously ill. Clinical observations and research refute the common assumption that a dying patient's sexuality ends with the diagnosis of terminal illness. Although this attitude is seldom verbalized, its existence is reflected in most care givers' avoidance of the subject. The few studies recorded in the literature indicate that sexuality continues to be an important part of many patients' lives although drive and rate of performance may be reduced. We need to take the first step and acknowledge the sexual rights and needs of seriously ill patients and their partners. Our actions might help patients to take their own essential first step: a statement of their difficulties.

BIBLIOGRAPHY

Amelar, R. D. and L. Dubin "Sexual Responses to Disease Processes," *Journal of Sex Research*, 4(4):257–264, November 1968.

—— and ——: "Impotence in the Low-Back Syndrome," *Journal of the American Medical Association*, **216**:520, April 19, 1971.

Apitbol, M. and J. Davenport: "Sexual Dysfunction After Surgery for Cervical Carcinoma," *Journal of Obstetrics and Gynecology*, **119**:181–189, May 15, 1974.

Bakker, Cornelis B. et al.: "Heart Disease and Sex: Response to Questions," *Medical Aspects of Human Sexuality*, 4(6):24, June 1971.

Barton, David: "Sexually Deprived Individuals," *Medical Aspects of Human Sexuality*, 6(2):88, February 1972.

Beeson, P. and W. McDermott: *Textbook of Medicine*, Saunders, Philadelphia, 1975, pp. 581–583, 1486–1487.

Belt, Bruce G.: "Some Organic Causes of Impotence," *Medical Aspects of Human Sexuality*, 7(1):152, January 1973.

Bernstein, William C.: "Sexual Dysfunction Following Radical Surgery for Cancer of Rectum and Sigmoid Colon," *Medical Aspects of Human Sexuality*, 6(3):156, March 1972.

Blumer, Deutrich: "Changes of Sexual Behavior Related to Temporal Lobe Disorders in Man," *Journal of Sex Research*, 6(3):173–180, August 1970.

Brand, L. and N. I. Kemorita: "Adapting to Long-Term Hemodialysis," *American Journal of Nursing*, 66:1778–1781, August 1966.

Calderone, M. S.: "Sex Education and the Physician," *Postgraduate Medicine*, 47: 100–104, February 1970.

Castelnuovo-Tedesco, Pietro: "Talking with Patients About Their Sexual Problems," *Medical Aspects of Human Sexuality*, 2(6):21, June 1968.

Coley, Silas B., Jr.: "Sexual Activity as a Coping Mechanism," *Medical Aspects of Human Sexuality*, 7(3):40, March 1973. Commentaries by Sherwin S. Radin and P. D. Dormont.

Comarr, A. E.: "Sexual Function Among Patients with Spinal Cord Injury," *Urologia Internationalis*, 25(2):134–168, 1970.

Curtis, J., J. Eastwood, E. Smith, J. Storey, P. Veroust, H. de Wardener, A. Wing, and E. Wolfson: "Maintenance Haemodialysis," *Quarterly Journal of Medicine*, 38: 49–89, January 1968.

Davis, Hugh J. and J. Naughton: "Answers to Questions," *Medical Aspects of Human Sexuality*, 6(7):80, July 1972.

Davis, Kenneth G.: "Eros and Thanatos: The Not-So-Benign Neglect of Sexuality, Death and the Physician," *Texas Reports on Biology and Medicine*, 32(1):43–48, Spring 1974.

Dengrove, Edward: "Sex After Major Urologic Surgery," *The Journal of Sex Research*, 4(4):265–274, November 1968.

Dlin, B. M. and A. Perlman: "Sex After Ileostomy or Colostomy," *Medical Aspects of Human Sexuality*, 6(7):32, July 1972.

——, ——, and F. Ringold: "Psychosexual Response to Ileostomy and Colostomy," *American Journal of Psychiatry*, 126:3, September 1969.

Drellich, Marvin G.: "Sex After Hysterectomy," *Medical Aspects of Human Sexuality*, 1(3):62, November 1967.

Dyk, R. and A. Sutherland: "Adaptation of the Spouse and Other Family Members to the Colostomy Patient," *Cancer*, 9(1):123–138, 1956.

Eliot, R. S. and G. F. Melody: "Answers to Questions," *Medical Aspects of Human Sexuality*, 8(1):135,221, January 1974.

Ellenberg, Max: "Impotence in Diabetics: A Neurologic Rather than Endocrinologic Problem," *Medical Aspects of Human Sexuality*, 7(4):12, April 1973.

——: "Answers to Questions," *Medical Aspects of Human Sexuality*, 8(6):137, 156, June 1974; 8(7):39, 57, July 1974.

Epstein, Arthur W.: "Disordered Human Sexual Behavior Associated with Temporal Lobe Dysfunction," *Medical Aspects of Human Sexuality*, 3(2):62, February 1969.

Ervin, Clinton V., Jr.: "Psychologic Adjustment to Mastectomy," *Medical Aspects of Human Sexuality*, 7(2):42, February 1973.

Ford, Amasa B. and Alexander P. Orfirer: "Sexual Behavior and the Chronically Ill Patient," *Medical Aspects of Human Sexuality*, 1(2):51, October 1967.

Gray, H. Twembly: "Sex After Radical Gynecological Surgery," *The Journal of Sex Research*, 4(4):275–281, November 1968.

Greenberg, Ernest: "Effects of Testosterone in Women with Breast Cancer," *Medical Aspects of Human Sexuality*, 8(2):134, September 1975.

Griffith, E. R., M. A. Tomko, and R. J. Timms: "Sexual Function in Spinal Cord-injured Patients: A Review," *Archives of Physical Medicine and Rehabilitation*, 54:539–543, December 1973.

Hellerstein, Herman K. and Ernest H. Friedman: "Sexual Activity and the Postcoronary Patient," *Medical Aspects of Human Sexuality*, 3(3):70, March 1969.

Jacobson, L.: "Illness and Human Sexuality," *Nursing Outlook*, 22:1, 50–53, January 1974.

Jaffe, Lois: "Sexual Problems of the Terminally Ill," in Harvey Gochros and Jean Gochros (eds.), *The Sexually Oppressed*, Association Press, New York, 1977.

Kass, Irving, Katherine Updegraff, and Robert B. Muffley: "Sex in Chronic Obstructive Pulmonary Disease," *Medical Aspects of Human Sexuality*, 6(2):32, February 1972.

Kinsey, A. C., W. B. Pomeroy, and C. E. Martin: *Sexual Behavior in the Human Male*, Saunders, Philadelphia, 1948.

——, ——, ——, and P. H. Gebhard: *Sexual Behavior in the Human Female*, Saunders, Philadelphia, 1953.

Klagsburn, Samuel C.: "Communications in the Treatment of Cancer," *American Journal of Nursing*, 71(5):944–948, May 1971.

Leshner, Martin, Herbert L. Fine, and Wanda Sadough: "Sexual Adjustment in a Chronically Ill and Physically Disabled Population: A Pilot Study," *Archives of Physical Medicine and Rehabilitation*, 52:311–317, June 1971.

Leviton, D.: "The Significance of Sexuality as a Deterrent to Suicide Among the Aged," *Omega*, 4(2):163–174, 1973.

Lyons, A. S. and M. J. Brokmeier: "Mechanical Management of the Ileostomy Stoma," *Surgical Clinics of North America*, 52:979–990, August 1972.

Malin, Joseph M. and B. M. Dlin: "Answers to Questions," *Medical Aspects of Human Sexuality*, 6(11):125, 171, November 1972.

Massie, Henry N. and Albert S. Lyons: "Answers to Questions," *Medical Aspects of Human Sexuality*, 6(5):10, 194, May 1972.

Masters, William H. and Virginia E. Johnson: *Human Sexual Inadequacy*, Little, Brown, Boston, 1970.

Melody, George F.: "Gynecologic Illness and Sexual Behavior," *Medical Aspects of Human Sexuality*, 2(10):6, October 1968.

Mourad, Mahmoud and Chiu Wu Shung: "Marital-Sexual Adjustment of Amputees," *Medical Aspects of Human Sexuality*, 8(2):46, February 1974.

Nahmias, Andre J.: "Answers to Questions,–Venereal Contraction of CA by Males," *Medical Aspects of Human Sexuality*, 7(5):228, May 1973.

Olin, H. S.: "A Proposed Model to Teach Medical Students the Care of the Dying Patient," *Journal of Medical Education*, 47:564–567, July 1972.

Peretz, D.: "Development, Object-Relationships and Loss," in Bernard Schoenberg et al. (eds.), *Loss and Grief*, Columbia Univ. Press, New York, 1970.

Pinderhughes, Charles A., E. Barrabee Grace, L. J. Reyna, and Ruth T. Anderson: "Interrelationships between Sexual Functioning and Medical Conditions," *Medical Aspects of Human Sexuality*, **6**(10):52, October 1972.

Proger, Samuel, et al.: "Viewpoints on Sex Activity for Post-Coronary Patients," *Medical Aspects of Human Sexuality*, **2**(2):22, November 1968.

Romano, M.: "Sexual Counselling in Groups," *The Journal of Sex Research*, **9**(1):69–78, 1973.

Sadoughi, W., M. Leshner, and H. Fine: "Sexual Adjustment in a Chronically Ill and Physically Disabled Population: A Pilot Study," *Archives of Physical Medicine and Rehabilitation*, **52**(7):311–317, July 1971.

Schon, Martha: "The Meaning of Death and Sex to Cancer Patients," *Journal of Sex Research*, **4**(4):288–302, November 1968.

Siddiqui, J. and D. N. S. Kerr: "Complications of Renal Failure and Their Response to Dialysis," *British Medical Bulletin*, **27**:153–159, May 1971.

Smith, JoAnn Kelley: *Free Fall*, Judson Press, Valley Forge, Pa., 1975.

Tyler, Edward A.: "Sex and Medical Illness," in Alfred M. Freedman and Harold I. Kaplan (eds.), *Comprehensive Textbook of Psychiatry*, 2d ed., Williams and Wilkins, Baltimore, 1974.

Wahl, C.: "Psychiatric Techniques in the Taking of a Sexual History," in C. Wahl (ed.), *Sexual Problems: Diagnosis and Treatment in Medical Practice*, Free Press, New York, 1967.

Woodburne, C.: *A Survey of Adjustment of Chronic Renal Failure and Intermittent Hemodialysis with Particular Attention to Sexual Adjustment*, M.S. in Nursing, University of Wisconsin, 1973.

Yamamoto, Joe: "Answers to Questions,–Refusal of Sex Following Bereavement," *Medical Aspects of Human Sexuality,* **7**(1):199, January 1973.

Chapter 32

Adaptation to Open Heart Surgery: A Psychiatric Study of Response to the Threat of Death

Harry S. Abram

Heart surgery, if only because of its newness and mystery, is an overwhelming ordeal. It is an even greater mental and spiritual ordeal than a physical one. As a great mystery to the patient, it is one that he can't face alone; shouldn't face alone (15).

Psychological response to cardiac surgery has interested psychiatrists, psychologists and surgeons for more than a decade. With advancement in this surgical field, the importance of postoperative psychological adjustment and the frequency of major psychiatric disturbances have become apparent. The recent implementation of the "heart-lung machine" or extracorporeal circulation has widened these fields considerably. This paper is concerned with the cardiac patient's reaction to open heart surgery and the realistic threat to life with which each is faced at the time of operation.

In 1952 Bliss and associates(5) reviewed the records of 37 adult patients undergoing mitral surgery. Of these patients 16 percent were "sufficiently anxious and depressed to merit comments by physicians and nurses" postoperatively. Fox and associates(10) in 1954 studied intensively the long-term and emergency defenses of

Read at the 121st annual meeting of the American Psychiatric Association, New York, N.Y., May 3–7, 1965.

This work was supported in part by Public Health Service grant FR-05131 from the National Institutes of Health.

Reprinted from *American Journal of Psychiatry*, **122**:659–668, December 1965.

32 patients having mitral surgery. Nineteen percent had "obvious emotional disturbances" following the operation. His group observed "the most important psychotherapeutic influence was, of course, the successful outcome of the operation," and "all of these patients reacted to the cardiac operation in terms of death or survival and the heart symbolized the life of the whole person."

Two years later Kaplan(13) concentrated on the long-term adjustment of 18 patients who had had mitral commissurotomies. Seventeen percent experienced psychotic symptoms postoperatively. Kaplan noted the manner in which the patients adjusted psychologically "depended upon their total personality organization and their life situation." Excellent physical results did not always lead to a healthy psychological adjustment; even after "alleviation of the (heart) disease . . . they (the patients) are then faced with anxiety-laden problems which they had previously been able to avoid because of their heart ailments."

The psychological meaning of mitral surgery and the reactions of 24 patients with mitral stenosis were well studied by Meyer and associates(17) in 1961. They described vividly the "catastrophe reaction" immediately following mitral surgery, which will be discussed in greater detail later in this paper. They concluded in a similar fashion to Fox's study that operating on the heart "partakes of the touching, manipulating, and cutting of an organ that, even by the most ignorant or the most unsophisticated subject, is viewed as the be-all and the end-all of life itself."

Three recent studies also worthy of note have dealt statistically with larger groups of heart surgery patients. Knox(14) in 1963 reviewed retrospectively 50 patients undergoing mitral surgery and 40 patients prospectively with preoperative and postoperative interviews. In the retrospective study, 32 percent manifested some form of psychiatric syndrome postoperatively, ranging from 14 percent with hysterical symptoms to 2 percent with confusional states and another 2 percent with organic brain damage. In the prospective portion of the report 15 percent developed postoperative symptoms in the form of hysteria. Knox states that prolonged dependency needs and sexual maladjustment along with other indices were often found preoperatively in those patients developing hysterical symptoms postoperatively. Combining both the retrospective and the prospective study, 4.4 percent developed "severe psychiatric disorder" postoperatively. Egerton and Kay(8) evaluated 90 adults and 36 children who underwent open heart surgery. Some 41 percent of the adult group developed delirious symptoms postoperatively. More recently, Blachly(4) has observed the occurrence of "post-cardiotomy delirium." Of 139 patients surviving open heart surgery, 57 percent had psychotic reactions postoperatively.

This study is the third dealing with the psychological aspects of open heart surgery. Although the work of Egerton and Blachly deals with larger series of patients, little attention is given to the *individual* reaction of the patient to the stress of surgery. This paper is concerned directly and intimately with such reactions. As such it is more closely related to the studies of Fox and Meyer, which emphasize the psychological factors involved in the response to closed (non-extracorporeal circulation) heart surgery.

METHOD

During the six-month period of November 1963 to April 1964, 23 patients at the University of Virginia Hospital scheduled for open heart operations were interviewed preoperatively and followed postoperatively by the investigator. Two of these patients were not interviewed preoperatively because of lack of time but were followed postoperatively. The investigator acted as psychiatric consultant and was one of a team of consultants composed also of a cardiologist and neurologist who evaluated each patient preoperatively and postoperatively. The number of patients was limited by the time the investigator could allow for this study.

Preoperative interviews usually took place 24 to 48 hours prior to surgery and lasted approximately one hour. The interview technique was not rigidly structured and attempted mainly to develop the patient's life history, his attitudes toward his heart disease and the approaching surgery, his general personality structure and typical defense mechanisms for dealing with and handling anxiety. Postoperatively follow-up consisted of daily visits after surgery until time of discharge. Some patients were seen after discharge from the hospital for further interviews or corresponded with the psychiatrist by mail.

RESULTS

Of the 23 patients interviewed and upon whom open heart surgery was performed, 8 expired at the time of operation or shortly thereafter. A ninth patient died several months postoperatively and after further heart surgery. The patients ranged between the ages of 16 and 62, the average being 44 years. Eight were female and fifteen male. Thirteen had total aortic replacements, 1 an aortic scraping, 3 closure of interatrial septal defects, 2 mitral and aortic valve replacements, 2 mitral valve replacements, 1 pulmonary valvuloplasty and 1 diversion of an anomolous pulmonic vein drainage. All utilized the pump oxygenator. From a psychiatric viewpoint, 3 patients or 16 percent of those patients not expiring at the time of operation developed severe psychotic episodes postoperatively; one patient became severely depressed, another severely anxious. These findings are summarized in Table 1.

Preoperative Observations   In the preoperative psychiatric interview the two most common reactions to stress of the approaching operation were (1) denial of the imminent threat to life facing the patient (33 percent); or (2) a breakthrough of the anxiety with its full expression during the interview (38 percent). The following illustrates a patient with *severe preoperative anxiety, a death omen and resignation to death prior to surgery*.

Case 16   Mr. R. R., a 53-year-old, separated, childless, ex-garage owner was admitted to the cardiovascular surgical service with a year's history of syncopal attacks and a diagnosis of aortic stenosis. A medical student working with the patient noted, "The examiner cannot help feel that the patient has symbolically closed the doors

Table 1 Description of 23 Open Heart Surgery Patients

Patient	Age	Sex	Diagnosis	Preoperative reaction to stress	Operation*	Postoperative cardiac status	Major postoperative psychiatric complications
1 G.A.	43	F	Mitral insufficiency	Anxiety	Mitral valve replacement	Improved	None
2 E.B.	33	M	Aortic insufficiency	Anxiety	Aortic valve replacement	Expired	Severe anxiety
3 M.C.	56	F	Atrial septal defect	Not remarkable	Closure septal defect	Improved	None
4 J.D.	30	M	Mitral & aortic insufficiency	Not remarkable	Mitral & aortic valve replacement	Expired	None
5 R.F.	43	M	Aortic stenosis & insufficiency	Anxiety	Aortic valve replacement	Expired	Cardiac psychosis
6 L.G.	45	M	Aortic stenosis & insufficiency	Anxiety	Aortic valve replacement	Improved	None
7 F.H.	54	F	Aortic stenosis	Not remarkable	Aortic valve replacement	Improved	None
8 M.H.	57	F	Aortic stenosis	Denial	Aortic valve replacement	Expired†	—
9 M.J.	16	M	Aortic stenosis insufficiency	Anxiety	Aortic valve replacement	Improved	None
10 J.L.	32	M	Atrial septal defect	Not remarkable	Closure septal defect	Improved	None
11 R.M.	36	M	Aortic stenosis	Denial	Aortic valve replacement	Improved	None
12 A.M.	60	M	Aortic stenosis, aneurysm ascending aorta	Denial	Aortic valve replacement, resection aneurysm	Expired†	—
13 A.N.	44	M	Aortic insufficiency, bicuspid aortic valve	Anxiety	Aortic valve replacement	Expired (after further hospitalizations and surgery)	None
14 B.N.	50	F	Mitral insufficiency	Denial	Mitral valve replacement	Improved	Depression
15 B.P.	34	M	Aortic insufficiency, mitral insufficiency and stenosis	Denial	Aortic & mitral valve replacement	Expired†	—
16 R.R.	53	M	Aortic stenosis	Anxiety	Aortic valve replacement	Expired†	—
17 H.S.	35	M	Atrial septal defect	Not remarkable	Closure defect	Improved	None

*All operations utilizing pump oxygenator.
†Expired at time of surgery or shortly afterward.

Table 1   Description of 23 Open Heart Surgery Patients (Cont.)

Patient	Age	Sex	Diagnosis	Preoperative reaction to stress	Operation*	Postoperative cardiac status	Major postoperative psychiatric complications
18 P.W.	40	M	Congenital aortic valve, aneurysm ascending aorta	Denial	Aortic valve replacement, resection aneurysm	Improved	None
19 C.G.	54	M	Aortic stenosis	Anxiety	Aortic valve scraping	Improved	None
20 M.M.	62	M	Aortic stenosis	Denial	Aortic valve replacement	Improved	None
21 M.D.	46	F	Pulmonic stenosis	—†	Pulmonary valvuloplasty	Improved	Cardiac delirium
22 M.F.	42	F	Anomalous pulmonary drainage	Depression	Diversion pulmonic drainage to left atrium	Expired (shortly after discharge)	None
23 M.B.	56	F	Aortic stenosis	—†	Aortic valve replacement	Improved	Cardiac psychosis

*All operations utilizing pump oxygenator.
†Patient not evaluated preoperatively.

behind him (closed down business, etc.). He has no close relatives and comes here with great resignation. It is my hope this resignation is not negative." During the psychiatric interview 24 hours prior to surgery, it was obvious the patient was highly anxious. He had been up since 2:00 a.m. after having awakened with arm pain and severe anxiety. He expressed concern that his anxiety was getting out of control and that he would go "mental." He spoke of superstitious thinking that he had never experienced before. Specifically he had noticed for the past two consecutive days blackbirds roosting outside his hospital window. He then went on to comment that blackbirds rarely come near to buildings and usually stay out in the field. These blackbirds represented to him a "good sign" and furthermore he would not sign the operative permit unless they returned that evening. Shortly after these comments he spoke of having made out his will. There were no other remarkable features detected during the interview and no evidence of any psychotic process.

The following day he underwent surgery with aortic valve replacement. Postoperatively the patient did well throughout the first night but early the next morning he became restless with increasing respiratory rate and decreasing venous and blood pressure. In spite of heroic maneuvers, including cardiac massage, he expired within a few hours. Whether or not the blackbirds did actually return is unknown. But it is of interest the patient reversed or perhaps denied the omen of the blackbird, usually interpreted as a death symbol into a "good sign."

Postoperative Observations In the immediate postoperative period the most common and perhaps consistent finding was the "catastrophe reaction" described by Meyer(17). These patients present a picture of complete apathy and fatigue after having gone through a severe stress and survived. Meyer states these patients resemble in their appearance "the photographed faces of survivors of civil disaster. the countenances of these patients present staring and vacant expressions of seeming frozen terror. Immobile, apathetic, and completely indifferent to their fate, they respond to inquiries in monosyllables devoid of affect." In the present study it was noted that after a few days this syndrome usually disappeared, followed by a mild depression and then a gradual lifting of the affect. However at times the reaction did not subside and the patient became psychotic. This state was discussed by Meyer in another paper(16) dealing with the catastrophe reaction in which the apathy and withdrawal are "accompanied by harrowing repetitive dreams and phantasies which appear to be derivatives or reproductions of phases of the operative experience . . . the patient is in a state of excitement, associated with ideas of depersonalization, and visual hallucinations."

Two patients in this series developed psychotic reactions similar to the depersonalization and visual hallucinatory state described above. In this paper the investigator uses the term *cardiac psychosis* to describe this syndrome and to distinguish it from the apathetic stage of the catastrophe reaction. These psychoses were characterized by transient but recurring sensory hallucinations or illusions without disorientation to time, place or person. They were not typical of the usual postoperative delirium and apparently different from the delirium described by Blachly(4) in that the patients were well oriented and had closer ties with reality. Except for the absence of disorientation, the transient quality of the psychoses with periods of several remissions during a 24 hour period was similar to postoperative delirious states or acute delirium associated with brain damage in which there are bouts of confusion interspersed with periods of lucidity. For example:

Case 22. Mrs. M. B., a 56-year-old housewife, was admitted to the University of Virginia Hospital for the first time with a history of a strep throat and a febrile illness in her teens followed by an asymptomatic period until two or three years prior to admission. At that time she developed substernal chest pain on exertion, relieved by rest. Six months prior to admission she noticed ankle swelling; five months later, she had an episode of acute pulmonary edema. Diagnosis on admission was aortic stenosis, secondary to the rheumatic heart disease, inactive and congestive heart failure. The patient was not seen preoperatively by the psychiatrist, but no other physician observed any abnormality in her mental status.

During her operation, the aortic valve was replaced with a Starr-Edwards valve prothesis utilizing extracorporeal circulation. She tolerated the operation well and continued to do so in the recovery room until six days postoperatively when one of the recovery room nurses noted, "Patient is evidently experiencing auditory hallucinations—says she hears daughter's husband pages over p.a. system, has been smelling strange gas all day." That afternoon she was seen by the psychiatrist. She was oriented in all spheres but was convinced that she would be taken back to the operating room for more surgery and that "new machines" had been brought into her room to do her harm. Her "hallucinations" were in actuality illusions with misinterpretations of various stimuli about her. There were indeed voices coming over the loudspeaker system, odors about, and various monitoring systems in use to gauge her pulse, heart functioning, and other physiologic measurements. The psychiatrist explained the situation to her and offered to stop by daily to see her. For the next three days she continued to be suspicious and fearful. The psychotic symptoms then subsided and did not recur for the rest of her hospital stay, which was uneventful.

When interviewed nine months postoperatively she spoke vividly of her experiences in the intensive care unit. Her affect was brighter and more appropriate. She had returned to her work as a clerk in a local court house and physically was doing quite well. Nevertheless she still had not given up completely her illusions. She spoke of the gas, the machines, the p.a. system, and wondered what the purpose of their use in the ICU had been. These doubts did not seem to occupy a significant part in her life, but she was not convinced it was her "imagination" as her husband said it was. When her misinterpretation of reality was re-explained to her by the psychiatrist she accepted his interpretation with some but not complete relief of her doubts. She spoke of the reassuring aspects of the psychiatrist's visits during her stay in the ICU and the beneficial qualities of his "standing beside" her during these frightening episodes. She reiterated her awareness of her surroundings during the delusional and illusionary period, saying that she always knew where she was.

Each of these patients had a neurological evaluation which was essentially negative except for the mental status as described.

DISCUSSION

When one considers the mortality of this series of patients, the threat of death is a situation with which each of these patients was faced. One may ask, "How much were these patients actually told about their chances to survive surgery?" Was their denial and anxiety related to what they had been told by their physician or was it based on factors outside of their awareness or by subliminal or nonverbal cues? As to what had actually been told the patients, the investigator can only surmise from what the physician and the patient told him. In all probability the patient was given an honest account of his prognosis but the risks of surgery were minimized. If such were the case the threat to life was recognized also from other factors, perhaps related to cues the patients picked up from the personnel caring for them or from unconscious factors.

Anxiety reactions to impending death have been well described by Biegler(2), who states, "There is an unconscious awareness on the part of the patient of his impending death and . . . this is reacted to with anxiety that may be repressed." Weisman and Hackett(21) speak of "middle knowledge" in the dying patient who is aware he is dying even though those about him deny it: "For the majority of dying patients, it is likely that there is neither complete acceptance nor total repudiation of the imminence of death."

In another but similar context Tolstoy describes the attitude of the dying patient and the physician treating him in *The Death of Ivan Ilych*(19): "Ivan Ilych knows quite well and definitely that all this is nonsense and pure deception, but when the doctor, getting down on his knee, leans over him, putting his ear first high then lower, and performs various gymnastic movements over him with a significant expression on his face, Ivan Ilych submits to it all as he used to submit to the speeches of the lawyer, though he knew they were lying and why they were lying."

It is important to note in this series of patients that each had been seriously ill with chronic severe cardiac disease and not infrequently had had bouts of congestive heart failure, precordial pain, etc. Most looked upon surgery as potentially life-saving or death-producing.

As commented on by Fox(10) and Meyer(17), the meaning of heart surgery to the patient seems to lie directly with the threat of cessation of the organ realistically and symbolically associated with continuation of life. Several patients in the present study expressed fears of their heart "not starting up again" after repair of the diseased valve. Another wondered if he would be alive while his heart was stopped and he was on "the pump." Mr. E. B. and Mr. R. R., both of whom died postoperatively, expressed a fear of going insane. These patients may well have been expressing their concern about impending death. Weisman and Hackett(21) comment, "The fear of dying may also represent itself in psychological terms as a fear of insanity."

The etiology and exact nature of the "cardiac psychosis" remains unclear, but it seems likely as described by Meyer(16) that it is an extension or a part of the catastrophe reaction. An important factor mentioned by Meyer and also by Egerton(8) is the role of sensory stimulation and deprivation in the formation of the postoperative psychotic symptoms. Egerton comments, "Apart from brief visiting periods and times of staff care, for a few days the patient's visual fields are restricted to white acoustic tiling viewed through the oxygen tent. Many patients remarked on the monotony of the ceiling, and visual hallucinations were often initially manifested by the appearance of patterns on the ceiling or of faces protruding from the small, regular holes in the tiling."

. The similarity of this description and Meyer's patients with dreams, phantasies, depersonalization and hallucinations in the two cases in this paper described as "cardiac psychosis" is of interest and not dissimilar from patients with poliomyelitis in tank-type respirators described by Solomon and associates(18). In their series, "The mental abnormalities began after the patient had been in the tank respirator for 24–48 hours or longer, and were characterized by well-organized visual and auditory hallucinations and delusions reacted to in different ways and to different degrees." In these cases there were no "febrile, anoxic, toxic or metabolic derangements," and an "imposed structuring of stimuli" was postulated as the etiology of this order.

In 1938 Cobb and McDermott(6) discussed 16 cases of postoperative psychosis who were not suffering from the usual delirium. These patients were well oriented but developed transient hallucinations and paranoid delusions. The authors comment:

It is of especial interest that all of these patients are foreigners, and most of them have language difficulty. They feel truly outlandish (in the real sense of the word) and they act that way. The environment is new and strange, the customs of the hospital are nothing like those in their homes. Even the speech is difficult to understand. Many of them were brought to the hospital after an entirely inadequate explanation. Once on the ward, the busy staff looked after them well, but the doctors did not make an effort to find out if the patient really knew before the operation what it was all about, just what the procedure would be and why it was necessary. Then came the operation; normal fears were exaggerated by loneliness and strangeness. After operation when drugs cause dreaminess and confusion, these people all get panic feelings, ideas of persecution and punishment and even delusions and hallucinations. The duration of the psychosis is from one to several weeks and the delusions, hallucinations and ideas of persecution that at first look schizophrenic seem to clear up fairly quickly, go over into a diffuse anxiety state with depression and then disappear entirely.

It is suggested that careful psychologic preparation for the operation by means of interpreter or better a priest who speaks the patient's language, would make postoperative psychoses less likely to occur.

Thus Cobb and McDermott were discussing a form of sensory deprivation in patients following general surgery leading to a postoperative psychosis quite similar to the "cardiac psychosis" described in this study.

The intensive care unit (ICU) at the University of Virginia Hospital, which is apparently not dissimilar from such units in other hospitals, is a sterile, barren room save for four beds for postoperative patients, a multitude of machines required for maintenance of the patient's life and various physiologic measuring devices. The patients often associated the ICU with severe discomfort, waking up after surgery, tracheotomies, intravenous fluids, the cardiac pacemaker and the monitoring devices. Several believed that they improved only after leaving the ICU and looked upon going back there as a death warrant. The apparatus in this unit, the hushed tone of doctors and nurses hustling about in an urgent fashion caring for critically ill patients, the starkness and sterility of the room and the placement of tubes in every conceivable orifice leave ample grounds upon which to base paranoid delusions. As one physician stated, "We take over every function of the patient in his breathing, urinating, defecating and eating. I believe these patients become panicky over our taking away these privileges."

Although all these procedures are lifesaving and the ICU is designed to care for in the most efficient manner the patient returning from major surgery, the patients often reversed this meaning. That is, believing that leaving the ICU led to recovery obviously reversed the situation in that the patient was only allowed to leave after he stabilized physically. But psychologically speaking, the patients often did improve after being placed back in an environment in which they were more familiar, where the patients were not as critically ill and in an atmosphere of less urgency.

The problem arises as to how much the patient experiences sensory deprivation and how much is actually sensory overstimulation. Blachly(3) comments, "These patients have just the opposite of sensory impairment, they have a fantastic amount of sensory input in the form of pain, noise from respirators, cardiac monitors, nurses and residents, etc., talking, multiple needle punctures, frequent examinations ad nauseum."

The patient in all probability experiences *both* deprivation and stimulation. The latter, however, consists of stimuli which are foreign, incongruous and dystonic to the patient; i.e. the monitoring systems, respirators, etc., in the intensive care unit. These devices, in spite of their necessary life-saving functions and their reassuring qualities to some patients, are perceived by others, especially those patients with poor reality ties, as threatening and ideal objects upon which to project their fears. The deprivation comes from the immobility of the patient and his estrangement from a familiar environment. Often for several days and at times longer the patient lies on his back, propped up and constrained by pain, urinary catheters and intravenous fluids.

It should be added that some investigators believe the mental changes seen after heart surgery are due to organic changes. Zaks(22) performed a series of psychological tests on patients before and after closed mitral and aortic surgery. He concluded "clinically observed . . . psychiatric disturbances in patients undergoing mitral commissurotomy do not appear to be of a purely functional nature . . . psychiatric problems are triggered off by certain psychological functions which appear to be related to organic changes in the course of heart disease and mitral valve surgery."

Dencker and Sandahl(7) in their study of mental disturbances after closed heart surgery for mitral disease conclude that the "operation as such is not responsible for the postoperative psychosis" and that it may be due to "an early cerebral injury of rheumatic type predisposing to mental disease." Blachly(4) also ascribes the psychotic reactions of his patients after open heart surgery to organic causes, the etiology of which is unclear in his report. Several possibilities are given, such as alterations in the serum protein from use of the pump oxygenator or a defect in the catecholamine metabolism giving rise to a product similar to LSD.

A recent report, however, by Herbert and Movius(12) using psychological testing on patients having closed mitral commissurotomies does not corroborate Zaks' findings. Their results are not compatible with those of others reporting postoperative CNS damage. Egerton(8) also reported negative results for intellectual dysfunction on psychological tests given to his series of patients before and after open heart surgery. From a neurological viewpoint a variety of cerebral disorders have been reported after open heart operations by Gilman(11).

In conclusion, the question arises as to the role of the psychiatrist in the care of the heart surgery patients and certain prophylactic measures which could possibly prevent some of the severe postoperative psychotic reactions reported in this and other papers. As reported elsewhere(1), certain preoperative psychological factors, namely the excessive amount of preoperative anxiety, the use of denial as a major defense mechanism and unrealistic expectations for the proposed surgery, were found to be valid prognosticators of untoward postoperative psychological reactions in general surgical procedures. Because of the high mortality in this present series of patients these factors could not be further elucidated and verified except to note that preoperative anxiety and denial were common findings.

With regard to the threat to life with which each patient was faced and the actual number of deaths in a large proportion of the patients, the psychiatrists did play an active role in their care. Eissler(9) writes, it is a "clinical fact—which as far as I know, is not disputed by anyone—that the psychiatrist has his rightful place at the side of the deathbed." Often in this group of patients the family and the patient looked to the psychiatrist as the most available member of the cardiovascular surgical team. Although he was not involved in the actual surgical procedure and did not go into details of the operation or the prognosis with the patient or family, he could give them certain information about the operation and at times keep the family informed of the patient's progress. In addition to listening to the patient's concerns about and fears of surgery and death, the psychiatrist had relatively close contact with the family postoperatively, not infrequently listened to their outpourings of grief in the case of death and experienced some of their feelings himself.

A relatively common finding was the lack of information given the patient preoperatively as to what could be expected postoperatively, especially his experience in the intensive care unit. From a preventive viewpoint such an explanation, with a carefully detailed preview of waking up with an endotracheal tube in place, possibly being on a respirator, being catheterized and on intravenous feeding and fluid maintenance, should be given in an attempt to relieve or allay postoperative anxiety. The use of cardiac monitoring and other physiologic measuring devices could also be described to the patient to reduce the possibility of paranoid projection upon these instruments. At times a preoperative visit to the ICU would be in order. Undoubtedly such measures would not entirely eliminate the postoperative psychoses and delirious states. But such explanations and attempts at establishing a doctor-patient relationship based on trust and honesty are backed by sound clinical and humanitarian principles.

Weisman and Hackett(20) effectively utilized such a relationship in decreasing the incidence of delirium after cataract surgery. Cobb and McDermott(6) discuss a similar relationship. Possibly allowing the patient to talk about his fears of death or if it be the case permitting him to entertain in his awareness the longing to die may prevent a postoperative panic which disrupts somatic processes. Working with the caretaking personnel especially in the ICU and instructing them in the psychological aspects of the surgery and postoperative care may also be helpful. Certain physiologic factors, e.g., avoiding dehydration and insuring adequate pulmonary ventilation, have been stressed in the prevention of postoperative psychotic states and are of definite importance, yet the psychological meaning, both realistic and symbolic, of this surgery should also be considered in the patient's preoperative preparation and postoperative care.

SUMMARY

This report is a clinical study of 23 patients undergoing open heart surgery and how some responded to it. It is evident that these patients reacted to the operation as presenting not merely a symbolic but realistic threat to life. The presence of anxiety and the use of denial preoperatively are described. Two cases of postoperative "cardiac psychosis" are reported and their relationship to the "catastrophe reaction" and "post-cardiotomy delirium" commented upon. The intensive care unit is seen as a life-saving necessity in modern heart surgery but at the same time frequently perceived by the patient as psychologically threatening. Certain prophylactic psychological measures are discussed.

REFERENCES

1 Abram, H. S., and Gill, B. F.: Predictions of Postoperative Complications, New Engl. J. Med. 265:1123–1128, 1961.
2 Biegler, J. S.: Anxiety as an Aid in the Prognostication of Impending Death, Arch. Neurol. Psychiat. 77:171–177, 1957.
3 Blachly, P. H.: Personal communication.
4 Blachly, P. H.: Post-Cardiotomy Delirium, Amer. J. Psychiat. 121:371–375, 1964.
5 Bliss, E. L., Rumel, W. R., and Branch, C. H. H.: Psychiatric Complications of Mitral Surgery, Arch. Neurol. Psychiat. 74:249–252, 1952.
6 Cobb, S., and McDermott, N. T.: Postoperative Psychosis, Med. Clin. N. Amer. 22:569–576, 1938.
7 Dencker, S. J., and Sandahl, A.: Mental Disease after Operations for Mitral Stenosis, Lancet 11:1230, 1961.
8 Egerton, N., and Kay, J. H.: Psychological Disturbances Associated with Open Heart Surgery, Brit. J. Psychiat. 110:433–439, 1964.
9 Eissler, K. R.: The Psychiatrist and the Dying Patient. New York: International Universities Press, 1956.
10 Fox, H. M., Rizzo, N. D., and Gifford, S.: Psychological Observations of Patients Undergoing Mitral Surgery, Psychosom. Med. 16:186–208, 1954.
11 Gilman, S.: Cerebral Disorders after Open Heart Operations, New Engl. J. Med. 272:489–498, 1965.
12 Herbert, C. T., and Movius, H. J.: Psychological Deficits with Mitral Commissurotomy, J.A.M.A. 187:191, 1964.
13 Kaplan, S. M.: Psychological Aspects of Cardiac Disease, Psychosom. Med. 18: 221–233, 1956.
14 Knox, S. J.: Psychiatric Aspects of Mitral Valvotomy, Brit. J. Psychiat. 109:656–668, 1963.
15 Lawton, G.: Straight to the Heart: A Personal Account of Thoughts and Feelings While Undergoing Heart Surgery. New York: International Universities Press, 1956.
16 Meyer, B. C., and Blacher, R. S.: A Traumatic Reaction Induced by Succinyl Chloride, New York J. Med. 61:1255–1261, 1961.
17 Meyer, B. C., Blacher, R. S., and Brown, F.: A Clinical Study of Psychiatric and Psychological Aspects of Mitral Surgery, Psychosom. Med. 23:194–218, 1961.
18 Solomon, P., Leiderman, P. H., Mendelson, J., and Wexler, D.: Sensory Deprivation, a Review, Amer. J. Psychiat. 114:357–363, 1957.
19 Tolstoy, L.: "The Death of Ivan Ilych," in Ten Modern Short Novels. New York: G. P. Putnam's Sons, 1958.
20 Weisman, A. D., and Hackett, T. P.: Psychosis after Eye Surgery, Establishment of a Specific Doctor-Patient Relation in the Prevention and Treatment of 'Black-Patch' Delirium, New Engl. J. Med. 258:1284–1289, 1958.
21 Weisman, A. D., and Hackett, T. P.: Predilection to Death, Death and the Dying as a Psychiatric Problem, Psychosom. Med. 23:233–255, 1961.
22 Zaks, M. S.: "Disturbances in Psychological Functions and Neuropsychiatric Complications in Heart Surgery," in Cardiology, vol. 3. New York: McGraw-Hill Book Co., 1959.

Chapter 33

Survival by Machine: The Psychological Stress of Chronic Hemodialysis

Harry S. Abram

Chronic hemodialysis for terminal renal failure is an example of medical progress in which the patient faces new, and at times overwhelming, psychological stresses. Dependence upon machines for survival is a recurrent theme of man's response to artificial organs. In cardiac surgical patients, the patient experiences this dependence in the Intensive Care Unit with its mechanical respirators, electrocardiograms, and computerized monitoring devices. In postcardiotomy deliria, patients often project their feelings upon these devices and have illusory experiences in which they perceive the machines as menacing. Usually the ICU stay and this type of dependence on machines is of short duration. However, with dialysis it is chronic and lifelong in nature. Put in one form or another the patient must learn to "live with the machine." Through patients' thoughts and fantasies we can learn a great deal about this relationship with an inanimate object which becomes an essential part of the patient's life.

The clinical use of dialysis began in the early 1960s after innovations in heart surgery already foretold some of the problems and conflicts to be expected. In dialysis, however, the environment shifts from the intensive care to the renal or dialysis unit, and the patient's concern with acute threat of death shifts to concern with the prolonging of life by artificial means.

Reprinted from Rudolf H. Moos (ed.), *Coping with Physical Illness,* Plenum Book Co., New York, 1977, pp. 295–309.

THE PROLONGATION OF LIFE

If one regards operating on the heart as the paradigm of the acute threat of death, chronic hemodialysis represents a related but contrasting situation—the meaning of prolonging life by artificial means. The patient dying of irreversible renal failure does face death and is in or near the terminal stage of uremia when he begins dialysis. He usually reacts with euphoria after a few "runs" on the dialyzer. His sensorium and mental confusion clear, and his extreme lethargy and apathy dramatically diminish. Symbolically and realistically he has "returned from the dead." When he is mentally alert the dialysis may initially create anxiety, particularly when he is "hooked" to the machine and witnesses his own blood running through the clear plastic cannulae into and out of the dialyzer. Usually this anxiety is transient, particularly if someone explains the procedure beforehand and as the routine is established. However, one patient, with whom I worked, had an episode of depersonalization during an initial dialysis in which he hallucinated himself on the ceiling watching himself being dialyzed. He reacted with panic, screaming, "Oh, my God, I've got to get out of here! Let me out of here!"

However, once the patient becomes accustomed to the dialysis regimen, concern with living overrides fear of dying. This latter fear does return in later stages of dialysis and especially with the death of a fellow dialysis patient. But for the remainder of the patient's life (unless he receives a successful renal transplant) he wrestles at both conscious and unconscious levels recurrently with the question which he asks himself in one form or another, "Is a life on dialysis worth living?" Wright[29] outlined well the stresses, the losses, and the restrictions with which the patient (and his family) must contend. Particularly bothersome are the dietary and fluid constrictions, the care of the shunt and fears of its becoming infected or clotting, and a sense of bodily deterioration. Bone demineralization, pruritis, insomnia, and sexual impotence are concomitant problems. And above all the patient must learn to live with the dialyzer, the machine which sustains his life.

Chronic dialysis thus creates unique psychological situations which require further elucidation, namely: (1) dependency versus independency needs in the patient; (2) a relationship with an inanimate object (the dialyzer); (3) ambivalence over life and death; (4) the role of denial as a major defense mechanism; and (5) interpersonal conflicts related to the dialysis unit personnel and the dialysand's spouse.

DEPENDENCY-INDEPENDENCY CONFLICTS

Dependency upon the treatment regimen is a relatively constant finding among dialysis patients. Being "hooked" to the dialyzer has meaning not only in the sense of the patient being attached to it via his cannulae but in the sense of his being "addicted" to it. In reality he is dependent upon it for his life and upon the dialysis unit nurses and physicians. Keeping his shunt clean and staying on a constricted diet also impose dependency, as well as limitations being placed on his life by having to keep a certain proximity to a renal unit. The patient, however, receives conflicting messages. He must "cooperate" with the program (that is, be able to accept his dependency upon it), and at the same time be independent (lead a "normal" life by keeping up his work and family relations). He must attach himself or be attached to the dialyzer for approximately 30 hours a week. During the remainder of the week he must keep up a semblance of a "healthy" life, in spite of physical complications and symptoms. "Postdialysis lethargy" is a particular problem when the patient must return to work after a "run" on the dialyzer when he is apt to feel weak and "washed out" (as a patient phrased it). This dual message ("be dependent and independent") gives rise to conflicts, which the patient handles in a variety of ways.

The patient may react through accepting the dependency and independency requirements. He follows the treatment program and is able to return to society as an active citizen. If, however, he is threatened by the dialysis situation and has unresolved dependency needs, he reacts either by becoming excessively dependent and unable to give up the "sick role" or rebels against the problem and refuses to accept the regimen. With excessive dependency the patient becomes demanding during dialysis and has difficulties outside of the unit with his work and family. It usually requires three to six months for the patient to resolve this conflict and return to his premorbid pattern of living. For the patient who does not resolve it, he may have continued difficulties giving up his role as patient to return to the workaday world. On the other hand, the patient who is too threatened by dependency cannot accept the program. He refuses to stay on his diet, takes poor care of his shunt, is grouchy with the nurses, and comes late to the dialysis unit for his treatments.

De-Nour[13] discusses dependency in chronic dialysis in a somewhat similar vein but with more emphasis upon repressed aggression resulting from the enforced dependency.

RELATIONSHIP WITH THE DIALYZER—
DISTURBANCES IN BODY IMAGE

A patient[1] wrote of his experience with dialysis and feelings about the dialyzer: "Though my contact with the machine is for only thirty hours a week, it is seldom, if ever, completely out of my mind. It maintains a powerful, almost frightening hold on my life. Were it not for the kidney I wouldn't be here to write this and yet I find it impossible to make friends with the monster."

Cooper[11] describes a thirty-five year-old woman who developed a hypomanic psychosis associated with chronic dialysis. Much of her delusional system centered around the dialyzer: "She became wildly excited and irritable and threw a bottle of saline at the window. . . . She expressed considerable hatred of the machine, endowing it with human motives. She expressed the view that the machine somehow knew of her dependence for her life on it and enjoyed, patronizingly and sometimes contemptuously because of her weakness, a feeling of total power." He then interprets her reaction as follows: "The patient's attitude to the machine was exteriorized during the psychosis. She clearly resented her dependency upon it but also feared the pain it could bring her. She referred to it vehemently, almost as if it had human attributes, as 'that hateful thing,' 'I despise it,' and 'I sometimes feel like destroying it.' In fact, the patient threw a bottle of saline, intended for infusion, through a window; this can be seen as a symbolic act of destruction directed at the machine."

Although such psychoses are rare among dialysis patients, the above description of a dialysand's primary processes does give us insight into the unconscious meanings of this relationship between patient and machine. Another source is that of the dialysis patient's fantasies about himself and the dialyzer. Shea[27] describes an adolescent patient who incorporated the dialyzer into his body image as shown in his "mechanical appearing (figure) drawings," and Wright[29] notes the "umbilical" symbolism in which the dialyzer represents the placenta and the cannulae the umbilical vessels. (Glud and Blane[16] describe the tank respirator or "iron lung" in similar terms as "a source of security, a womblike structure which the patient fears to leave.") From a psycho-analytic viewpoint this fusion between patient and machine complicates the process of separation and individuation seen in the extreme symbiosis of the early infant-mother relationship as discussed by Mahler,[20] even though the relation is not truly a symbiotic one (as the machine receives no gratification from the patient).

It is of interest that Prugh and Tagiuri,[23] in their observations on the emotional aspects of respiratory care involving the "iron lung" in children with poliomyelitis, also note an incorporation of an artificial lung similar to Shea's adolescent. "Bill, a seven-year-old boy, was able to incorporate his chest respirator as part of his body image, using the acceptable and somewhat humorous fantasy that he resembled a 'man from Mars.'" The science fiction theme (that is, the "man from Mars" in the above quotation) also occurs with dialysis patients. Such fantasies as "zombies" (having arisen from the dead) or "androids" (science fiction robots who appear human) are not uncommon. A minister being dialyzed gave his first sermon after returning to the pulpit on "the rather simple story of Jesus raising someone from the dead" and de-scribed himself as a present-day Lazarus saved by "the miracle . . . of . . . advanced medical science." Another patient[10] spoke of his complexion as a "half olive color" and described himself as looking "like a candidate for a downtown morgue." He also fantasied conversations between himself and the dialyzer, and spoke of himself as a machine ("After all, I was kind of an experimental machine in a frontier world.").

Borgenicht, Younger, and Zinn[7] in an unpublished thesis on the psychological aspects of home dialysis give the following striking examples of "dehumanization and loss of identity to the dialysis machine."

> Mr. X said he thought the machine was "very funny" and that "the whole idea is very amusing to me. When I am on dialysis I am half-robot, half-machine." What he meant to say was "half-man, half-machine" or "half-robot, half-man," but the words he used are very revealing. The word "man" is omitted and he thinks of him-self as all machine.
>
> Mrs. Y, a patient, noted with annoyance that a doctor had once told her, "If you learn to run the machine, you'll get closer to it." "I don't want to be buddy-buddy with the machine," she said angrily, "It's a machine—if it does its job, I'll do mine."

Kemph[18] also describes a dialysis patient who "depicted himself quite graphically as 'a broken man, a disjointed man,' jerked about and completely controlled by the strings to his arms, a sick puppet. At this time he had a blood pressure apparatus on one arm and the dialysis tubes on the other."

A dialysis patient with whom I have worked intensively in psychoanalytic therapy free-associated during one session.

> We're sort of zombies . . . sort of close to death. . . . I guess we're like the living dead . . . somebody who should be dead but who isn't. . . . We're sort of just marking time. In essence we're dead anyway. I'll never have the feeling of being a whole human being. Even if I have a [kidney] transplant one of these days, I'll never get over the feeling I'm already dead.[4]

He also wondered if he would be held responsible for murder if he committed one, as he was kept alive by artificial means and actually died when he was accepted for dialysis. In his words he was "already dead" and his "death warrant . . . signed and sealed a year and a half ago" (when he began dialysis). Litin[19] also speaks of dialysis patients as having "Frankenstein fantasies" associating the cannulae or shunts with the tubes protruding from the monster's neck. As I note in an earlier paper,[3] "These associations (of zombies, etc.) were of special interest to me, as they corroborated some of my fantasies in working with some of these patients. At times while watching some of them being dialyzed, I had fantasies that they were in many aspects 'the living dead' who had to be 'revitalized' twice weekly by machines or that they were machines themselves (science fiction 'androids') in the shape of humans and dependent on other machines for their existence."

The patient thus *incorporates* the dialyzer and *projects* his feelings onto it. (We noted a similar but fleeting projection in ICU patients after open-heart surgery.) In addition to the mechanical aspects the dialysis patient's concept of his body has a defective, deathlike quality to it. My analytic patient condensed many of these feelings one day by exclaiming. "What a piece of junk I've become!" Searles[25] comments extensively on the schizophrenic's view of inanimate objects. He describes patients "who react to various *parts* of themselves as being nonhuman. It is as if such patients have particularly abundant reason for their anxiety lest they become wholly nonhuman, for parts of themselves have already, in their subjective experience of themselves, become so." With the dialysis patient there is also objective experience that a vital part of their existence is in fact nonhuman.

AMBIVALENCE OVER LIFE AND DEATH

In this section I shall deal directly with the prolongation of life, the patient's ability to adapt to the chronic stress of dialysis, and the problem of suicide among dialysis patients. In its most simplified and yet in its most complex form the question the patient asks himself is, "Is it worth living?" (under the restrictions and hardships of a dialysis program). For as Camus[9] most succinctly put it in his opening sentence of *The Myth of Sisyphus*, "There is but one truly serious problem and that is suicide. Judging whether life is or is not worth living amounts to answering the fundamental question of philosophy." Most patients on dialysis programs speak of suicide at one point or another. Most do not commit suicide, yet there are a certain number who do through various means either actively or passively kill themselves. The "passive" forms consist of withdrawing from dialysis programs and an inability or refusal to follow the medical regimen (e.g., adhere to the dietary and fluid restrictions, take proper care of the shunt), and the "active" form includes suicidal attempts through such means as cutting the shunt (thereby bringing about death through exsanguination), ovedosage, use of firearms, etc.

How often does the active and passive suicidal behavior occur? In a recent study[5] I report on the results of a questionnaire study which contains data on 3,478 dialysis patients in the United States. The following summarizes our findings: 29 patients withdrew from programs, 117 died from an inability or a refusal to follow the medical regimen, and 20 successfully committed suicide (another 17 attempted suicide but were not successful). There were also 9 "accidental" deaths from shunts falling apart, 37 "unexplained deaths," and 107 "accidents" (such as shunts falling apart) without death. Therefore, excluding "unexplained" and "accidental" deaths, 166 patients or approximately one out of every twenty ended their lives through active and passive suicidal behavior.

Here are some examples of these forms of suicide:

Death through Dietary Indiscretion

Rubini notes:

> We have had one suicide. He was a chap who, as a child, didn't like his teachers or his parents. As an adult he didn't like his bosses; they all told him what to do. After he was dialyzed two years, he didn't like dialysis either, as we tried to tell him what to do also. He picked the Easter weekend. He went on a tremendous feed, almost a Roman orgy. He started off in the San Francisco docks, where he purchased a number of kinds of shell fish and a jug of chianti. He went home, put a suckling pig on the spit; he partook of all these goodies and more. When admonished by his visiting mother, he retorted he knew better than his doctors how to take care of himself. He returned to the hospital with severe hyperkalemia, suffered a cardiac arrest and he died.[24]

Withdrawal from Program

An answer from our questionnaire and a newspaper clipping:

> Two people requested to be taken off dialysis. In both cases, the patients were in extremely poor physical health and were unable to be successfully rehabilitated; one because of eighth nerve damage secondary to Kanomycin which resulted in permanent vertigo and complete deafness and in the other case that of a physician with personality problems prior to dialysis—simply a failure to thrive on dialysis despite the best possible management. Both patients' requests to be withdrawn from dialysis were acceded to by the staff with some degree of relief on our part.

" 'It's Time to Die', Ailing Man Decides" read the headlines of an Associated Press release about a thirty-three-year-old dialysis patient. It describes his "wasting body and his demoralized mind." The article quotes his saying, "I'm taking myself off the machine. . . . I'm ready to die," and comments that "a day later, he signed a waiver removing himself from further treatment." He remarked, "When I signed the waiver I knew what kind of symbol that was, like signing your own certificate. . . ."

Active Suicide

Three terse responses from the questionnaire:

> One patient, a fifty-four-year-old man unhappy with maintenance dialysis in his second year of therapy, began playing with his shunt. He had two "accidental" falls fracturing his hip. Later, his shunt "opened" when he was alone at home and he exsanguinated.

> Sixty-four-year-old-male – walked into the cellar at 3:00–4:00 a.m., placed his arm in a bucket, and cut his shunt with a scissor. The patient exsanguinated.

> Patient with severe renal osteodystrophy, osteomalicic pain and multiple pathological fractures. Shot himself in head with a shotgun after three years of center dialysis.

Another response to the questionnaire brought up requesting a transplant as a suicidal maneuver, "There is also a group of patients who *request* high-risk (poorly matched) cadaver transplant. The usual statement is 'I'll try anything rather than this' (dialysis)."

Beard speaks of the dilemma of the dialysis patient as "fear of death and fear of life": "The fear of dying and the fear of living were an integral part of the whole problem of renal failure and its treatment. To these patients, their major concerns were involved with this dilemma. To them, working out some solution to this dilemma was their primary task. To these patients, the whole matter of chronic renal failure, hemodialysis, and kidney transplantation meant dealing with this dilemma."[6]

Thus the dialysis patient struggles with his life and ambivalent feelings about it. Psychotherapy is often crucial, especially to allow the patient to become aware of and work through the ambivalence. Depressions often are concurrent with physical complications, both in the patient and in a fellow patient. One of the major defenses for coping with these conflictual feelings about life and death is denial, and it is to this mechanism that we now turn our attention.

DENIAL

As with the dependency conflicts associated with dialysis, denial is a universal finding in psychological studies of chronic hemodialysis. Nemiah[21] defines denial as "a mechanism of defense in which the facts or logical implications of external reality are refused recognition in favor of internally defined, wish-fulfilling fantasies." With this definition "external reality" represents the dialysis regimen and its implications and the "wish-fulfilling fantasies" the wish not to be ill. Such denial not only involves the patient but his caretaking personnel as well. In one form or another they ask,

"Why should dialysis be upsetting? It doesn't really affect you. It's a little inconvenient but that's all."

Short and Wilson[28] describe in detail the roles of denial in chronic hemodialysis. They note:

> The capacity for denial in these patients is phenomenal, but what are they denying? Previously, it was pointed out that these patients accept their condition and the inevitability of their outcome. What is denied is that it is happening now. When their bones become bowed from osteomalacia, and they go from a cane to a walker, and then to a wheelchair, they continue to expect and to hope that this process will be reversed. When clotting, bleeding, or infections occur at the cannula site, they accept this as a singular occurrence, only to have it happen again. . . .
>
> In view of the foregoing, it would appear that increasing denial would be an inevitable consequence of chronic hemodialysis. However, in actuality, it may be necessary that these patients be allowed to maintain their capacity to repress in order to cope with their life situation.

Hackett[17] makes a similar point (i.e., the necessity and actual beneficial aspects of denial) in his work with coronary care patients. Denial is so commonly found among dialysis patients that psychotherapeutic intervention is often extremely difficult or impossible. And indeed if denial is so strong it is best left alone. Denial becomes dangerous, however, when the patient refuses to accept dialysis, that is, when the wish not to be ill leads to a massive psychotic denial and a break with reality. Such denial occurred in four patients whom I studied. Two had "religious conversions" in which they became convinced their kidney failure was cured by God and that dialysis was no longer necessary, and a third after using massive denial since the beginning of his dialysis became transiently psychotic, developed a hysterical dysphonia (in which he could not "speak" of his troubles) and gradually declined to a state of invalidism and death. This patient shortly before his psychotic break was interviewed by a local newspaper reporter. In the newspaper article he states, "I could go on indefinitely (with dialysis) . . . the 'machine' hasn't changed my life much at all. People don't look at me as an invalid. I'm simply a whole man who needs treatment. I still work and raise a family. I guess I'm pretty normal. . . . I've learned to live with it and appreciate it" (speaking of the dialyzer). The fourth, a woman from a primitive background, refused dialysis from the onset, as she did not want to uproot her family to move to our dialysis center.

Short and Wilson also stress that denial occurs in the families of dialysis patients, the community, and the caretaking personnel. In particular the dialysis physician affirms there is "nothing wrong" with his patient, thereby compounding the patient's denial. For example, Norton[22] writes of dialysis, "When a vital biological organ fails and is adequately replaced by a workable and relatively convenient socially devised and maintained organ, the person tends on the whole to go on living in much the same manner as he did before his loss. Having been given a social reprieve from a biological death he acts like a living person rather than one dying." In response to the suicide questionnaire discussed earlier, one physician answered, "The problems appear little different than in a nondialyzed population." Another stated, "You will be making an error if you equate inability to stay on the diet with a 'death wish' or suicide. Patients have problems with the diet and other facets of dialysis because it represents a limitation of their freedom or because they cannot comprehend the necessity of close cooperation." I believe such examples of blanket denial on the physician's part are related to his emotional investment in the success of his dialysis program which prevents his stepping back and viewing objectively what is happening to his patients.

INTERPERSONAL RELATIONS

It is of interest that few studies deal directly with the spouse of the dialysis patient, especially as the spouse is so intimately involved and in home dialysis is responsible for the patient's treatment (i.e., attaching him to the dialyzer, etc.). As impotence and infertility in male dialysis patients and infertility in women patients are frequent complications, the lack of work in this area is all the more surprising. Aside from Shambaugh's[26] reports of his group work with the spouses of dialysis patients, there is little available material in the area. The unpublished thesis of Borgenicht[7] and his colleagues comments extensively on the marital interactions of home dialysis patients, and it is indeed unfortunate that this work is not available to a larger audience.

Shambaugh paints a rather dim picture of the spouse's response to the dialyzed partner. In his group therapy sessions with spouses (some of whom operated their partner's dialysis machines themselves) over an eight-month period, denial and guilt were common findings.

Hostility and murderous impulses toward the sick partner were quite prevalent in the group (for example, "A husband fantasied taking an axe to the kidney machine"). And although the group worked through some of these intense feelings, denial ("reluctance to face the horrible facts") and a number of deaths among the sick partners eventually resulted in the group's disbanding. Indeed, the intensity of the group's reaction and the dialysis physicians' response to Shambaugh's report (requesting he discontinue his group meetings) may account for there being so few studies in this area. However, Borgenicht's paper corroborates his work, as do isolated reports of dialysis deaths brought about by "carelessness" on the part of the spouse responsible for setting up the dialysis equipment for his partner. Borgenicht describes a death in a patient with rather serious marital discord as occurring after her husband "used the wrong dialysate in the dialysis machine." In reply to the suicide questionnaire mentioned earlier a physician remarked in an item dealing with "accidental" deaths, "The 'accidental' death may have been deliberately done by the patient's wife."

Many of the same reactions exhibited by the spouses occur with the dialysis team. As the reader is by now aware, denial is present among patient, spouse and personnel. With the latter I have already noted some physicians' responses to the suicide questionnaire, the reaction to Shambaugh's findings, and remarks such as Norton's. In spite of the multiple and independent reports of the psychological and physical hardships of dialysis, some dialysis physicians tenaciously hold on to the idea there is nothing traumatic about dialysis, that it is "a way of life" or no different from adaptation to any chronic illness. One dialysis physician refused to let a psychiatrist talk with his patients as he feared "it would upset them." Such physicians look upon the expression of any feelings, especially negative ones, as harmful and to be avoided. And indeed the conspiracy of denial in the patient, family, and physician can make psychiatric intervention or exploration extremely difficult or impossible. "Cooperativeness" is also stressed by dialysis physicians. Often "cooperative" describes the uncomplaining patient who passively accepts all that comes his way and even "thanks" nurses and physicians for procedures which are painful and unpleasant. As noted earlier Brown[8] discontinued therapy in "uncooperative" patients, and apparently patients have been taken off of dialysis in other centers for similar reasons. Therefore complaints are discouraged, and the patient quickly perceives that negative attitudes are not tolerated. Some dialysis patients fear rejection by the unit and believe (perhaps correctly in some instances) that if they are not "good" patients their dialysis will be terminated.

Although interaction between doctor and patient is important, the dialysis nurse actually spends more time with the patient and the intensity of this relationship may create more of a problem (Abram,[1] Fellows[15]). With the patient coming to the dialysis unit twice weekly for 15 hours the remainder of his life, intense transference and countertransference reactions develop. De-Nour[13] and Cramond et al.[12] both discuss this area and the problems of possessiveness and withdrawal which occur in nurses and patients. Nurses are frequently frustrated by the patient who will not let them take care of him, the patient who becomes demanding, or the negativistic patient. Sexual advances by a patient are also threatening, and in some units nurses report male patients becoming exhibitionistic or openly masturbating. I have found group therapy helpful with the renal unit nurses to help them understand their patients' reactions and not be threatened by them. For example, understanding the demanding patient as one with excessive dependency needs, or sexual advances as a symptom of the patient's fear of impotency and a regressive phenomenon in which he is looking for "mothering" from the nurse can be reassuring and prevent her rejecting the patient entirely. Nurses often identify with their patients and have dreams of themselves being dialyzed. The following is an example:

I had a dream just today about cannulae and the kidney. I didn't ever think I would this soon after starting to work with them. Anyway, I barged in unexpectedly on a class at a college and started talking about the artificial kidney. I told the teacher that I "just had to tell these people all about the kidney." So I did—I had cannulae in my leg by the way. I woke up just after leaving the classroom, but the teacher was running after me and yelling, "You forgot to show them your cannulae."

In summary, chronic dialysis serves as a paradigm not only of man's response to a chronic illness but to a treatment which requires dependence upon an artificial device for survival. As such, it has some similarities to use of the "iron lung" in patients with respiratory poliomyelitis and also serves as an example of how patients may react to artificial organs. With chronic dialysis certain psychological conflicts are highlighted, and we are given an unusual opportunity to look at such aspects as the patient's relationship to a machine, the role of dependency and independency in chronic illness, the use of denial as a major defense mechanism and interpersonal relations involving patient, family, nurse, and physician. An editorial in the *Journal of the American*

Medical Association[14] speaks of the problems in chronic dialysis which may prove pertinent to other transplanted and artificial organs.

> An unknown number of people are today alive and working under biweekly hemodialysis who would otherwise be dead. Even committed to their slavery to a machine, it is understandable that life may be sweet, in its limited way. The submission, with the reaper smiling grimly behind every movement, knowing that his turn will come, does not lead to a placid temperament and easy acceptance. To the contrary, the person who lives successfully with hemodialysis lives in a state of suppressed inner turmoil from which there can never be an escape except in death. The history of those who have lived with and at the mercy of hemodialysis confirmed the difficulty of the position. . . .
>
> The man who lives on borrowed time lives uneasily, and the latest medicosurgical creations of borrowed time must eventually be questioned in terms of the moral result, as well as their physical result. They may be creating nothing, except something of that which philosopher Unamuno called the "too long" life.

REFERENCES

1 Abram, H. S. The nurse and the chronic dialysis patient. *A Dialysis Symposium for Nurses.* Philadelphia, April, 1968(a).

2 Abram, H. S. The psychiatrist, the treatment of chronic renal failure, and the prolongation of life: I. *American Journal of Psychiatry* **124**, 1351–8, 1968(b).

3 Abram, H. S. The psychiatrist, the treatment of chronic renal failure, and the prolongation of life: II. *American Journal of Psychiatry* **126**, 157–67, 1969(a).

4 Abram, H. S. Psychotherapy in renal failure. *Current Psychiatric Therapies* **10**, 86–92, 1969(b).

5 Abram, H. S., Moore, G. L., & Westervelt, F. B. Suicidal behavior in chronic dialysis patients. *American Journal of Psychiatry* **127**, 1199–1204, 1971.

6 Beard, B. H. Fear of death and fear of life. The dilemma in chronic renal failure, hemodialysis, and kidney transplantation. *Archives of General Psychiatry* **21**, 373–80, 1969.

7 Borgenicht, L., Younger, S., & Zinn, S. Psychological aspects of home dialysis. Unpublished, 1969.

8 Brown, H. W., Maher, J. F., Lapierre, L., Bledsoe, F. H., & Schreiner, G. E. Clinical problems related to the prolonged artificial maintenance of life by hemodialysis in chronic renal failure. *Transactions of the American Society for Artificial Organs* **8**, 281–91, 1962.

9 Camus, A. *The myth of sisyphus.* London: Hamish Hamilton, 1960.

10 Chadd, K., & Estlack, M. Transplant . . . A layman's account of a kidney transplant. Unpublished.

11 Cooper, A. J. Hypomanic psychosis precipitated by hemodialysis. *Comparative Psychiatry* **8**, 168–74, 1967.

12 Cramond, W. A., Knight, P. R., Lawrence, J. R., Higgins, B. A., Court, J. H., MacNamara, F. M., Clarkson, A. R., & Miller, C. D. J. Psychological aspects of the management of chronic renal failure. *British Medical Journal* **1**, 539–43, 1968.

13 De-Nour, A. K. Emotional problems and reactions of the medical team in a chronic hemodialysis unit. *Lancet* **2**, 987–91, 1968.

14 Editorial. On borrowed time. *J.A.M.A.* **195**, 13, 168, 1966.
15 Fellows, B. J. The role of the nurse in a chronic dialysis unit. *Nursing Clinics of North America* **1**, 577–86, 1966.
16 Glud, E., & Blane, H. T. Body-image changes in patients with respiratory poliomyelitis. *The Nervous Child* **11**, 25–39, 1956.
17 Hackett, T. P., Cassems, N. G., & Wishnie, H. A. The coronary-care unit: An appraisal of the psychological hazards. *New England Journal of Medicine* **279**, 1365–70, 1968.
18 Kemph, J. P. Renal failure, artificial kidney and kidney transplant. *American Journal of Psychiatry* **122**, 1270–4, 1966.
19 Litin, E. M. Discussion of three papers on man and the artificial organ. Read at the 123rd Meeting of the Amer. Psychiat. Assn., Detroit, Mich., May, 1967.
20 Mahler, M. On human symbiosis and the vicissitudes of individuation. *Journal of the American Psychoanalytic Association* **15**, 740–63, 1967.
21 Nemiah, J., *Foundations of psychopathology*. New York: Oxford University Press, 1960.
22 Norton, C. E. Attitudes toward living and dying in patients on chronic hemodialysis. Abstract, New York Academy of Sciences Symposium "Care of Patients with Fatal Illnesses," February, 1966.
23 Prugh, D. G., & Tagiuri, C. K. Emotional aspects of the respirator care of patients with poliomyelitis. *Psychosomatic Medicine* **16**, 104–28, 1954.
24 Rubini, M. I. Proceedings, the conference on dialysis as a practical workshop. New York: National Dialysis Committee, 1966.
25 Searles, H. F. *The non-human environment*. New York: International Universities Press, 1960.
26 Shambaugh, P. W., & Kanter, S. S. Spouses under stress: Group meetings with spouses of patients on hemodialysis. *American Journal of Psychiatry* **125**, 928–36, 1969.
27 Shea, E. J., Bogdan, D. F., Freeman, R. G., & Schreiner, G. F. Hemodialysis for chronic renal failure: IV. Psychological considerations. *Annals of Internal Medicine* **62**, 558–63, 1965.
28 Short, M. J., & Wilson, W. P. Roles of denial in chronic hemodialysis. *Archives of General Psychiatry* **20**, 433–7, 1969.
29 Wright, R. G., Sand, P., & Livingston, G. Psychological stress during hemodialysis for chronic renal failure. *Annals of Internal Medicine* **64**, 611–21, 1966.

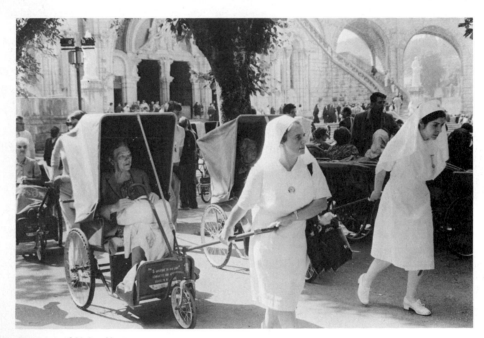

Courtesy of Helen Nestor

Part Eight

Care of the Dying Patient: Recent Developments

Chapter 34

The SHANTI Project:
A Community Model
of Psychosocial Support
for Patients and Families
Facing Life-Threatening Illness

Charles A. Garfield
Rachel Ogren Clark

INTRODUCTION

Recent advances in medical knowledge and technology have produced profound qualitative changes in the nature of dying and chronic illness. The increasing sophistication of therapeutic measures capable of prolonging life has lengthened the average time between the onset of fatal illness and the termination of life. That added time could be a great blessing, allowing the dying person and those he or she loves the possibility to renew their intimacy, be together, share their sorrow, anger, fears, and the joy that comes from the experience of their loving. This time is a potentially powerful opportunity for growth and resolution. However, because our culture has taught us to deny and camouflage dying and death, few of us—patients, families, friends, and medical personnel—know how to use this gift of time in a positive way. The majority of patients still face the dim prospect described by Aldous Huxley: "increasing pain, increasing anxiety, increasing morphine, increasing demandingness, with the ultimate disintegration of personality and a loss of the opportunity to die with dignity."

This paper was presented at the First (1976) and Second (1977) National Training Conferences for Physicians on Psychosocial Care of the Dying Patient sponsored by the Cancer Research Institute, University of California, San Francisco and at the American Psychological Association Annual Convention, San Francisco, 1977.

We organized the SHANTI Project as a response to the moribund realities of social distancing and emotional alienation. Our hope was to develop an effective model of health care intervention for dealing with some of the psychological and social needs of people facing life-threatening illness—patients, their families, and the professionals who serve them. In developing this model we had three specific aims: (1) to offer *direct community services* consisting of counseling and companionship for patients and families facing life-threatening illness, and grief counseling for survivors of a death; (2) to provide opportunities for *professional training and public education* on relevant issues that arise in ministering to the psychological and social needs of the dying and their families; and (3) to conduct substantive *research* to evaluate the impact of the SHANTI Project as a community service, using research methodology from clinical and social psychology and sociology.

WHAT HUMAN PROBLEMS COME TO OUR ATTENTION?

Who calls the SHANTI Project? Our basic operating principle concerning calls is that we will respond to requests for assistance from anyone dealing with a life-threatening illness.

In general, calls to the Project fall into two major categories: (1) requests for information and (2) requests for services. Calls for information come primarily from people who want to know how they can become volunteers in the Project, where they can attend professional training programs, or how they can get a SHANTI volunteer to address their group or provide inservice education.

> Following a call from the head nurse of a hospital coronary care unit, several volunteers visited the unit to discuss the SHANTI Project. The initial meeting was set up to explore the possibility of making referrals to the Project. Soon after the joint discussions began, it became clear that the nurses on the unit had personal issues to discuss. Many acknowledged the tremendous emotional stress of their work and spoke more about their own reactions than about the needs of their patients. The volunteers assumed the role of consultants and tried to point out the covert norms operating in the social system of this unit. For instance, one of the powerfully enforced contextual rules was that anyone expressing strong feelings related to patient care or requesting help with a given patient was less than fully competent. That is, although individual nurses paid lip service to the team approach and to cooperative endeavor, there were very stringently enforced rules about individual responsibility that practically excluded collaborative effort. Many nurses experienced considerable distress because they felt unable to request legitimate support even in near-emergency situations. One SHANTI volunteer pointed out that the senior nurses on the unit, who had less direct contact with patients, were enforcing these norms covertly while never admitting to them verbally. Each of the staff nurses admitted to strong negative feelings about particular senior nurses stemming from situations in which the staff nurse had been chastised for requesting assistance in what should have been a routinely collaborative task. One nurse, who had recently completed what she later described as a totally inadequate orientation, broke into tears when she realized that some of her "failures" were due not to incompetence

but rather to inadequate introduction to specific procedures. She received much support from her fellow staff nurses, who acknowledged that she had been victimized by an inappropriate orientation.

The nurses soon changed their request to the SHANTI Project and inquired about the possibility of having one or two volunteers serve as facilitators of a support group for staff nurses. A volunteer recommended that the meeting also be opened to senior nurses so that clear and direct communication could be established within the unit to the benefit of nursing staff and patients alike.

The nurses also spoke of their frustration in dealing with contradictory inputs from medical staff. For example, one specialist might recommend a set of procedures indicating an aggressive approach to therapy, while a second might conclude that there is nothing more to do for the patient. The nurses expressed tremendous dismay at having to deal with these contradictory opinions. Therefore, they said that another item on their agenda for these group support meetings would be the development of more effective communication with medical staff.

The calls for services are usually from one of four kinds of clients. First there are calls from *patients who desire inperson counseling, companionship, and emotional support from a volunteer.*

A SHANTI volunteer who had been regularly visiting an elderly patient in a nursing home learned that Becky, her client, was expected to die very soon. When the volunteer visited Becky it was clear that she was not fully aware of the severity of her condition, although physically she had deteriorated appreciably. Becky was confused about her medical status and was receiving little accurate information from her physician or the nursing staff. Her belongings had already been packed in cardboard boxes in expectation of her death. Her family and friends had not been notified about the gravity of the situation. With Becky's permission and encouragement, her volunteer called the physician, who had known his patient for many years, and requested that he visit with Becky. He promptly came and expressed to Becky and the volunteer his own sad feelings about the impending loss of his friend and patient. The volunteer called Becky's best friend, her younger brother, and her niece to tell them Becky was dying. During the next few hours, all three came to see Becky for the last time. None of them, however, felt comfortable staying more than a few minutes. The nursing staff was willing to allow the volunteer as much time as she needed, and she decided to stay with Becky throughout the night. They spoke at length and Becky revealed that she was aware of her situation because of the discussions with her doctor and the volunteer. She indicated that she felt far better now that the ambiguity of her condition had been reduced. She was able to say good-bye to several of the people most important to her and later that evening, with the SHANTI volunteer holding her hand, Becky died.

Many callers are quite specific about their needs. Some ask for a volunteer who can teach them relaxation techniques to help reduce their pain or anxiety; someone who can help them deal with breaking the news of their illness to other members of the family; someone who will listen without being frightened away like family and friends who change the subject at each mention of death or when fear or anger arises. Although occasionally the requests are for a limited number of visits, the vast majority of contacts have developed into close relationships between volunteer and patient, lasting from several weeks to many months.

The members of the SHANTI Project are aware of the value and effectiveness of peer counseling. Some of our volunteers are dealing with cancer, heart diesease, or other chronic life-threatening illnesses. They have been trained to counsel other patients and to apply what they learn from these interactions to their own situations. Peer counselors are often unusually effective because they have access to perspectives unavailable to the rest of us.

Barbara, a woman with seriously advanced uterine cancer, requested a counselor who was knowledgeable about her specific illness. When the opportunity to meet with a peer counselor was presented, Barbara agreed and an ongoing relationship was established. Because she was anticipating continuing chemotherapy treatments of the sort that her volunteer had also experienced, much useful exchange of information took place between volunteer and client. The volunteer agreed to accompany Barbara to her chemotherapy treatments, and encouraged her to discuss openly with her physician any aspect of the treatment or the disease that concerned her. The two developed an extremely strong bond based primarily on their joint efforts in fighting a common illness. Later, when Barbara's husband requested support, a second SHANTI volunteer was sent to assist him. This conjoint model, i.e., more than one volunteer working with a single family, has been employed quite successfully. This case is still in progress. The first volunteer, her own health permitting, intends to remain with Barbara throughout the course of her illness. The second volunteer is prepared to provide support to Barbara's husband and in the event of her death, to be available throughout the period of grief.

The second group of requests for service comes from people close to a patient. They may ask for a *volunteer to spend time with an entire family* in which one member is suffering from a life-threatening illness; or for a *volunteer to work with just one member of a patient's family—often a spouse*. The patients for whom these people are caring (1) have not requested the help of a volunteer, (2) live outside the geographical range of the SHANTI Project (whereas the relative lives in the San Francisco Bay Area), or (3) are already seeing another volunteer (in which case one volunteer would serve primarily as the patient's advocate and companion and the other as advocate and support for the patient's spouse or family).

Following an introductory call from a well-known oncologist in the Bay Area, Paula, the wife of a 35-year-old man with acute leukemia, called the SHANTI Project to ask for help. As a nurse, Paula recognized the importance of emotional support for cancer patients, but her husband, Jim, was not itnterested in talking with anyone, even his wife. Paula found the impact of living with the threat to Jim's impending death increasingly difficult to bear and had become extremely anxious and unsure of her ability to care for and relate to her husband. The side effects of Jim's chemotherapy treatments, remissions followed by recurrence of symptoms, the change from outpatient to inpatient status were all causing confusion for Paula and jeopardizing her relationship with Jim. Paula communicated all of this information during her initial phone call to the SHANTI Project, and requested a volunteer who could help her separate the realities of the situation from the morass of confusion. She especially wanted to plan a strategy for coping with her own feelings while re-establishing communication with Jim. Paula asked for a woman volunteer who was about her age and who understood Catholicism, as she felt her religion to be her primary source of support. A volunteer fitting that description was available and met with Paula that evening. After this initial meeting, the volunteer saw Paula often, sometimes accompanying her to the hospital to visit Jim. They spent many additional hours consulting by phone.

Upon realizing how important the volunteer was to his wife, Jim requested another volunteer as his own advocate. He had many unexpressed feelings that he felt he could not communicate to Paula. Most were related to his fear of death, his feelings about the possibility of survival, and his relationship with his parents and brother in Indonesia. Another volunteer was sent to serve as a primary support for Jim. As time progressed, the volunteer-client relationships evolved into a conjoint format in which the four individuals would meet together as well as in pairs. The help that Paula received in recognizing her own strength allowed her to make it possible for Jim to die at home as he wished. It also made it possible for her to be with him in a loving, calm, and supportive manner during his final hours, even though her pain was great. Both SHANTI volunteers were with Paula and Jim when he died.

More than 6 months later, and in the midst of grieving, Paula and her SHANTI volunteer still meet frequently. They are attempting to help Paula work through her grief and they discuss various aspects of their shared and separate experiences with Jim. They have become close friends and seem likely to continue their relationship throughout the grieving period and beyond.

It is important to recognize that the strain of an extended life-threatening illness can be enormous for patient and family and that few adequate emotional supports are available. Most dying people desperately want and need the presence and affection of those whom they love. Yet without caring support for themselves and validation of their rights and feelings, those loved ones, because of their own fear, sorrow, frustration, and sense of helplessness, often withdraw and become emotionally and physically inaccessible to the patient. The presence of emotional support can help generate that degree of hope and strength necessary for patient and family to deal with the seemingly overwhelming burdens of a terminal illness.

The third group of callers who request volunteers are *people who have survived the death of a family member or close friend.* They are often experiencing the trauma of separation including loneliness, profound sadness, and a sense of loss and disorientation.

Jane, a single parent, called the Project to request a volunteer to help her through her grief. Her only child, a 10-year-old boy, had died 2 weeks earlier after open-heart surgery that had a 90 percent chance of success. Jane had no family support, and while her friends were good listeners, they were unable to provide her with useful feedback. She needed to talk with someone who understood the psychological aspects of grief and who could point out that her reactions were normal. She was very relieved to learn that her feelings were not predictors of imminent and irreversible mental breakdown.

A volunteer whose primary expertise is grief counseling was selected and has spent many hours with Jane. At Jane's request, they have discussed the horror of watching her child attached to tubes and monitors and not being allowed to hold him and, even worse, the anguish of not being with her son when he died. This occurred because caring but misguided medical staff felt it would be too painful, and therefore sedated her heavily and put her to bed in a room down the hall. Jane has talked with her volunteer about the need to redefine her own identity (she has seen herself as a mother for 10 years, and suddenly is without a child to mother); about the changes in her lifestyle and perspective that have occurred now that no one depends upon her, waits for her, loves her completely; about letting go of any possibility of seeing her son grow to adulthood; about her sleeplessness, her loss of appetite, her inability to concentrate, and her sudden bouts with depression, all of which are typical symptoms of grief. Jane's volunteer provided loving and practical support throughout potentially suicidal situations brought on by the depths of existential despair. They were able to view the severe depression as a sign that Jane had accepted her son's death and was beginning the slow, undeniably painful process of adjusting to that sad reality.

Jane and her volunteer have agreed to work together for as long as they both feel that the relationship is a supportive one. In putting together the pieces of her life, Jane is attempting to map out her plans for the immediate future and, with the help of her volunteer, has developed a more satisfactory social life.

Unfortunately, survivors of a death must suffer their anguish in a death-denying society whose principal messages are: "Don't let it get you down"; "Cheer up"; "Be brave"; "Forget the past—it's over"; "Just throw yourself into living." These messages clearly say, "Don't show me your pain. It frightens me." Our culture encourages us to short-circuit emotional suffering at every opportunity. For the grieving person, this means there is little chance for working through the pain of loss, because what is in reality a psychological necessity is seen by others as morbid self-indulgence. SHANTI volunteers look upon grief counseling and continued emotional support for survivors as an integral function of their work. The Project offers help during the period of grieving to survivors of our own clients (those with whom we have worked prior to their deaths) and to survivors of persons with whom we had no contact before they died.

The fourth type of call for services consists of *requests for backup consultation and/or emotional support from people who work with the dying outside the usual institutional settings.* Private duty nurses who care for terminally ill patients at home, clergy who are called upon to counsel dying members of their congregations, teachers who work as home tutors to children with potentially terminal illnesses, visiting homemakers, and others who work along with the dying frequently encounter the psychological conflict and emotional anguish that accompany terminal illness. However, they often have no readily accessible colleagues with whom to discuss their reactions and feelings and the cumulative emotional impact of their work. SHANTI volunteers can share the personal understanding they have gained through similar contact with the dying as well as general information on specific issues related to dealing with life-threatening illness.

HISTORY AND OPERATION OF PROJECT

In June 1974, Dr. Garfield and several colleagues were discussing possible alternative support systems for the dying. They talked of hospices and the expense and organizational expertise that would be needed to form such an institution in the Bay Area. They also explored the feasibility of using volunteer counselors to provide support for those dealing with life-threatening illness. Dr. Garfield was hoping to find an alternative requiring less long-term planning and fewer financial demands, a way to bring help to people *now*. Stewart Brand, who developed the *Whole Earth Catalog*, came up with the uniquely simple concept that formed the functional basis of the SHANTI Project. Brand's suggestion was to make it possible to reach a group of volunteers at one central telephone number who had the interest, ability, and time to work with the dying. These volunteers, when contacted, would go out into the community to visit with patients in their homes, in hospitals and nursing homes, or in any other mutually agreeable location.

On February 1, 1975, an answering machine was attached to a telephone in the home of Rachel Ogren Clark, codirector of the SHANTI Project. Anyone who wants to use our service can call and leave a message. Mrs. Clark returns the calls, discusses the client's situation and needs in detail, and then relays that information to the SHANTI volunteer best equipped to meet the needs of the caller. That volunteer then sets up a time to meet the client, and hopefully begins an ongoing, one-to-one supportive relationship. We accept only firsthand referrals, which means that we work only with those people who themselves request a volunteer. There is only one exception to this principle of operation: if a person is too ill to talk on the phone we will accept a referral from nursing, medical, and social work staff or family member if we are assured that the patient has knowledge of the Project and has asked to see a volunteer. This policy usually prevents situations in which patients agree to see a volunteer when they would really rather not.

A psychologist from an oncology unit at a major hospital called the Project to request a volunteer for Steven, a terminally ill man with lung cancer. It was learned that, in 2 weeks time, Steven would be leaving for an extended-care facility. The psychologist realized that a volunteer who could provide continuity of care might be a valuable asset to his patient. Steven was having tremendous difficulty acknowledging the emotional impact of his illness. He was extremely frightened by the prospect of dying and the flood of powerful feelings it threatened to release. After clearly determining Steven's interest and obtaining his permission, the psychologist introduced the SHANTI volunteer to Steven, and the three of them engaged in conversation. When Steven left the acute-care hospital for the extended-care facility, the volunteer accompanied him and continued to visit throughout his stay at the new institution. Later, when Steven returned home, he asked his volunteer to continue visiting him. The volunteer was able to provide ongoing support for Steven as well as periodic feedback to the staff members of the acute-care and extended-care facilities. The volunteer will remain with Steven until he dies, and then will be available to Steven's wife for grief counseling, should she request it.

Initial calls to the Project are recorded and volunteers keep notes on all contacts with their clients. These records are kept confidential and are used only for purposes of evaluating our work. To date, the telephone service has worked efficiently and our intention is to continue this mode of operation.

THE SHANTI VOLUNTEERS

SHANTI volunteers are client advocates. The word *advocate* literally means "supporter, favorer, and friend." It also means "Holy Spirit" and "Spirit of Truth." In serving as a client advocate, the SHANTI volunteer is not bound by a rigid definition of his or her role as are most professionals and family members. Each volunteer becomes an advocate through a commitment to doing what needs to be done as determined by both patient and volunteer. At times, volunteers serve their client as companion and friend; at other times they consult with medical and nursing staff or family members; and at still other times they clean ashtrays or make phone calls. The SHANTI volunteer is not a professional psychotherapist or member of the clergy, although some function elsewhere in these capacities. However, each volunteer must sometimes deal with psychological and spiritual issues in the interests of the client. Volunteers are aware of the importance of knowing when to contact specific health professionals, for example, psychotherapist, physician, nurse, social worker, or clergy. While patient advocacy often calls for a high tolerance for ambiguity, it allows for a considerable flexibility in the service of client and family. As volunteers learn to avoid the trap of addiction to action and thereby discover the art as well as the science of helping another human being, they frequently find that "the experience of being cared for may benefit the patient more than the direct effect of the care" (Quint, 1967). This heightened advocacy and resulting increases in functional latitude make it easier to maintain the compassionately caring and empathetic attitude that impelled most volunteers to enter the Project in the first place.

Volunteers realize that approaching the patient as a willing advocate, and possessing considerable expertise in the psychosocial aspects of life-threatening illness maximize their likelihood of providing meaningful emotional support. Because they consider themselves to be guests in the hospital rooms or homes of their clients, volunteers recognize that their sustained presence may be directly connected with their physical, emotional, and spiritual utility. For many volunteers, an additional revelation has been that caring for another human being can be as emotionally rewarding for the helper as for the recipient.

The SHANTI Project is committed to providing continuity of care for all clients. Once a client-volunteer relationship is established, the SHANTI volunteer's primary allegiance is to the client rather than to any single institutional setting. The volunteer continues to work with his or her client whether the client is at home, agrees to a series of hospitalizations, or is moved to an extended-care facility. This continuity of care is one of the major factors differentiating the SHANTI Project from other existing social services.

Volunteers come to the client's bedside not as singular experts in life-threatening illness but as advocates wishing to cooperate as fully as possible with professional staff. As facilitators of communication between their client and various health professionals, volunteers are often in a position to offset the all-too-frequent lay perception that hospital professionals are insensitive automatons performing esoteric physiological rites on the bodies of their patients. They can recound experiences in which professional staff emerged as kind, sensitive human beings forced to work under extreme stress, and who possessed vital information about the client's emotional needs. The volunteers remain open to full cooperation with staff in the service of the client's needs.

Most people approach helping services in one of three ways—through self-initiated action, through the advice of others (physician, nurse, family, friends, the clergy), or by coercion. Because the SHANTI Project only accepts firsthand referrals, health professionals and others can only obtain the services of a patient advocate by first familiarizing themselves with the Project and then making relevant information known to the patient. A clear, concise explanation by a health professional about the SHANTI Project as well as about other community resources, allows a patient to evaluate his or her own needs and then decide on the advisability of contacting the Project.

As the Project has progressed, we have learned to predict what kinds of people will make the most effective volunteers. All prospective volunteers send us a statement describing why they want to work with patients and families facing life-threatening illness. They are subsequently invited to an interview in which one or two experienced volunteers and the codirectors of the Project meet with each prospective SHANTI volunteer. In addition to an evident sense of compassion, we look for many qualities, among them a high tolerance for ambiguity; an ease in talking about dying (as evidenced by discussion that is personalized rather than predominantly philosophical); the ability for introspection as reflected in extensive self-knowledge; a healthy sense of self-confidence; a high tolerance for frustration; a degree of psychological mindedness; a sense of humility that allows one to view sharing in someone else's dying as a joint process with learning occurring on both sides; the ability to speak and understand various metaphors (religious, cultural, or symbolic); and relevant professional training in counseling, psychology, social welfare, nursing, or medicine. SHANTI volunteers do not pretend to be totally altruistic; all admit that the work brings them valuable rewards and enhances their personal growth. However, a prospective volunteer who sees working with the dying primarily as one more event in a series of personal-growth experiences would not be accepted into the Project; neither would someone whose religious convictions included the need to proselytize. Other characteristics that would exclude a prospective volunteer from the Project are a powerful need to control and a strong belief that there is a right way to die.

Each SHANTI volunteer makes a commitment to work at least 1 year with the Project, and expects to spend 8 to 10 hours per week with clients. We consider individualized training, supervision, and support necessary for all volunteers. Each initiates their potential association with the Project by attending a training seminar before being accepted into the program. Among the various training seminars offered by the SHANTI Project is a 5-day national conference conducted yearly. The training programs are designed to supply prospective volunteers with information about the Project so that we may be assured that they are familiar with both the skills required of volunteers and the basic orientation of the Project.

Although all volunteers attend one or more prerequisite training seminars before coming to work for the Project, we view volunteer training as an open-ended process. We try to facilitate frequent contact between experienced Project members and new volunteers. Ongoing training takes place at regular weekly meetings in which volunteers freely share professional and personal expertise in an unusually supportive emotional milieu seldom found elsewhere. We generally follow case-conference format, occasionally inviting guest consultants to speak on training issues of particular interest. In addition to the weekly meetings, all volunteers have easy access to the Project's co-directors and staff throughout the week. This contact is encouraged so that volunteers are free to contact those in supervisory positions whenever necessary. The directors also meet frequently with volunteers to maintain an awareness of the particular needs, skills, and development of each volunteer.

The idea behind the SHANTI Project was a new concept, and the perseverance of the SHANTI volunteers has made it a workable one. The volunteers are a heterogeneous group, both in philosophical orientation and in personal background and experience. Almost every religious belief (including nonbelief) is represented among the volunteers. Many come from the helping professions: social workers, psychologists, teachers, gerontologists, and the clergy. Others are housewives, architects, students, artists, secretaries, and musicians. Their ages range from 22 to 73. What our volunteers have in common is the willingness, emotional strength, training, and sensitivity to confront humanely the realities of death and dying without resorting to the evasion and denial so often apparent. Almost all the volunteers have experienced profound personal loss and have gained considerable psychological maturity as a result. They are hardworking, deeply committed people—sometimes prone to compassionate overwork—who have exhibited the courage to provide consistent support to clients faced with the enormous emotional burdens resulting from serious illness. At present the volunteers are providing more than 3,000 hours of counseling per month—services that did not exist prior to the establishment of the SHANTI Project.

To say we are pleased with what we have learned and done would be an understatement; to say we have completed our development would be incorrect. We will continue our efforts and encourage all those interested in the SHANTI Project to contact us at 1137 Colusa Avenue, Berkeley, California 94707.

BIBLIOGRAPHY

Quint, Jeanne: *The Nurse and the Dying Patient*, Macmillan, New York, 1967.

Chapter 35

Hospice Care
in Terminal Illness

Robert Woodson

WHAT IS HOSPICE?

Hospice is a concept whose time has come.[1] It involves the skilled and compassionate care of dying patients and their families. Pioneered successfully throughout England and Europe for centuries as a place of rest for travelers on their way, the hospice is becoming a major medical innovation throughout America and Canada in the treatment of the terminally ill. It is an innovation in the sense that until only recently the specialized palliative care of the dying patient was left largely to chance or to the charge nurse. Consciousness raising efforts by Elisabeth Kübler-Ross[2] and others to sensitize American medical practitioners to the denial of death syndrome and the death with dignity notion did much to alleviate any further need for placing dying patients in rooms at the ends of hospital corridors where they could die in peace, alone.

Today there are some three dozen programs throughout America and Canada where the dying patient may receive this highly specialized palliative care. They are called hospices. Patterned largely after England's world famous St. Christopher's Hospice in Sydenham, these hospices all have the same common goal: to keep the patient pain-free, comfortable, and fully alert during the final phases of his illness and his life.

[1] Alice Heath, Founder, Santa Barbara Hospice, Inc.
[2] Elisabeth Kübler-Ross, *On Death and Dying*, Macmillan, New York, 1969, pp. 1–37.

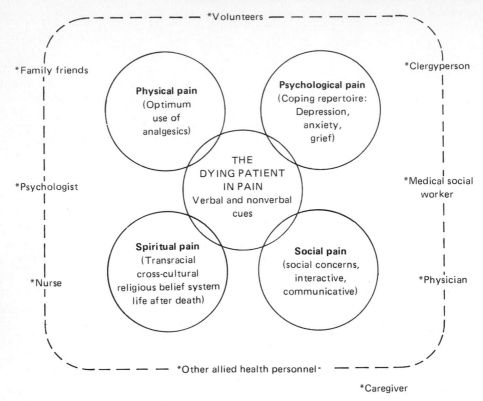

Figure 1   The hospice pain model.

This goal is achieved through a highly sophisticated—although basic—scientific and artistic system of palliative care developed over the years largely by Cicely Saunders and her hospice staff. The system includes the following major components.

A FOURFOLD APPROACH TO PAIN CONTROL

In terms of the hospice concept pain may be either physical, psychological, social, spiritual, or any combination of these four (see Figure 1). The task of the skilled clinician in alleviating pain is to tease out through careful observation and examination of the patient specifically which of the four components of pain are present, active, in what combination, and to what degree. Once the combination has been determined, then the *appropriate* combination of intervention strategies can be initiated.[3] Since pain control measures must be adjusted to each individual patient's needs, his own particular social-cultural response to pain, including his own unique autoplastic pain process, must also be considered in any initial assessment. Pain control then, in terms of the hospice approach, becomes one of pain management involving several forms of

[3] Dr. T.S. West, personal interview, St. Christopher's Hospice, Sydenham, England, October 3, 1975.

intervention all aimed at keeping the patient completely pain-free, comfortable, and fully alert until the moment of death. How is this achieved?

Physical Pain

Physical pain can be defined as that constant or occasional discomfort ranging from a mild toothache—and dying cancer patients do get toothaches—to the severe and chronic debilitating pain so familiar to those who have treated the advanced-stage cancer patient. In her paper, "The Treatment of Intractable Pain in Terminal Cancer,"[4] Cicely Saunders states that "pain itself is the strongest antagonist to successful analgesia and if it is ever allowed to become severe, the patient will then increase it [pain] with his own tension and fear."[5] Once the patient has been allowed to continually experience the severe physical pain associated with his illness, he becomes anxious and fearful that he will never again be pain-free. This generalized anxiety and loss of confidence in the caregivers' ability to lower the patient's pain threshold in turn increases the patient's susceptibility to pain and he becomes trapped in the all too frequent downward spiral of the intractable pain syndrome.[6]

Since physical pain influences and is influenced by the three other kinds of pain, a careful assessment of the possible symptoms that trouble the patient must first be made. Once an assessment has been made—which is by itself a highly specialized art— the appropriate intervention strategies can be initiated. This usually starts with the immediate removal of *all* the annoying symptoms of the patient's already diagnosed cancer. The goal, it must be remembered, is to keep the patient pain-free, comfortable, and mentally alert until death occurs. The success in achieving this goal is not so much a question of the specific drugs used as it is of the principles underlying their use. Several cardinal principles of controlling physical pain in the terminally ill cancer patient have emerged over the last two decades, primarily through the work of Cicely Saunders and her colleagues with thousands of dying cancer patients, at both St. Joseph's Hospice and St. Christopher's Hospice.[7]

These cardinal principles include the following: (1) the successful management of the cancer patient's pain is both an art and a science; (2) the concept of addiction does not apply in the care of the terminal cancer patient; and (3) there is a need for great flexibility in both the variety of drugs used and in their dosage levels. The skillful management of the terminal cancer patient's physical pain is an art in and of itself. It is an art in the sense that it involves (1) the careful assessment of the patient's symptoms, and this often includes an assessment by other members of the care team, (2) the selection of the appropriate drugs administered at an optimum dosage, and (3) the sensitivity to appreciate the fact that, in the final stages of treatment, the dying cancer patient's needs change rapidly and the medication regimen must keep pace with these

---

[4] Cicely Saunders, "The Treatment of Intractable Pain in Terminal Cancer," *Proceedings of the Royal Society of Medicine,* 56(3):1-7, March 1963. Hereafter referred to as Saunders, "Intractable Pain."

[5] Ibid, p. 2.

[6] Dr. Cicely Saunders, personal interview, St. Christopher's Hospice, Sydenham, England, October 3, 1975.

[7] Saunders, "Intractable Pain," pp. 1-7.

changes. The science of treating the patient's physical pain needs includes (1) solid mastery of the drugs used in palliative care and (2) a genuine clinical understanding of their interactions and side effects. It is only through a skillful blending of both the art of knowing how to listen with the third ear to the patient in pain and the science of seeing with the third eye what his or her needs are that the full and proper care of a dying patient can be achieved.[8]

The question of addiction is not an issue in the hospice treatment of the dying cancer patient for two main reasons: (1) the concerns that physicians frequently express regarding accidental addictions are based primarily on an inappropriate application of the medical school model emphasizing the treatment/cure/get well dimension of medical practice that carries little or no validity when applied to the care of the dying. It is a fact of medical practice that patients sometimes do become drug-dependent, especially if they have had a long and difficult recovery from a curable/treatable illness, and this dependency sometimes poses a medical management problem. It is also a fact of life that not all patients have curable diseases, and not all of them get well; some do in fact die, no matter how many analgesics are given or are withheld. They die just the same, with or without the medication. The solution to the concern over addiction seems obvious, yet the issue will undoubtedly continue to be debated in the lecture halls of academic medicine and in the hospitals where the hospice concept has not yet achieved full and complete adoption. (2) Interestingly enough, dying patients are almost never emotionally dependent on their drugs[9] in contrast to findings by researchers using the drug-addiction models depicted in standard medical and pharmacological texts, which have been mainly constructed from data collected on the youthful offender, the diversion of the chronic drug user, and so on. The data base upon which these models have been built, moreover, has totally ignored the whole area of the dying cancer patient's medication needs.

The models used in assessing addiction factors of terminally ill patients are neither valid nor reliable. Dying patients frequently display a surprising amount of dosage reduction behavior once their pain has been brought under control.[10] The central issue is one of care vs. cure and since the dying cancer patient is not going to be cured it seems logical that he or she be cared for compassionately.

There are undoubtedly several drugs that can be employed in the successful treatment of physical pain and its related symptoms. While many physicians have their own special set of favorite drugs, there is a decided need for greater flexibility in the variety of drugs (and dosage levels) used in treating physical pain. The pharmacology of cancer, pain control, and related symptomology has mushroomed in the past decade and the variety of analgesics available for treating the mild, moderate, and severe pain that is so much a part of the cancer patient's clinical course is at times overwhelming. While 30 mg of a particular analgesic may seem high, 60 mg may indeed be the appropriate optimum dosage level when one considers the nature of the illness and the special needs of the individual patient. There is no easy formula.[11]

[8] Ibid.
[9] Ibid., pp. 2–3.
[10] Dr. T.S. West, op. cit.
[11] Ibid.

In treating the advanced-stage cancer patient's physical pain, it is important to remember that analgesics should be given *regularly*, usually every 4 hours. "The aim is to titrate the level of analgesia against the patient's pain, gradually increasing the dose until the patient is pain free."[12] The next dose is given *before* the effects of the previous one have worn off and "before the patient may think it necessary."[13] The notation "P.R.N." on an analgesic medication order, therefore, is inappropriate since this suggests that the patient will ask for his pain medication when he feels he needs it. Since not all terminal cancer patients request pain medication when they experience discomfort for fear of bothering the nurse or of violating a socially acceptable norm, and since the goal of comprehensive pain management involves preventing pain from *occurring,* analgesics are given routinely.[14]

The following adopted drug schedule is presented as *one* example of *some* of the approaches used at St. Christopher's[15] in dealing with physical pain and its related symptomology.

Mild Physical Pain
1   Dextropropoxyphene with paracetamol: 2 tabs every 4 hours or
2   Paracetamol: 2 tabs every 4 hours.
These are also used as adjuncts to stronger analgesics and are often useful in bone pain.

Moderate Physical Pain
1   Dipipanone 10 mg with cyclizine 30 mg, 1 to 2 tabs every 4 hours. This is a useful analgesic of medium strength and is especially valuable with outpatients or if the patient prefers a tablet to a mixture.
2   Diamorphine and cocaine elixir (B.P.C.), MACS solution in U.S.

B.P.C.			U.S.	
Diamorphine HCl	5 to 10 mg		Morphine	10 mg
Cocaine	10 mg		Cocaine	10 mg
Alcohol (90%)	1.25 ml		Ethanol	20 mg
Syrup	2.5 ml		Simple Syrup qsad	5 ml
	Chloroform water to 10 ml			

Unless transferring from another potent narcotic analgesic, the initial dose given is 5 mg. This is given with a phenothiazine, usually as a syrup. Prochlorperazine 5 mg in 5 ml is the one usually added, chlorpromazine 12.5 to 25 mg in 5 ml if sedation is required. These potentiate the effect of diamorphine, and also act as antiemetics and tranquilizers. For outpatients, prochlorperazine or chlorpromazine syrup can replace syrup in the standard mixture when a stable level of analgesia is obtained.
3   Phenazocine 5 mg, 2 to 3 tabs every 4 hours. This is a useful strong analgesic, especially if the patient dislikes the diamorphine and cocaine elixir, or prefers a tablet.

---

[12] "Drugs Most Commonly Used at St. Christopher's Hospice," unpublished paper, St. Christopher's Hospice, Sydenham, England, January 1975, p. 1. Hereafter referred to as "Drugs, St. Christopher's."
[13] Ibid.
[14] Saunders, "Intractable Pain," p. 2.
[15] "Drugs, St. Christopher's," pp. 1–3.

Severe Physical Pain   Diamorphine and cocaine elixir, 10 to 40 mg, or even 60 mg, every 4 hours is usually effective. If this does not control the pain the patient should be transferred to injections of diamorphine every 4 hours, starting with half the previous oral dose and increasing it until the pain is controlled. The analgesic effect of diamorphine is shorter when given by injection, especially at higher doses. Sometimes therefore it may be necessary to inject the patient every 3 hours.

The phenothiazine should continue to be given, either orally or by injection. Diamorphine alone can be given subcutaneously.

Physical Pain and Vomiting   The diamorphine and cocaine elixir with phenothiazine may be tolerated and prove effective. However, it may be necessary to give injections of diamorphine and a phenothiazine for a few days; this may need to be prolonged in the case of intractable vomiting, obstruction, or if the patient cannot swallow. Oxycodone pectinate suppositories (30 mg) (1 to 2 every 8 hours) are occasionally used with outpatients to avoid the regular injections of analgesics. (In the United States oxymorphone 5 mg suppositories are used.)

Nausea and Vomiting   Probably the phenothiazines are the most useful drugs. Prochlorperazine 5 to 10 mg, promazine 25 mg, or chlorpromazine 25 mg are all useful antiemetics and are listed in ascending order of sedative effect.

They may be given every 4 hours in syrup or as a suspension in the case of promazine. Alternatively, they may be given in tablet form or by I.M. injection. Prochlorperazine suppositories (25 mg) and chlorpromazine suppositories (100 mg) are useful if oral preparations are not tolerated and injections are impracticable—for example, if the patient is at home. These are normally given every 8 hours. If these prove inadequate it is probably better to add a further antiemetic of a different type rather than to increase the dose. Cyclizine 50 mg orally or I.M. (intramuscularly), B.D. (twice daily), is often useful, as is metaclopramide 10 mg, especially if given about 1 hour A.C. (before meals).

Obstructive Vomiting   It is usually possible to control the pain and vomiting caused by malignant large bowel obstruction in its terminal phase by the use of adequate analgesics and by a combination of antiemetics. In these cases tabs of dioctyl sodium sulfosuccinate 100 mg, 1 to 2 T.D.S. (3 times per day) are sometimes used until it appears that obstruction is complete. Tabs Lomotil 2 Q.D.S. (4 times per day) may have a place in the control of painful colic.

Psychological Pain

The dying patient experiencing psychological pain is frequently the frightened or anxious patient, the lonely or depressed patient, or the hurt and angry patient. As he begins his final stage of growth by anticipating his own death, the terminally ill patient often endeavors to set things in balance by attempting to maintain a kind of

[16] The term *equifinality* was introduced in the late 1950s by general systems theorists in an attempt to provide biomedical researchers with a more *dynamic* as opposed to *static* definition of living or "open" systems.

psychological homeostatis of equifinality[16] with his inner emotional self and *his* perception of the immediate environment. This imbalance or loss of control over his or her life, especially the now new experience of learning how to die, usually calls up a repertoire of coping behaviors aimed chiefly at reducing the stresses of dying and at regaining control over one's life. An early attempt to understand this was presented by Elisabeth Kübler-Ross in her work on a stage theory of dying (denial, isolation, anger, bargaining, depression, and acceptance).[17]

The hospice approach to treating the patient in psychological pain, like its approach to treating the patient in any of the other three kinds of pain, is concerned first of all with the notion that *anxiety, depression,* and *agitation*—three terms for affective disorders that abound in the psychiatric literature—are normal, fight-flight reactions to coping with dying and death. When viewed as *normal*, given the nature of the illness, as opposed to *abnormal*, as current psychiatric diagnostic procedures would have one believe, depression, anxiety, and agitation take on a very different kind of emotional pain profile. They take on an affective domain pain profile, which, when viewed through the hospice model, suggests that amelioration of the dying patient's psychological pain may best be achieved through a careful analysis of the primary emotional sequelae operating at that particular moment, along with their accompanying secondary symptoms, and then through initiation of the appropriate combination of chemotherapeutic (antianxiety and antidepressive) and psychotherapeutic (clergyperson, therapist, family, friends, etc.) agents.

Thirty minutes of cathartic grieving with a family member, nurse, or skilled therapist can have profound positive effects on a dying patient's depression and concomitant anxiety. Five milligrams of diazepam or fifty of a phenothiazine may do little more than add one additional order the attending pharmacist has to fill and the nurse has to administer. The key to intervening in order to alleviate psychological pain in the dying patient as suggested by the hospice approach is to first acknowledge that in any organic disease or dysfunction there is *always* an emotional pain component operating in concert with or in opposition to the other three types of pain associated with terminal disease. The treatment intervention strategy used in combating psychological or emotional pain must be considered, moreover, in a framework that goes beyond the conventional unidimensional concepts of reactive depression and acute anxiety reaction, and must include a clinical appreciation for the delicate balance between psychological pain, social pain, spiritual pain, and physical pain, and quite possibly existential pain as suggested so eloquently in Martin Buber's concept of the I-thou.[18]

The following chemotherapeutic agents have been proven useful in treating the advanced cancer or psychological pain of dying patients.[19] Their success in removing the symptoms of the stresses associated with the dying process, namely anxiety and

---

[17]Elisabeth Kübler-Ross, op. cit, pp. 38–137. See also Elisabeth Kübler-Ross(ed.), *Death: The Final Stage of Growth,* Prentice-Hall, Englewood Cliffs, N.J., 1975, p. 161.

[18]Martin Buber, *I and Thou,* 2d ed., Scribner's, New York, 1958, pp. 3–137. See also Avery D. Weisman, "Misgivings and Misconceptions in the Psychiatric Care of Terminal Patients," *Psychiatry,* **33**:72, February 1970. The author visited St. Christopher's Hospice in Sydenham, England, in October 1975 through a special grant from the Smythe-Sollenberger family to observe firsthand the care provided patients in that facility.

[19]"Drugs, St. Christopher's," pp. 4–5.

depression, lies not so much in their pharmokinetic properties, but in their appropriate combinations and dosages offered within an atmosphere of genuine caring and concern for the patient's well-being.[20]

Depression (1) Attention to physical and mental distress; (2) antidepressants: amitriptyline 10 to 25 mg T.D.S. if mild sedation is also required, or 25 to 50 mg nocte; imipramine 10 to 25 mg T.D.S. if sedation is not required. Patients with malignant disease should usually be started on a small dose, e.g. 10 mg T.D.S., as larger doses sometimes precipitate confusion in debilitated patients.

Anxiety (1) Tabs diazepam 2 to 5 mg T.D.S.; (2) tabs promazine 25 mg T.D.S. or chlorpromazine 25 T.D.S.; (3) I.M. or I.V. diazepam 10 mg is of use in acute panic states or prior to some procedure that distresses the patient, e.g. catheterization.

Confusion In mild confusion chlorpromazine 10 to 25 mg Q.D.S. may be adequate. In severe restlessness and confusion, injection chlorpromazine 25 to 100 mg may be needed or injection methotrimaprazine 25 to 50 mg. These may be given with opiates or in conjunction with diazepam if necessary.

Insomnia Nonbarbiturate sedatives are preferred, chloral glycerolate (chloral hydrate in the United States), tabs dichloralphenazone (ethchlorvynol in the United States), or tabs nitrazepam (flurazepam in the United States). It is sometimes useful to add chlorpromazine 25 to 50 mg either with the hypnotics or in the early evening.

Social Pain

Social pain may be defined in two ways: (1) it may be defined as a patient's mild-to-severe discomfort with man's inhumanity to man—a common theme in the history of all technocratic civilizations; or (2) it may be defined as simply a patient's discomfort with the level and intensity of his or her interpersonal relationships, especially if one is in the process of dying. Extensive research by Colin Murray Parkes[21] and others concerned with the process of anticipatory grief, grief, grief work, and bereavement has clearly documented the importance of the need for the dying patient and his or her family to finish any unfinished interpersonal business including learning how to say good-bye to one another for the last time.

This unfinished interpersonal business becomes of immense importance in the final days of the dying patient's life. Should the dying patient be denied the opportunity to resolve or attempt to resolve such interpersonal business, i.e., to put some kind of closure on his or her social/interpersonal relationships with family and close friends, it can cause tremendous social pain for both the patient and his or her family. This kind of pain frequently appears as a passive-depressive presenting set of symptoms that all too often gets diagnosed as psychological pain and is inappropriately treated with an

[20] Dr. T.S. West, personal interview, London, England, October 9, 1975.
[21] Colin Murray Parkes, "The First Year of Bereavement: A Longitudinal Study of the Reaction of London Widows to the Death of Their Husbands," *Psychiatry*, **33**:444–467, November 1970.

antidepressive agent, which in turn only further separates the dying patient from his need to resolve, with the help of those around him, any pressing social/interpersonal concerns with family and friends. This does not mean that it is necessary or even desirable to hold a party around the patient's deathbed—although some cultures do it routinely—but that well-timed, well-planned selective social interaction is a vital and necessary part of appropriate social pain intervention. Since the dying patient and his family (and this could include his adopted family of medical caregivers) in their transactions with one another over a period of time have worked out a highly patterned, balanced system of social exchange, which constitutes a unit of care,[22] full consideration must be given to the social concerns of the dying patient and his family when any assessment is made regarding the nature and level of their verbal and unverbalized social pain.

The hospice approach in dealing with social pain, as determined by the patient's needs, is to facilitate (in the necessary and proper doses) *quality* social interaction. This helps the patient live more fully until he or she dies. Through the process of preventing the takeover of social pain (isolation) the caregiver performs the vitally important function of preventive psychiatry of providing additional opportunities for the grieving process to begin, i.e., anticipatory grief, before the patient dies. This also affords the caregiver with another opportunity to participate in a rich and personally rewarding experience in caring. As far as the man's inhumanity to man theme of social pain is concerned, it is already being dealt with right here and now on a one-to-one basis with any dying patient fortunate enough to have a caregiver who knows about social pain in the broader context and who will hear him or her out.

Spiritual Pain

To date there is no clear-cut definition of what constitutes spiritual pain, particularly as it relates to the dying. Spiritual pain is as different for each patient as is the patient's specific religious, racial, or cultural background. When Alaskan Indians die, for example, they "exhibit a willfulness about their death,"[23] as demonstrated by their active participation in its planning and in the time of its occurrence, that shows a remarkable power of personal choice. They frequently initiate their final dying rituals by calling their whole family and their close friends together, and then, when everyone is assembled, they tell the story of their life and pray for all the members of their family.[24] Spiritual pain for the Alaskan Indian might be the fear, or the reality, of not being able to participate in his or her own dying process because of the effect of sleep-producing drugs or the existential crisis of dying alone, without the comfort of meaningful praying, singing, and interacting with family and friends before death.

In sharp contrast to man's Westernized view of dying and death, Hindus and Buddhists see death and dying as anything but "the endless time of never coming back,"[25]

---

[22] Edward F. Dobihal, "Talk or Terminal Care?" *Connecticut Medicine,* 38:366, July 1974.

[23] Murray L. Trelease, "Dying Among Alaskan Indians: A Matter of Choice," in Elisabeth Kübler-Ross (ed.), *Death: The Final Stage of Growth,* Prentice-Hall, Englewood Cliffs, N.J., 1975, p. 33.

[24] Ibid., p. 34.

[25] J. Bruce Long, "The Death That Ends in Hinduism and Buddhism," in Elisabeth Kübler-Ross (ed.), *Death: The Final Stage of Growth,* Prentice-Hall, Englewood Cliffs, N.J., 1975, p. 53. Hereafter referred to as Long, "Hinduism and Buddhism."

or "the absence of presence."[26] Hindus view death as both a necessity and a blessing—
a necessity in the sense that "without the establishment of an operative balance
between the workings of the powers of birth and death, the world of living beings
would soon choke to death on the excessive creativity of the creator himself."[27]
Buddhists, by contrast, see death and dying as "a cutting off of the life-force or a total
nonfunctioning of the physical body and the mind."[28] This life-force[29] is not destroyed at death, but is temporarily displaced to continue to function in another
(unspecified) form. Every birth is a rebirth in linear fashion according to Buddhist
doctrine, occurring immediately or 49 days after death.[30] Hindu doctrine holds that
"it is an individual's *Karma* that is the fundamental cause of birth and death . . . and
for the time being, until all creatures have liberated themselves from the law of rebirth,
a provision must be made both for the coming-to-be and the passing-away of things,
for the sake of the well-being of the world"—a blessing.[31]

Although Hindus and Buddhists are not in concurrence on whether there is a real
self that survives from one lifetime to the next, both belief systems generally agree
that "the most effective method of *conquering* [italics added] death is to accept death
as the chief fact of life and as the main signal that all the things you hoped for will be
utterly destroyed in due course and that once you come to be able to neither long for
nor fear death, you are beginning to transcend both life and death and coming into
unity with the Changeless Absolute."[32]

Spiritual pain for the practicing Buddhist or Hindu—should he or she ever have
any—might be as expressed in the sermon of the thirteenth-century Zen master Dogen:

> To find release you must begin to regard life and death as identical to Nirvana
> neither loathing the former nor coveting the latter. It is fallacious to think that
> you simply move from birth to death. Birth, from the Buddhist point of view, is a
> temporary point between the preceding and succeeding; hence, it can be called
> "birthlessness." The same holds for death and deathlessness. In life there is nothing
> more than life, in death nothing more than death: we are being born and dying at
> every moment.[33]

Jewish tradition, on the other hand, specifically views the period of dying (*Goses*)
and terminal illness (*Shechiv Mera*) as a time when loved ones should surround, comfort, and encourage the patient.[34] Jewish law provides for death with dignity and

---

[26] Ibid. See also, Richard Lamerton, "Care of the Dying 7," *Nursing Times,* **69**:88 January 18,
1973.

[27] Ibid., p. 64.

[28] Ibid., p. 65.

[29] It is interesting to note how frequently the term *life-force* or the notion of life-force appears
in the recorded transcripts of psychiatric patients undergoing therapy, even dying ones.

[30] Long, "Hinduism and Buddhism," p. 65.

[31] Ibid., p. 64.

[32] Long, "Hinduism and Buddhism," p. 71.

[33] Ibid., p. 70.

[34] Rabbi Zachary I. Heller, "The Jewish View of Death: Guidelines for Dying," in Elizabeth
Kübler-Ross (ed.), *Death: The Final Stage of Growth,* Prentice-Hall, Englewood Cliffs, N.J., 1975,
p. 39.

meaning by "allowing the dying person to set his house in order, bless his family, pass on any message to them he feels important, and make his peace with God."[35]

> The deathbed confessional is viewed as an important element in the transition to the world to come. The dying patient is to be instructed to recite the confessional according to the limitations of his physical and mental condition. "And one says (to the patient), 'Many have confessed and have not died and many who have not confessed have died, as a reward for your confession you will live, and whoever confesses has a portion of the world to come.'" (Yoreh Deah 378)

> This deathbed scene is thus structured to give the terminally ill and dying patient an outlet for expression of natural concerns and anxieties, yet within a reassuring framework which never attempts to be deluding.[36]

> Each of these procedures—repentance, confession, the ordering of one's material affairs, the blessing of family, and ethical instruction—takes into account the theological, practical, and emotional needs of the terminal patient. They enable the patient to express fears, find comfort and inner strength, and communicate meaningfully with those close to him.[37]

> Contemporary programs to alleviate the distress of terminally ill and dying patients are very much in consonance with teachings of the Jewish tradition which stress the normalcy of these events of the life cycle. The patient's emotional equilibrium is maintained, with the continued support of family and community, who perform the mitzvah of "Bikkur Cholim"—visiting the sick with a sensitivity nurtured by their religious tradition. When death, the natural end of human existence, inevitably does come it is accepted as the degree of human mortality by the Eternal and Righteous Judge.[38]

Spiritual pain then, for the dying Jewish patient, could include any accidental thwarting of his or her reconciliation with God, any blocking of confession, or any interference with the ordering of the patient's material affairs, the blessing of family, and the passing on of ethical imperatives as laid down in the finest of Jewish law and tradition.

Regardless of the form (unspecified anxieties, etc.) or function (passive or active existential crises) of spiritual pain, it must be recognized as such and treated appropriately by the appropriate person (not by drugs)—which may or may not be the hospital chaplain, visiting priest, rabbi, or resident Zen master. The important point is that clergymen or clergywomen by virtue of their particular religious teachings and training are highly skilled listeners, especially in those times of profound spiritual silence that are an inherent part of the dying patient's experience as he moves through the various stages of his illness. They are unquestionably the key caregivers and supporters of patients experiencing spiritual pain. The clergyperson's role in relieving spiritual pain and effecting a kind of spiritual healing is simply to be present, to minister to the spiritual/religious needs of the patient and his family and to meet the related spiritual

---

[35] Ibid., p. 38.
[36] Ibid., p. 40.
[37] Ibid., p. 41.
[38] Ibid., p. 43.

needs of the medical caregivers on a P.R.N. basis. The clergyperson's job, unlike that of the immediate hospice staff, does not end with the patient's death, but continues through the period of the funeral and the ensuing grief work done by the patient's family long after the 6-month follow-up by the medical social worker.[39]

The clergyperson may choose to work either directly with the patient and his or her family through the religious medium of confession, communion, prayer, etc., or indirectly through other members of the care team as a counselor/consultant, or both. The approaches and the options are as varied as are the patients. To be able to *see* and *hear* (diagnose) the dying patient in spiritual pain and to minister to that pain by hearing confession, offering communion, praying with the patient, or by participating in his singing rituals (as in the case of the Alaskan Indians) is to reduce that patient's suffering and alleviate his or her pain—a worthy calling for a man or woman of the cloth and a vital function in the case of the dying.

PHILOSOPHICAL AND ORGANIZATIONAL COMPONENTS OF HOSPICE CARE

In addition to the fourfold approach to pain control so central to the hospice concept there are eight other major components or characteristics of hospice care that distinguish it from other programs of terminal care. These eight components comprise the basic philosophical and organizational framework of an authentic hospice program and are described briefly below.

The Provision of Care by an Interdisciplinary Team

The successful care of the dying patient and his or her family must utilize an interdisciplinary team approach. Interdisciplinary or multidisciplinary team care must not by a synonym for fragmented care in which the bewildered patient does not know who is in charge or who is dealing with which problems (see Figure 2). Authentic hospice care mandates that the multidisciplinary team sit down together at regular conferences, usually weekly, to work out a plan of care for the patient and his or her family and to learn something of each other's specialized (professional) language code. This is of particular importance when the team comprises members with divergent racial and cultural backgrounds. The team includes the dying patient, his immediate family, his primary physician, his nurses, the medical social worker, volunteers, and appropriate clergypersons.

Service Availability to Home Care and Inpatients on a 24-Hour-a-Day, 7-Day-a-Week, On-Call Basis with Emphasis on Availability of Medical and Nursing Skills

Although most Americans (98 percent) now die in either a hospital or extended-care facility (i.e., nursing home), the increasing trend among more and more Americans is toward dying at home in their own bed surrounded by loved ones, as was the custom in this country before the turn of the century. In order to provide hospice care for

[39]Colin Murray Parkes, op. cit.

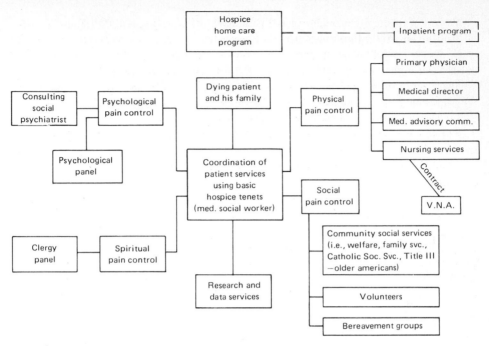

Figure 2 Hospice psychosocial model of direct care services using the multidisciplinary team

those choosing to die at home, 24-hour-a-day, 7-day-a-week skilled and supportive services—with an emphasis on visiting nurses and homemaker services—must be available to patients and their families. All too often medical emergencies occur at night and on weekends when nursing or medical services are scarce.

Such was the case of a husband who reluctantly placed his wife in a convalescent home for the final 3 months of her life because the stresses of coping with the unavailability of inhome nursing service were overwhelming. Upon admitting his wife to the facility, he recalled with vivid horror the time her gastrostomy tube fell out at 3:00 a.m. one weekend and how he desperately tried replacing it according to telephone instructions from an unknown emergency room physician. Although actual case examples like this one are fortunately in the minority, they do occur. The availability of a 24-hour-a-day, 7-day-a-week nursing service not only eliminates the possibility of such unfortunate events from occurring, but also allays the already burdened family's fear that no one will be there to help when it is needed most.

Home Care Service in Collaboration with Inpatient Facilities

A true hospice program has both a strong home care program and an inpatient facility or back-up beds of some kind. Since there are already some three dozen hospices throughout the British Isles and Europe, each with its own unique program of home care, there is little need for constructing a rationale for building more hospices. In America, however, there are presently no free-standing inpatient hospice facilities, although there are a growing number of home care programs with limited numbers of back-up beds, or specialized hospice type units within existing hospitals and extended-care facilities. While these back-up bed arrangements present a special set of problems (i.e., reimbursement, visiting hours, presence of pets at the patient's bedside, room design, coordination of care team, etc.), these arrangements are deemed by many hospice authorities as only temporary until more appropriate *care* guidelines are incorporated into the legal, medical, and economic policies and regulations governing the bulk of health care facilities in the United States.

Other alternatives, of course, include building hospices and then linking them up with existing community-based home health agencies (HHAs)—the result, a bonafide hospice program. Until such true hospice programs become a reality in America, the trend over the next several years will be toward developing strong home care programs, using volunteers extensively, and establishing a system of back-up beds in one or two local hospitals that agrees to accept *any* medical insurance carried by the patient and agrees to take an *active* role in meeting the special needs of the patient and family placed in its care. It is in this particular component of hospice care that most of the necessary legislative changes will occur, the greatest modifications in our system of health insurance will be seen, and about which no doubt the liveliest of academic discussion will ensue.

The Patient and Family Together Regarded as the Unit of Care

It is a fundamental principle of hospice care that nothing we do as caregivers should serve to separate someone who is dying from his or her family and, even though there will undoubtedly be moments of difficulty and despair, it is of paramount importance that the family come through to the end together. Because most people in America die in hospitals or extended-care facilities, the traditional and familiar home setting with all its comforting presence is absent from the process. The absence of family members—including children and grandchildren—and the familiar home setting more often than not works to the social and psychological demise of the patient long before he or she dies physically. Maintaining meaningful interaction for the advanced cancer or dying patient with his family, through either face-to-face social exchange, telephone conversations, letters, audio-tape cassettes, or other electronic means helps the patient—especially the older patient—stay in touch with life until he dies. It is therefore vital that the family be the unit of care and receive full and proper attention.

A Bereavement Follow-Up Service

In a genuine hospice program, care does not end with the death of the patient but is extended to provide a program of emotional support for the surviving family members during their bereavement. Families must be visited on both a regular and an emergency basis right through the time of death of the family member and on into the mourning period. Because the social and psychological loss of a loved one can sometimes be so emotionally devastating to surviving family members—particularly spouses—assistance must be given in an attempt to prevent any further unnecessary suffering.

In the first year after the loved one's death, for example, there is a documented vulnerability of the survivors to illness[40] as reflected in a 40 percent increase in the mortality rate of widows. Other less well studied (consequently less-understood) illnesses include increased alcoholism, reactive depression, cardiac dysfunction, psychotropic drug addiction, and long-term detrimental effects to children caused by the loss of a parent, especially if the death was sudden and unexpected. Research by Colin Murray Parkes[41] and others suggests that simple friendly visits by *trained* caregivers with the survivors gives them an opportunity to *express* (not *ventilate*) their grief and discuss the terminal illness including the death itself, and that this can go a long way toward mitigating the ill effects of bereavement.

The first few bereavement visits are typically made by the primary nurse who was involved in the direct care of the patient before his or her death. This provides the family with a caregiver who was close to the patient when he or she died and provides the family with someone who can discuss with them such often-asked questions as, "Should we have kept her at home?" "Should we have taken him to the hospital?" "Was it worth continuing with that unpleasant treatment for so long?" "Should we have pressed him to continue with chemotherapy?" "Why didn't she go to the doctor as soon as she felt the lump?" Many of these questions can easily be answered in the course of frank and open discussions. Ideally, much of this follow-up bereavement counseling—which in one sense is a very specific form of preventive psychiatry—could be done by adequately trained volunteers. The need in this aspect of hospice care is great, the possibilities many.

Extensive Use of Volunteers as an Integral Part of the Hospice Care Team

Fundamental to the continued success of any hospice program is the extensive use of trained volunteers. While the wise use of volunteers has in the past been conspicuously absent in the United States from the care of the dying and their families, there is at present a resurgence of interest in the use of volunteers for such purposes (as evidenced by the emergence of the professionally trained volunteer) and this has provided a welcome change in our thinking about and in our care of the dying. Trained volunteers provide two primary services to patients and their families: (1) they provide such vital household services as helping with transportation, light housework, shopping, babysitting, laundry, letter writing, etc., and (2) perhaps even more vital, they provide friendship to the dying and to the family by giving of themselves in a basic, person-to-person sort of way that seems to help keep the patient and his or her family from falling through the many psychological and social cracks professionals pride themselves on successfully filling.

There are many models of volunteer programs for the terminally ill and the one that will undoubtedly serve as the key model for training volunteers for most hospice programs in the United States and Canada is the highly successful SHANTI Project. According to its founder, Charles Garfield, the project "was developed on a shoestring

[40]Thomas H. Holmes and Richard H. Rahe, "The Social Readjustment Rating Scale," *Journal of Psychosomatic Research*, 11:213–218, August 1967.
[41]Colin Murray Parkes, op. cit.

budget and in just 2 years of operation has provided emotional support to thousands of patients and families facing a life-threatening illness."[42] Its success as a training model for volunteers interested in working with the fatally ill and their families is grounded in the notion that, through caring counseling and emotional support during a time of severe illness or grief, the presence of another human can be helpful in generating the emotional strength needed to cope with sorrow and stress.

Volunteers are indeed the vital thread that ties the whole hospice program together and extensive use of them is absolutely essential if the full and proper care of the dying and their families is to be achieved and if the label "hospice care" is to be applied in describing the services rendered.

Central Administration and Coordination of Services

It is essential that a hospice program have its own autonomous central administration and system of coordination of patient services. All too frequently well-intentioned community health care agencies join forces to provide care for the terminally ill and their families only to learn later that much of their success is highly dependent on how smoothly the simple logistics of record keeping, team leadership, distribution of supplies and caregivers, communication, etc. are carried out. Many acute-care hospitals and extended-care facilities are now employing personnel whose specific function is to coordinate inpatient and home care services in order to ensure some measure of continuity of care for the patient once he or she is discharged from active treatment. This is a step in the right direction toward providing a comprehensive program of terminal care, but it must be well conceived (i.e., it must use a general systems theory approach) and carried out by dedicated caregivers with the thought in mind that it is only a first step in moving toward a *completely* centralized administration and system of coordination of services for the dying.

Knowledge and Expertise in the Control of Symptoms (Physical, Psychological, Social, Spiritual)

At the outset of this chapter, we identified the four types of pain frequently experienced by terminally ill patients and their families and suggested some rather specific intervention strategies caregivers could employ in their work with the dying and the bereaved. It was also stated that the role of the hospice caregiver in alleviating the patient's pain—which is in some way *always* tied to the family's ability to deal with pain, or to the stresses associated with an impending loss (death) of a family member—was to tease out through careful observation and inquiry the specific pain components operating at that moment and to then apply the appropriate intervention(s).

For many medically oriented caregivers this suggests that all pain has its beginnings in a physical trauma of some sort. While real *physical* pain must be respected as such and adequate analgesics given (e.g., the Brompton mixture, etc.) in addition to competent nursing care (e.g., bowel, bladder, oral, and skin care, etc.) to ensure the patient's complete physical comfort during the final days of his or her life, not all pain has its origin in human tissue. The pain associated with terminality is often psychosocial and

---

[42]Personal interview, Santa Barbara, Ca., October 9, 1976.

spiritual in origin and it can indeed become intense enough to hurt and to cause such specific secondary physical symptoms as blood in the urine or stool, nonspecific tachacardia, migraine, spastic colon, TMJ disorders, and a whole range of other psychosomatic illnesses.

One such example is that of a 32-year-old male of Latin descent who was referred to the author not long ago for therapy when his urologist could find no physical or clinical basis for the presence of blood in the patient's urine (the symptom). Upon only one visit it was learned that the man's ex-wife[43] was dying of cancer and because he had been asked by her to tell their son about her illness he had become uptight and resented having to be the one to tell his oldest boy about his mother's impending death. It is a clinically documented fact that when sphincter muscles become constricted or tight (probably due to stress) they can cause tissue irritation pain and even bleeding.

It took no major mental exercise on the patient's part to begin to understand the what and when (not why) of his passing blood and within a few days his urine content returned to normal and during a follow-up telephone conversation a week later he reported having easier bowel movements and no more constipation. In this particular case the patient was male, in his 30s, a father, once divorced, although remarried, and, as he himself indicated, uptight no doubt as a direct consequence of being placed in the position of having to impart the information of his ex-wife's illness to their son and of worrying about the effect all this would have on his present marriage and his two children. There are literally thousands of cases like this one and, although it was easily handled, it clearly underscores the principle that psychological pain is a distinct and unique category of pain quite different in origin, coding, usage, and treatment, from the category of physical pain and physical pain control. A demonstrated knowledge and expertise in symptom control is central to the whole concept of hospice care and if these skills are appropriately applied they can have profound effects on the *quality of life* for the dying.

BIBLIOGRAPHY

Abram, Harry S.: "Psychological Responses to Illness and Hospitalization," *Psychosomatics,* **10**:218–224, July–August 1969.

Amacher, Nancy Jean: "Touch Is a Way of Caring," *American Journal of Nursing,* **73**: 852–54, May 1973.

"At Home with Death," *Newsweek,* January 6, 1975, pp. 43–44.

Baer, Eva, Lois Jean Davitz, and Renee Lieb: "Inferences of Physical Pain and Psychological Distress: I. In Relation to Verbal and Nonverbal Patient Communication," *Nursing Research,* **19**:388–392, September–October 1970.

Baqui, Mufti, Rabbi B. Joseph Hackney, and Rabbi M. Levenstein Bow: "Jewish and Muslim Teaching Concerning Death," a St. Joseph's Hospice occasional paper, London, England.

---

[43] Given the data that many Americans are children of divorced parents and, according to current statistics, will themselves stand a good chance of being divorced, it is important that this be kept in mind when any assumptions are being made about the makeup of a particular patient's family.

Barnett, Kathryn: "A Theoretical Construct of the Concepts of Touch as They Relate to Nursing," *Nursing Research*, 21:102–110, March–April 1972.

Barton, David, Joseph H. Fishbein, and Frank Stevens Jr.: "Psychological Death: An Adaptive Response to Life-Threatening Illness," *Psychiatry in Medicine*, 3:227–236, July 1972.

Brodsky, Carroll M.: "The Pharmacotherapy System," *Psychosomatics*, 11:24–30, January–February 1970.

Bronzo, Anthony and Gerald Powers: "Relationship of Anxiety with Pain Threshold," *Journal of Psychology*, 66:181, July 1967.

Buber, Martin: *I and Thou*, 2d ed., Scribner's, New York, 1958.

Cook, Mark, Lalljee Cook, and G. Mansur: "Verbal Substitutes for Visual Signals in Interaction," *Semiotica*, 6(3):212–221, 1972.

Cramond, W. A.: "The Psychological Care of Patients with Terminal Illness," *Nursing Times*, 69:339–343, March 15, 1973.

Craven, Margaret: *I Heard the Owl Call My Name*, Dell, New York, 1973.

Cronk, Hilary M.: "The Business of Dying," *Nursing Times*, 68:1100, August 31, 1972.

Crowther, Clarence Edward: "Care Versus Cure in the Treatment of the Terminally Ill," unpublished doctoral dissertation, University of California, Santa Barbara, December 1975.

de Groot, M. H. L.: "The Clinical Use of Psychotherapeutic Drugs in the Elderly," *Drugs*, 8:132–138, 1974.

Dobihal, Edward F.: "Talk or Terminal Care?" *Connecticut Medicine*, 38:364–367, July 1974.

Driver, Caroline: "What a Dying Man Taught Doctors About Caring," *Medical Economics*, 50:81–86, January 22, 1973.

"Drugs Most Commonly Used at St. Christopher's Hospice," unpublished paper, St. Christopher's Hospice, Sydenham, England, January 1975.

Ekman, Paul and Wallace V. Friesen: "The Repertoire of Nonverbal Behavior—Categories, Origins, Usage and Coding," paper presented at the University of California Medical Center, Langley Porter Neuropsychiatric Institute, San Francisco, October 1967.

Enelow, Allen T., (ed.): *Depression in Medical Practice*, Merck, Sharp & Dohme, West Point, Pa., 1971.

Feifel, Herman, (ed.): *The Meaning of Death*, McGraw-Hill, New York, 1959.

Feinstein, Alvan R.: "Biologic Dependency, 'Hypothesis Testing,' Unilateral Probabilities, and Other Issues in Scientific Direction vs. Statistical Duplexity," *Clinical Pharmacology and Therapeutics*, 17:499–513, April 1975.

Formby, Father John, Reverend Michael Hickey, and Reverend A. Gordon Jones: "Christian Teaching Concerning Death," a St. Joseph's Hospice occasional paper, London, England.

Gladman, Arthur E.: "The Role of Non-Verbal Communication in the Development and Treatment of Emotional Illness," *Psychosomatics*, 12:107–110, March–April 1971.

Goldberg, Harold L.: "Sleep Disturbances Accompanying Clinical Depression/Anxiety," Clinical Cassette Series, Pfizer, New York, 1972.

Gordon, Audrey: "The Jewish View of Death: Guidelines for Mourning," in Elisabeth Kübler-Ross (ed.): *Death: The Final Stage of Growth*, Prentice-Hall, Englewood Cliffs, N.J., 1975, pp. 44–51.

Hart, Betty and Ann W. Rohweder: "Support in Nursing," *American Journal of Nursing,* **59**:1398–1401, October 1959.

Heller, Rabbi Zachary I.: "The Jewish View of Death: Guidelines for Dying," in Elisabeth Kübler-Ross (ed.), *Death: The Final Stage of Growth,* Englewood Cliffs, N.J., 1975, pp. 38–43.

Hinkle, Lawrence E., Jr.: "The Concept of 'Stress' in the Biological and Social Sciences," *The International Journal of Psychiatry in Medicine,* **5**:335–357, Fall 1974.

Hinton, John: *Dying,* Penguin, Baltimore, 1972.

Hoffman, Esther: "Don't Give Up on Me!" *American Journal of Nursing,* **71**:60–62, January 1971.

Huszar-Bronner, Judith: "The Psychological Aspects of Cancer in Man," *Psychosomatics,* **12**:133–138, March–April 1971.

Johnson, Betty Sue: "The Meaning of Touch in Nursing," *Nursing Outlook,* **13**:59–60, February 1965.

Joyce, C. R. B.: "The Issue of Communication Within Medicine," *Psychiatry in Medicine,* **4**:357–363, October 1972.

Kavanaugh, Robert E.: *Facing Death,* Penguin, Baltimore, 1972.

Kram, Charles and John M. Caldwell: "The Dying Patient," *Psychosomatics,* **10**:293–295, September–October 1969.

Krant, Melvin J. and Ned H. Cassem: "Anxiety/Depression: Terminal Disease," *PROBE* Audio-Tape Series, Wallace Pharmaceuticals, Cranbury, N.J., 1973.

Kron, Thora: "How We Communicate Nonverbally with Patients," *Nursing Research,* **68**:21–23, November 1972.

Kübler-Ross, Elisabeth: *On Death and Dying,* Macmillan, New York, 1969.

———: "What Is It Like to Be Dying?," *American Journal of Nursing,* **71**:54–61, January 1971.

———: *Questions and Answers on Death and Dying,* Macmillan, New York, 1974.

———: *Death: The Final Stage of Growth,* Prentice-Hall, Englewood Cliffs, N.J., 1975.

Lamerton, Richard: "Care of the Dying 2," *Nursing Times,* **68**:1544–1545, December 7, 1972.

———: "Care of the Dying 3," *Nursing Times,* **68**:1578, December 14, 1972.

———: "Care of the Dying 4," *Nursing Times,* **68**:1642–1643, December 28, 1972.

———: "Care of the Dying 5," *Nursing Times,* **79**:16, January 4, 1973.

———: "Care of the Dying 7," *Nursing Times,* **69**:88–89, January 18, 1973.

———: "Drugs for the Dying: The Treatment of Terminal Pain," *St. Bartholomew's Hospital Journal,* **79**(1):353–354, 1975.

Lazarus, Richard S.: "Psychological Stress and Coping in Adaptation and Illness," *The International Journal of Psychiatry in Medicine,* **5**:321–333, Fall 1974.

Liegner, Leonard M.: *St. Christopher's Hospice—Site Visit Report: Care of the Dying Patient, 1974,* Columbia University, Department of Radiology, College of Physicians and Surgeons, New York, 1974.

Long, J. Bruce: "The Death That Ends Death in Hinduism and Buddhism," in Elizabeth Kübler-Ross (ed.), *Death: The Final Stage of Growth,* Prentice-Hall, Englewood Cliffs, N.J., 1975, pp. 52–72.

MacKinnon, Bernard L.: "Death and the Doctor," *The Journal of the Maine Medical Association,* **63**:169–171, August 1972.

McNulty, Barbara: "The Needs of the Dying," lecture given to the Guild of Pastoral Psychology, Sydenham, England, January 1969.

———: "Care of the Dying," *Nursing Times,* **68**:1505–1506, November 30, 1972.

Miller, Sara and Stuart Miller: *First Report of the Program in Humanistic Medicine 1972–1973*, Institute for the Study of Humanistic Medicine, San Francisco, 1973.

Morison, Robert S.: "Dying," *Scientific American*, **229**:55–74, September 1973.

Mount, Balfour M.: "Death and Dying: Attitudes in a Teaching Hospital," *Urology*, **4**:741–747, December 1974.

———: "Death—A Part of Life," *CRUX, A Quarterly Journal of Christian Thought and Opinion*, **11**(3):3–13, 1973–1974.

Mowbray, R. M.: "The Hamilton Rating Scale for Depression: A Factor Analysis," *Psychological Medicine*, **2**:272–280, August 1972.

Nadelson, Dr. Theodore: "Anxiety/Depression: Clues to Their Recognition," *PROBE* Audio-Tape Series, Wallace Pharmaceuticals, Cranbury, N.J., 1972.

Nolen, William A.: "Fewer Pills and More Conversation," *PRISM*, **1**:29–81, October 1973.

Parkes, Colin Murray: "Effects of Bereavement on Physical and Mental Health—A Study of the Medical Records of Widows," *British Medical Journal*, **2**:274–279, August 1964.

———: "The First Year of Bereavement: A Longitudinal Study of the Reaction of London Widows to the Death of Their Husbands," *Psychiatry*, **33**:444–467, November 1970.

———: "Psycho-Social Transitions: A Field for Study," *Social Science and Medicine*, **5**:101–115, April 1971.

———: "Components of the Reaction to Loss of a Limb, Spouse or Home," *Journal of Psychosomatic Research*, **16**:343–349, August 1972.

Pozos-Bonilla, Randolfo: "The Santa Barbara Hospice: An Anthropological Perspective on the Planning and Development of Special Services for the Terminally Ill," unpublished paper, University of California, Berkeley, Department of Anthropology, May 1975.

Rees, W. Dewi: "The Distress of Dying," *Nursing Times*, **68**:1479–1480, November 23, 1972.

Rogers, Carl R.: "The Characteristics of a Helping Relationship," address delivered at the APGA Convention, St. Louis Missouri, March 31–April 3, 1958.

Saunders, Cicely: "The Treatment of Intractable Pain in Terminal Cancer," *Proceedings of the Royal Society of Medicine*, **56**:1–75, March 1963.

———: "Watch with Me," *Nursing Times*, **61**:1615–1617, November 26, 1965.

———: "The Need for In-Patient Care for the Patient with Terminal Cancer," *Middlesex Hospital Journal*, **72**:1–6, February 1973.

———: "The Need for Institutional Care for the Patient with Advanced Cancer," unpublished paper, St. Christopher's Hospice, Sydenham, England.

———: "Terminal Care," in K. D. Bagshane (ed.), *Medical Oncology*, Blackwells, Oxford, 1973.

Scott, Patrician Cumin: *Some Information for Those Caring for Patients*, St. Christopher's Hospice, Sydenham, England, 1974.

Simpson, Michael A.: "What Is Dying Like?" *Nursing Times*, **69**:405–406, March 29, 1973.

Strode, Orienne Elizabeth: Program Bulletin for "Human Dimensions in Medical Education," The Center for Studies of the Person, La Jolla, Ca., Summer 1975.

St. Christopher's Hospice Annual Report, Sydenham, England, 1973–1974.

Tanner, E. R.: "A Time to Die," a St. Joseph's Hospice occasional paper, London, England.

Thompson, Captane P.: "Prevention in Psychiatry," *Nursing Times,* **61**:1620–1621, November 26, 1965.

Torrey, E. Fuller: *The Mind Game: Witchdoctors and Psychiatrists,* Bantam, New York, 1973.

———: *The Death of Psychiatry,* Penguin, Baltimore, 1974.

Trelease, Murray: "Dying Among Alaskan Indians: A Matter of Choice," in Elisabeth Kübler-Ross (ed.), *Death: The Final Stage of Growth,* Prentice-Hall, Englewood Cliffs, N.J., 1975, p. 33.

Twycross, Robert G.: *The Dying Patient,* Christian Medical Fellowship Publications, London, 1975.

Watts, Alan W.: *Psychotherapy East and West,* Ballantine, New York, 1961.

Weisman, Avery D.: "Misgivings and Misconceptions in the Psychiatric Care of Terminal Patients," *Psychiatry,* **33**:68–75, February 1970.

West, T. S.: "Approach to Death," *Nursing Mirror,* **139**(15), October 10, 1974.

Whybrow, Peter C.: "The Use and Abuse of the 'Medical Model' as a Conceptual Frame in Psychiatry," *Psychiatry in Medicine,* **3**:333–342, October 1972.

Zung, William K. and Thomas H. Wonnacott: "Treatment Prediction in Depression Using a Self-Rating Scale," *Psychiatry,* **2**:321–329, October 1970.

Chapter 36

The Brompton Mixture: Effects on Pain In Cancer Patients

R. Melzack
J. G. Ofiesh
B. M. Mount

There is convincing evidence that pain perception is not simply a function of the amount of physical injury but is also determined by the level of anxiety, expectation and other psychological variables.[1] It is therefore apparent that brain activities subserving these psychological processes are important in determining the quality and intensity of perceived pain. The gate-control theory of pain[2] provides a conceptual model for incorporating these cognitive contributions to pain experience. The theory suggests that the amount of input transmitted from peripheral fibres to the brain is determined by sensory input from the body as well as by brain activities that exert a descending influence on the gate system. When the amount of input to the brain exceeds a critical level, the ensuing pain experience[3] comprises three dimensions: (1) the sensory-discriminative dimension of pain, (2) the powerful motivational drive and unpleasant affect that trigger the organism into action and (3) the evaluative or cognitive dimension.

Cancer pain is best understood within such a framework. Lesions of different kinds of tissues may produce pain that varies in intensity, duration and temporal pattern.

We are grateful to Miss Michele Hornby and Miss Judydale Hymovitch for their invaluable assistance, and Dr. Ina Ajemian and Dr. John Scott for their help in carrying out the study.

This study was supported by grant A7891 from the National Research Council of Canada.

Reprinted from *CMA Journal*, **115**:125–128, July 17, 1976.

Moreover, the pain is greatly influenced by psychological factors such as the knowledge of impending death, fear of disfigurement by the disease, and worries about financial or family matters related to prolonged illness.[4,5] These factors affect the sensory, affective and evaluative dimensions of pain.[3]

There is convincing evidence that the Brompton mixture,[6] an oral narcotic (usually morphine) preparation given with a phenothiazine, provides a powerful method for the control of pain.[5,6] Morphine acts at many neural levels,[7] including the brain stem, where it excites inhibitory fibres,[8] and can block or modulate pain signals throughout the nervous system. Morphine and the phenothiazines also decrease anxiety and despair and would therefore be expected to diminish the affective and evaluative components as well as the sensory dimension of pain. Because the Brompton mixture is given every 4 hours in the attempt to maintain continuous control over pain, this therapy also diminishes the fear or expectation of pain, thereby decreasing pain still further.

The effectiveness of the Brompton mixture has been established at St. Christopher's Hospice,[5,6] which also provides its patients with an understanding staff and all possible comforts and psychological support. However, because there have not been adequate tools to measure pain, it has been difficult to gauge the magnitude of the effect of the mixture, its relative effects in different hospital environments, or how it compares with traditional methods of pain control in cancer patients. The recent development of the McGill-Melzack Pain Questionnaire to measure clinical pain[9] has given us an opportunity to examine these aspects of the effects of the Brompton mixture on pain in cancer patients.

PATIENTS AND METHODS

Patients

Palliative Care Unit (PCU) During this study 143 patients were registered in the PCU at the Royal Victoria Hospital, Montreal, a ward specializing in the care of the terminally ill. Ninety of these patients received the Brompton mixture. Of the remainder, many had relatively little pain, which could be kept under control with codeine or another mild or medium-strength, orally administered analgesic. Others were unable to receive oral medication for a variety of medical reasons; indeed, many died within hours of arrival.

Of the 90 patients who received the Brompton mixture the pain could not be controlled in 8 (9 percent): 1 had severe bladder spasms, 2 had sharp nerve-root pain that radiated into the legs, and 5 complained of severe pain, a major component of which was their despair and anguish at their impending death. These patients were treated with additional or other methods in the attempt to achieve physical and psychological comfort.

Eighty-two of the 90 patients received the Brompton mixture on a continuing basis, and 26 were chosen at random to receive the pain questionnaire. The mean number of questionnaires given to the patients during their stay in the PCU was 4.7 (range, 1 to 16).

Wards and Private Rooms   During the study 238 patients on general hospital wards or in private rooms were given the Brompton mixture. The ward rooms consisted of four-bed standard accommodation on the general medical and surgical wards. The private rooms consisted of single-bed accommodation. As in the PCU group, the pain required additional or other treatment in about 10 percent of the patients. The remainder received the Brompton mixture on a continuing basis, and 66 (46 ward patients and 20 private patients) were chosen at random to receive the pain questionnaire. The mean number of questionnaires given to the ward patients was 4.6 (range, 1 to 20) and to the private patients, 7.7 (range, 1 to 49).

Measurement of Pain

Pain was measured by means of the McGill-Melzack Pain Questionnaire (Figure 1), which was developed as an experimental tool for studies of the effects of various methods of pain management.[9] The three major indices measured were (1) "present pain intensity" (PPI), or overall pain intensity, measured on a scale of 0 to 5 (0 = none, 1 = mild, 2 = discomforting, 3 = distressing, 4 = horrible, and 5 = excruciating); (2) "number of words chosen" (NWC) from 20 sets of qualitative words, with two to six words per set, that describe the sensory, affective and evaluative properties of pain; and (3) "pain rating index.. (PRI), the sum of the rank values of all the words chosen (based on the positions of the words in each set).

Procedure

Each patient selected for the study was informed that he was being given a drug—the Brompton mixture—to control pain and that it was important to evaluate the intensity and kind of pain he felt in order to determine the proper dosage of the drug. Each patient was instructed as follows: "I will read several groups of words that express feelings and sensations. If any of these words describe what you feel right now, please tell me and I will make a mark at the side of the appropriate word. Choose only one word in each group, the one that best expresses how you feel. Omit any groups that are not appropriate."

The questionnaire was generally completed in about 10 minutes. At first more time was required to explain the meaning of some of the words. Occasionally patients asked to have certain groups reread to be certain of the decision that a word was appropriate. When the patient felt no pain a zero was recorded and the list of descriptors was not read.

While a standard approach was followed in the PCU setting (as to the ingredients of the Brompton mixture and the method of administering it), there was greater variability in time and dose scheduling in the wards and private rooms.

After the first 8 months of the study an analysis of the data indicated differences in pain control among the PCU, ward, and private patients. Consequently, it was impressed on the staff associated with all three groups of patients that it was essential to administer the Brompton mixture every 4 hours, even if the patient claimed he was not in pain or if it meant waking him to provide medication.

McGill - Melzack Pain Questionnaire

Patient's Name _____ Date _____ Time _____ am/pm
Analgesic(s) _____ Dosage _____ Time Given _____ am/pm
Dosage _____ Time Given _____ am/pm

Analgesic Time Difference (hours): +4 +1 +2 +3
PRI: S_____ A_____ E_____ M(S)_____ M(AE)_____ M(T)_____ PRI(T)_____
(1–10)   (11–15)   (16)   (17–19)   (20)   (17–20)   (1–20)

1 FLICKERING	11 TIRING
QUIVERING	EXHAUSTING
PULSING	12 SICKENING
THROBBING	SUFFOCATING
BEATING	13 FEARFUL
POUNDING	FRIGHTFUL
2 JUMPING	TERRIFYING
FLASHING	14 PUNISHING
SHOOTING	GRUELLING
3 PRICKING	CRUEL
BORING	VICIOUS
DRILLING	KILLING
STABBING	15 WRETCHED
LANCINATING	BLINDING
4 SHARP	16 ANNOYING
CUTTING	TROUBLESOME
LACERATING	MISERABLE
5 PINCHING	INTENSE
PRESSING	UNBEARABLE
GNAWING	17 SPREADING
CRAMPING	RADIATING
CRUSHING	PENETRATING
6 TUGGING	PIERCING
PULLING	18 TIGHT
WRENCHING	NUMB
7 HOT	DRAWING
BURNING	SQUEEZING
SCALDING	TEARING
SEARING	19 COOL
8 TINGLING	COLD
ITCHY	FREEZING
SMARTING	20 NAGGING
STINGING	NAUSEATING
9 DULL	AGONIZING
SORE	DREADFUL
HURTING	TORTURING
ACHING	PPI
HEAVY	0 No pain
10 TENDER	1 MILD
TAUT	2 DISCOMFORTING
RASPING	3 DISTRESSING
SPLITTING	4 HORRIBLE
	5 EXCRUCIATING

PPI_____ COMMENTS:

CONSTANT
PERIODIC
BRIEF

ACCOMPANYING SYMPTOMS:
NAUSEA
HEADACHE
DIZZINESS
DROWSINESS
CONSTIPATION
DIARRHEA
COMMENTS:

SLEEP:
GOOD
FITFUL
CAN'T SLEEP
COMMENTS:

FOOD INTAKE:
GOOD
SOME
LITTLE
NONE
COMMENTS:

ACTIVITY:
GOOD
SOME
LITTLE
NONE

COMMENTS:

Figure 1 McGill-Melzack Pain Questionnaire, adapted for study of the Brompton mixture. Descriptors fall into four major groups: sensory, 1 to 10; affective, 11 to 15; evaluative, 16; and miscellaneous, 17 to 20. The rank value for each descriptor is based on its position in the word set. The sum of the rank values is the "pain rating index" (PRI). The "present pain intensity" (PPI) is based on a scale of 0 to 5.

RESULTS

Questionnaire Scores

The mean PPI and PRI scores for the PCU, ward and private patients are shown in Table 1. Statistical analysis revealed no significant difference between ward and private patients in the effects of the Brompton mixture on their pain. However, the patients in the PCU had significantly less pain than those in the wards and in private rooms. By means of the median test,[10] comparison of PCU patients with ward and private patients revealed significant differences in both the PPI and the PRI values. Pain scores for all three groups were remarkably low. Since a PPI score of 1 represents mild pain, it is clear that most ward patients had mild pain, private patients had mild to discomforting pain, and PCU patients had mild pain or none at all. The Brompton mixture, then, had a powerful effect on perceived pain in patients in all groups, but a significantly greater effect on patients in the PCU.

The percentages of patients with pain at various levels are shown in Table 2. The mean PPI score for each patient was assigned to one of four categories: no pain (0 to 0.9), mild (1 to 1.9), discomforting (2 to 2.9) and distressing, horrible or excruciating (3 to 5). In the first three groups the pain may be considered to be bearable, whereas in the last category it may be considered to be unbearable. The mean PRI scores for the patients were similarly assigned to one of four groups. Since the PRI scores for all patients ranged from 1 to 29 the scores were divided into four intervals comparable to those for the PPI. The percentages of patients in each group are approximately the same on the basis of the PPI and the PRI scores. On the basis of the PPI it is apparent that all patients in the PCU who received the Brompton mixture had bearable pain.

Table 1   Mean "Present Pain Intensity" (PPI) and "Pain Rating Index" (PRI) Values for Patients in the Palliative Care Unit (PCU), Wards and Private Rooms

	Patient category		
Variable	PCU (n = 26)	Ward (n = 46)	Private (n = 20)
Sex			
Male	11	25	7
Female	15	21	13
Mean age (yr)	53	54	59
Mean dose of morphine (mg) in			
Brompton mixture	13.3	13.2	10.5
Mean PPI*	0.3	1.1	1.3
Range	0–2	0–4	0–3
Mean PRI*	1.0	5.6	6.9
Range	0–13.6	0–29	0–28

*Differences between means for PCU and both ward and private patients were significant by two-tailed tests based on the median test.[10] P values were as follows
 PCU v. ward: PPI, P < 0.01; PRI, P < 0.05.
 PCU v. private: PPI, P < 0.01; PRI, P < 0.01.
 PCU v. ward + private: PPI, P < 0.001; PRI, P < 0.02.

Table 2 Percentages of Patients with Mean Pain Scores within Specific Ranges of the PPI and PRI

	PPI scores and % of patients			
	0-0.9	1-1.9	2-2.9	3-5
PCU (n = 26)	84	8	8	0
Ward (n = 46)	54	26	7	13
Private (n = 20)	50	15	25	10
	PRI scores and % of patients			
	0-5.9	6-11.9	12-17.9	18-29.9
PCU (n = 26)	92	4	4	0
Ward (n = 42)*	64	17	7	12
Private (n = 19)*	53	26	5	16

*Smaller numbers because patients who were able to make a decision on their level of pain on a scale of 0 to 5 but whose vocabulary was too limited to complete the PRI portion of the questionnaire were excluded.

Among the ward and private patients, about 10 to 15 percent of those taking the mixture continued to have unbearable pain.

These data exclude the 9 to 10 percent of patients in all three groups whose pain could not be controlled with the Brompton mixture alone and who required additional or other methods to achieve physical and psychological comfort. If these patients are included in the overall analysis it may be concluded that the Brompton mixture was effective in controlling pain in 90 percent of patients in the PCU and 75 to 80 percent of patients in wards or private rooms.

The effectiveness of the Brompton mixture is indicated further in Table 3. In an earlier study[9] all patients that attended the outpatient pain clinic at the Royal Victoria Hospital were administered pain questionnaires. Sixteen had pain associated with

Table 3 Mean PPI, "Number of Words Chosen" (NWC) and PRI for Cancer Patients Observed in an Outpatient Pain Clinic, the PCU, Wards and Private Rooms

	Mean age (yr)	Mean PPI	Mean NWC	Mean PRI[†]				
				S	A	E	M	T
Pain clinic (n = 16)	56	2.8	8.8	17.3	2.3	4.1	2.3	26.0
PCU (n = 5)*	53	1.0	2.9	3.6	0.5	1.0	0.3	5.4
Ward (n = 20)*	54	1.5	5.1	6.1	1.7	1.7	2.3	11.7
Private (n = 12)*	59	1.6	4.8	6.4	1.1	1.4	2.0	11.0

*Patients (21 from PCU, 26 from wards and 8 from private rooms) who reported total absence of pain are excluded from this analysis.
†PRI scores for sensory (S), affective (A), evaluative (E), miscellaneous (M) and total (T) categories.

cancer. Their scores for PPI, NWC and PRI are shown in Table 3, along with those of the PCU, ward and private patients. All patients who obtained total pain relief with the Brompton mixture were omitted from this analysis. Thus, Table 3 permits comparison of treatments among cancer patients who were in pain at the time of administration of the questionnaire. The patients seen at the pain clinic were all ambulatory and received a variety of oral analgesics and tranquilizers. Their pain levels were therefore influenced by a variety of medications (such as codeine and propoxyphene) and were presumably lower than they would have been in the absence of any medication. Nevertheless, the ward and private patients who received the Brompton mixture had consistently lower scores than the cancer patients receiving other medications (and presumably in less advanced stages of the disease). The scores of the patients in the PCU were lowest of all. Moreover, the Brompton mixture clearly produced low scores in all three dimensions of pain—sensory, affective and evaluative.

Morphine Dosage

The average dose of morphine in the Brompton mixture was calculated for all the patients in the study. It was found that 78 percent received morphine doses of less than 20 mg, while 22 percent received 20 mg or more. The mean dose for all patients was 12.3 mg (Table 1).

The average dose of morphine was generally raised if the patient's pain was not brought under control. However, dosage was carefully adjusted according to the patient's need and there was no evidence of habituation to the morphine, thus confirming Twycross's observations in an earlier study.[6] Once a satisfactory morphine dose was determined for a patient, his pain scores remained virtually constant, with only minor fluctuations, rarely exceeding one PPI interval. This constancy was noted particularly in patients who were observed over a period of several weeks, and one for as long as 40 days. Moreover, sequential assessments at 1, 2, 3 and 4 hours after mixture administration showed no fluctuations in the pain. Once the adequate dose was determined and pain was under control, the pain remained at the same level. This is consistent with observations of patients who received the Brompton mixture for periods as long as a year without dose escalation.

It became apparent early in the study that, in attempting to prescribe the lowest effective dose of morphine, physicians were often reluctant to increase the dose when needed. As the physicians became more comfortable with the method of treatment, the mean prescribed doses tended to increase slightly. Data obtained during the first 8 months of the study are compared with the data of the entire study in Table 4. The mean morphine doses for the entire study were slightly higher than those for the first 8 months and the pain levels were accordingly lower. As noted above, morphine tolerance, with its attendant dose escalation, was not observed.

Domiciliary Care

Several PCU patients who took part in the study were permitted to go home once their pain and other medical problems were brought under control, and they used a home recording card[9] to record their pain at prescribed periods 4 times a day. There

Table 4 Comparison of Pain Scores During the First 8 Months and the Total 18 Months of the Study

	Mean dose of morphine (mg) in Brompton mixture	Mean PPI	Mean PRI	% of patients in 3 PPI ranges		
				0–1.9	2–2.9	3–5
First 8 months						
PCU (n = 9)	12.4	0.7	1.9	88	12	0
Ward (n = 16)	11.9	1.6	9.4	53	18	29
Private (n = 11)	9.9	1.0	5.0	55	36	9
Total 18 months						
PCU (n = 26)	13.3	0.3	1.0	92	8	0
Ward (n = 46)	13.2	1.1	5.6	80	7	13
Private (n = 20)	10.5	1.3	6.9	65	25	10

was usually a remarkable consistency in the PPI scores on the cards. If there was a change in the score it could be immediately detected by the visiting nurse. If the score showed a radical change the patient was immediately readmitted to hospital until the pain was brought under control (assuming no other major change in the patient's condition).

DISCUSSION

The results show clearly that the Brompton mixture provides a powerful tool for the control of pain in most patients with cancer. Its effectiveness was evident in all three groups of patients and was especially impressive in the PCU group. Since the doses of morphine and other ingredients were comparable for the three groups, the reasons for the significantly greater effectiveness of the Brompton mixture in the PCU group requires explanation. The primary reason, we believe, was the psychological impact of the unit itself. The presence of a highly concerned staff and the help of volunteers who provided comfort and good cheer, as well as all the other amenities of the unit, must undoubtedly have had a strong psychological effect on the pain. Since the PCU is comparable to St. Christopher's Hospice, the data confirm Twycross's observations[5,6] of the powerful analgesic properties of the Brompton mixture in the context of a highly supportive and comforting environment.

The results of this study are consistent with the gate-control theory of pain.[2] They provide convincing evidence of interacting psychological and physical effects on pain. The Brompton mixture, moreover, does not act on only a single dimension of pain but has a strong effect on the sensory, affective and evaluative dimensions together. The purpose of the PCU is to enhance the quality of life of a terminally ill patient; the Brompton mixture appears to contribute significantly to this goal. It diminishes pain to a striking extent in most patients. Once pain is bearable, social interaction and personal understanding[4] become possible. It is only in the absence of unbearable pain that a desirable quality of life can be achieved.

The lowering of the pain scores during the second part of the study, compared with the first 8 months, can be attributed primarily to the increased morphine dose, to more strict adherence to the 4-hour regimen of administration of the mixture, and to more consistent inclusion of the phenothiazine with the mixture. However, it may also be due in part to an enhanced placebo effect since the results of the first half of the study were encouraging, and the staff's enthusiasm for the mixture may have raised the patients' belief in its effectiveness.

The results show that the PCU provides powerful psychological support to patients suffering pain associated with terminal cancer. The psychological support, together with the Brompton mixture, is capable of reducing pain to bearable levels in most patients. There is no reason to believe that the results showing greater effectiveness of the PCU than care in wards or private rooms were biased by selection of the patients who received questionnaires. Roughly 10 percent of patients in all three groups had severe pain that could not be controlled by the Brompton mixture and had to receive additional or other treatment. Of the remaining patients, the samples from the three groups were chosen at random. The mean ages of the patients, it was found at the conclusion of the study, were approximately the same, and the mean doses of morphine were also about the same for the three groups. Although the dose of the phenothiazine was not regulated rigidly, it varied within a narrow range—too narrow to explain the large differences between the PCU group and the ward and private groups. The questionnaire itself provides objective measures of pain, and the high correlations between PPI and PRI scores found in an earlier study[9] were also found in this study.

The validity of the results is further indicated by the fact that the PCU patients had less pain than either the ward or private patients considered separately. Selection or sampling bias in these control groups was unlikely since each came from hospital populations with different socioeconomic and educational backgrounds. Conversely, it is reasonable to assume that the patients in the PCU did not have less pain initially than those in the other two groups. Indeed, the patients sent to the PCU tended to be those with the most troublesome pain. These factors should have militated against greater relief in PCU patients than in the two other groups. The differences, therefore, are even more striking and underscore the power of the combination of the Brompton mixture and psychological support provided by a hospital service such as the PCU.

REFERENCES

1 Melzack, R.: *The Puzzle of Pain*, Harmondsworth, England, Penguin, 1973.
2 Melzack, R., Wall, P. D.: Pain mechanisms: a new theory. *Science* **150**:971, 1965.
3 Melzack, R., Casey, K. L.: Sensory, motivational and central control determinants of pain: a new conceptual model (chap. 20), in *The Skin Senses,* Kenshalo, D. (ed.), Springfield, Charles C. Thomas, 1968, p. 423.
4 Kübler-Ross, E.: *On Death and Dying*, New York, Macmillan, 1969.
5 Twycross, R. G.: Principles and practice of the relief of pain in terminal cancer. *Update* **5**:115, 1972.
6 Idem: Clinical experience with diamorphine in advanced malignant disease. *Int J Clin Pharmacol* **9**:184, 1974.

7   Jaffe, J. H., Martin, W. R.: Narcotic analgesics and antagonists (chap. 15) in *The Pharmacological Basis of Therapeutics,* 5th ed, Goodman, L. S., Gilman, A. (eds.), New York, Macmillan, 1975, p. 245.

8   Akil H., Mayer, D. J., Liebeskind, J. C.: Antagonism of stimulation-produced analgesia by naloxone, a narcotic antagonist. *Science* **191**:961, 1976.

9   Melzack, R.: The McGill Pain Questionnaire: major properties and scoring methods. *Pain* **1**:277, 1975.

10 Siegel, S.: *Nonparametric Statistics,* New York, McGraw-Hill, 1956.

Chapter 37

Use of the Brompton Mixture in Treating the Chronic Pain of Malignant Disease

B. M. Mount
I. Ajemian
J. F. Scott

THE NATURE OF CHRONIC PAIN

It is in treating acute pain that most physicians gain experience in the use of analgesics. Acute pain is reversible. It warns us of a problem that needs attention. It can therefore be viewed as linear, with a beginning and an end. Chronic pain, however, can be characterized as a vicious circle with no set time limit. The fearful anticipation of its perpetuation leads to anxiety, depression and insomnia, which in turn accentuate the physical component of the pain.[1] Leshan[2] suggests that meaninglessness, helplessness and hopelessness are characteristic of the unreal nightmare world in which the patient with chronic pain lives every day. Saunders[3] has coined the term "total pain" to describe the all-consuming nature of chronic pain and our need to attack all of its components—physical, psychological, financial, interpersonal and spiritual. For the patient with advanced malignant disease, pain forcibly reminds him of his prognosis and thus further accentuates his total agony.

Reprinted from *CMA Journal*, **115**:122–124, July 17, 1976.

AIMS OF TREATMENT

The aims of treatment of the intractable pain of advanced malignant disease include the following:

1. *Identifying the cause:* Clarification of the cause is an essential first step in symptom control and may often lead to specific forms of therapy (e.g., radiotherapy for a localized bony metastasis, estrogens in carcinoma of the prostate, or purgatives in pain due to constipation).

2. *Preventing pain:* The aim is to anticipate and prevent pain rather than treat it. This requires the *regular* administration of appropriate amounts of analgesic. Waiting for pain to reappear (as with "p.r.n." orders) only accentuates the problem of pain control. "The physician should not wait until the pain becomes agonizing; no patient should ever wish for death because of his physician's reluctance to use adequate amounts of potent narcotics."[4]

3. *Erasing pain memory:* As the anxious anticipation and memory of pain is lessened by successful pain prevention, the amount of analgesic required will frequently decrease.

4. *An unclouded sensorium:* Many patients feel trapped between perpetual pain on the one hand and perpetual somnolence on the other. The balance, a pain-free state without sedation, requires careful individual regulation of analgesic dose according to the patient's needs.

5. *Normal affect:* The ability of a patient to relate to his environment with a normal affect, neither euphoric nor depressed, is an obvious treatment aim.

6. *Ease of administration:* Oral administration of analgesics can allow a patient to retain a degree of independence and mobility that he cannot have when analgesics are given parenterally. Cachexia may also make regular parenteral medication difficult and painful.

USE OF NARCOTICS

The current North American anxiety surrounding the use of narcotics for the intractable pain of advanced malignant disease is summarized in the following points: "Giving narcotics is bad management. Narcotics give you 'ups and downs' producing addiction and destroying the personality. They depress cortical function."[5]

Our experience suggests that with attention to detail none of these statements need be true, and that all of the treatment aims outlined may be achieved with few exceptions.

With moderate to severe chronic pain, only the narcotic analgesics provide adequate control. Milder analgesics should always be tried for less severe pain and may be helpful in combination with more potent drugs. A wide variety of agents is available; Catalano[6] presents a good recent review.

THE BROMPTON MIXTURE

In our experience the Brompton mixture is effective in most cases of severe pain and as a liquid has advantages over tablets for oral administration:

1 The dosage can be easily adjusted to meet the patient's need.
2 Many patients have dysphagia, either functional or due to local disease, and find a syrup easier to swallow than a tablet.

The Brompton mixture is used when non-narcotic and milder narcotic preparations are ineffective. Lengthy anticipated survival is *not* a contraindication because, with care in adjusting the dosage to meet the patient's need, the mixture may be used for periods of many months to several years without dose escalation.

Although generations of British physicians have gained familiarity with variants of the oral narcotic mixture bearing the name of the Brompton Chest Hospital, it was not until 1973 that this formulation was recognized in the "British Pharmaceutical Codex."[7] The important experience of Saunders and her coworkers[3,8] at St. Christopher's Hospice and St. Joseph's Hospice has led to a refinement and standardization of approach, which has been associated with greatly increased effectiveness in achieving the above aims of therapy. The standard mixture contains a variable amount of morphine, 10 mg of cocaine, 2.5 ml of ethyl alcohol (98 percent), 5 ml of flavoring syrup and a variable amount of chloroform water, for a total of 20 ml. The contributions to the effectiveness of this mixture of the small amount of cocaine and the stabilizing effect of the ethyl alcohol are uncertain. Further elucidation must await the results of trials aimed at simplifying the mixture.

For most patients the chronic pain of advanced malignant disease can be controlled with 5 to 20 mg of morphine per dose of the mixture, but small or elderly patients may require as little as 2.5 mg. The usual sequential doses of morphine given are 2.5, 5, 10, 15, 20, 30, 40, 60, 90 and 120 mg. This standard elixir is always given with a phenothiazine. The phenothiazines are potent antiemetics and are thus useful in countering vomiting, a frequent side effect of narcotics. Experience also suggests that they potentiate the narcotic analgesia. Prochlorperazine, 5 mg in 5 ml, is usually highly effective as an antiemetic, with little sedative effect. If restlessness or agitation is a feature, chlorpromazine, 10 to 25 mg, may be substituted. Twycross[9] has shown a shelf life of sustained effectiveness that exceeds 8 weeks.

Administration

In adjusting the dosage of narcotic and phenothiazine to achieve a pain-free state without sedation, a number of factors are important:

• The morphine elixir should be given in 20-ml doses with the phenothiazine every 4 hours around the clock because the serum half-life of morphine taken orally is about 4 hours. Occasionally a patient may require a 3-hourly schedule. The nighttime dose is omitted only when the patient can sleep through the night free of pain. Careful attention to exact dosage and timing will pay dividends in results.
• For most patients a pain-free state can be achieved by giving sequential increments in narcotic dose.[10] To treat excruciating pain one may elect to start with a higher narcotic dose, then make sequential decrements until analgesia without sedation is achieved (Fig. 1). In determining the dosage required, dose alterations should be made at intervals of 48 to 72 hours. During this period further analgesia can be achieved with the use of supplemental analgesics as required.

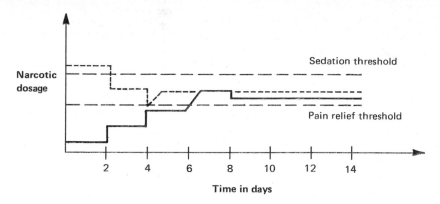

Figure 1 Alternative methods of dosage adjustment. Pain relief in the absence of sedation may be achieved with sequential increments in narcotic dose at intervals of 2 days (———). In a few cases the severity of the pain will require an initially high dose, followed by sequential decrements until the pain reappears (– – – –). A slight increase in dose provides analgesia without sedation (— —).

- In general, it is wise to change only one variable, the narcotic or the phenothiazine, at a time. Since the phenothiazines and morphine are synergistic, great care must be exercised. Small changes in either variable may produce profound changes in analgesia and sedation.
- Initiation of narcotic therapy will usually produce transient sedation lasting 48 to 72 hours. It is important to reassure both patient and family that pain can and will be controlled and that the initial drowsiness is temporary. Their confidence that control can be achieved will promote analgesia.
- Dispensing the morphine mixture and the phenothiazine syrup separately allows greater flexibility in adjusting dosage. Once a continuous pain-free state is achieved, they may be combined in dispensing for greater ease of administration.
- Careful observation of the patient's condition over a complete 24-hour period may suggest augmentation of one or two specific doses at periods of peak activity.
- If parenteral medication becomes necessary, the equivalent dose of morphine is one-half the previous oral dose. Thus, a patient whose pain has been controlled with 30 mg taken orally would then receive 15 mg intramuscularly.[8]
- The maximum effective oral dose of morphine is ill defined. Recent experience at St. Christopher's Hospice (C. Saunders: personal communication, 1975) suggests that continuing effectiveness may be obtained in some patients with oral doses of 90 mg or more; however, most patients' pain can be controlled with less than 30 mg q4h.

Adverse Effects

These basically are the adverse effects common to all narcotics and include the following:

Sedation When narcotic therapy is introduced transient sedation frequently occurs. The phenothiazine may exaggerate this effect. However, patients with advanced malignant disease often have other causes for somnolence (e.g., hepatic or renal insufficiency, or metastases).

Nausea and Vomiting   Routine use of a phenothiazine with the mixture counters this common side effect of all narcotics. If a patient is vomiting before therapy is instituted, control should first be achieved with parenteral medication and subsequently maintained with oral medication.

Constipation   The combined effects of poor dietary intake, dehydration, inactivity and narcotic therapy almost invariably lead to constipation. This should be prevented by using a combination of a stool softener and a bowel stimulant (e.g., dioctyl sodium sulfosuccinate and senna concentrate).

Tolerance-dependence   Evans[11] and Twycross[8] both reported that dependence (addiction) is not a problem when narcotics are used for the pain of malignant disease. Marks and Sachar[12] stated: "The excessive and unrealistic concern about the danger of addiction in the hospitalized medical patient is a significant and potent force for undertreatment with narcotics." It would seem, rather, that undertreatment with analgesic medication may encourage craving and psychological dependence. Progressive tolerance and escalating dosage requirements are often given as reasons for delaying the onset of narcotic therapy. Our own experience confirms that of Twycross[8] that a change in dosage requirement heralds a change in disease status rather than tolerance.

Other Adverse Effects   Extrapyramidal effects, orthostatic hypotension and other side effects of the phenothiazines must be watched for but they occur infrequently with suggested doses. Because of phenothiazine's synergism with morphine, a small dose of the former is often sufficient. Although cocaine may be highly toxic to habitual abusers, there is some question whether tolerance to cocaine develops.[13] The dose of cocaine used by us is similar to that used at St. Christopher's Hospice and is one-half the dose suggested in the "British Pharmaceutical Codex."[7] It has not led to important toxicity. Hypersensitivity reactions to morphine and to the phenothiazines are rare. When used as outlined above, the Brompton mixture provides convenient and uniform pain control without important adverse effects.

Case Reports

Three current cases illustrate the use of the Brompton mixture.

Case 1   A 70-year-old woman with breast carcinoma had received the Brompton mixture intermittently for more than 1 year at the time of this report (Fig. 2). It was initially instituted during radiation therapy for lower thoracic back pain due to spinal metastases. At that time she was bedridden and had a decubitus ulcer. Over the ensuing 40 weeks she was given progressively smaller doses of morphine in the mixture and felt well enough to walk short distances. Once she was pain-free the mixture was discontinued. She was mobilized and was able to walk with assistance. The ulcer healed. For 2 months (weeks 40 to 48) she was given a codeine and propoxyphene compound. At weeks 49 to 50 increasingly severe back pain related to progression of her disease led to reinstitution of therapy with the Brompton mixture, the dose of morphine temporarily being high. Radiation therapy again relieved the pain and the dose of morphine

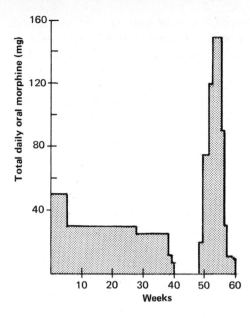

Figure 2 Therapy with the Brompton mixture in case 1.

was tapered. At 60 weeks the narcotic mixture was once again discontinued. No symptoms related to narcotic withdrawal were noted.

Case 2   A 52-year-old woman with lumbar back pain, weakness, lower limb edema and anemia related to disseminated carcinoma of the cervix had been managed with parenteral morphine for 6 weeks when she was transferred for further care to the Royal Victoria Hospital's palliative care unit. Therapy with the Brompton mixture was instituted and gave excellent results (Fig. 3). She is presently able to be up in a chair and is pain-free; the doses of morphine in the mixture are being decreased.

Case 3   A 78-year-old man with prostatic carcinoma was admitted to hospital with incapacitating back pain. Therapy with the Brompton mixture was instituted (Fig. 4). The prompt ensuing relief enabled his return home for 14 weeks. During this time he

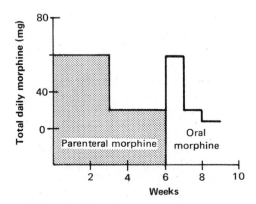

Figure 3 Therapy with parenteral morphine, then the Brompton mixture in case 2.

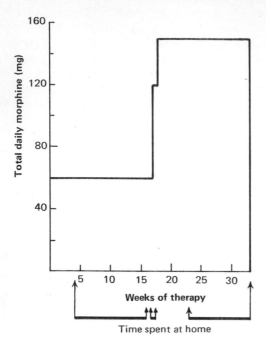

Figure 4 Therapy with the Brompton mixture in case 3.

was up and about and was able to enjoy his garden. He was then readmitted to hospital with increased pain and increasing spinal cord compression, resulting in paraplegia. Increasing the dosage again controlled his pain and he was able to be cared for at home for the final 10 weeks of his life.

These cases illustrate the use of the Brompton mixture for periods ranging from 9 weeks to more than 1 year. In all three there was complete pain control, increased mobility, and an absence of drug-induced somnolence, personality change or dose escalation.

Additional Measures

The Brompton mixture, to be effective against the "total pain" of advanced malignant disease, must be used in combination with other therapies. Symptom control may require additional measures such as radiotherapy, peripheral nerve or intrathecal block, neurosurgery, or physical measures such as splinting and passive exercises. Tricyclic antidepressants, benzodiazepines, anti-inflammatory agents (e.g., phenylbutazone), corticosteroids and hypnotics can all be useful in attacking the vicious circle of chronic pain. Environmental manipulation can also decrease pain. Melzack, Ofiesh and Mount, in their evaluation of the Brompton mixture (see Chapter 36) have suggested the importance of creating a pleasant, supportive environment in which a patient is able to communicate his concerns and where the resources of an interdisciplinary team are available to help in areas of interpersonal, psychosocial and philosophical need. Their study confirms our clinical experience that morphine, given in the form of the Brompton mixture with a phenothiazine, is a highly effective, flexible, safe and convenient means of controlling the chronic pain of malignant disease.

REFERENCES

1 Melzack, R.: *The Puzzle of Pain*, Harmondsworth, England, Penguin, 1973, p. 142.
2 Leshan, L.: The world of the patient in severe pain of long duration. *J. Chronic Dis.* 17:119, 1964.
3 Saunders, C.: *The Management of Terminal Illness*, London, Hosp. Med. Publ., 1967.
4 Jaffe, J.: Narcotic analgesics (chap. 15), in *The Pharmacological Basis of Therapeutics*, 4th ed., Goodman, L. S., Gilman A. (eds.), New York, Macmillan, 1970, p. 254.
5 *Drug and Pain Management*, Leinbach composite videotape no. 3, Seattle, U. of Washington CCTV services, 1974.
6 Catalano, R.: Medical management of pain caused by cancer. *Semin. Oncol.* 2: 378, 1975.
7 *British Pharmaceutical Codex*, London, Pharmaceutical Pr., 1973, p. 669.
8 Twycross, R.: Clinical experience with diamorphine in advanced malignant disease. *Int. J. Clin. Pharmacol.* 9: 184, 1974.
9 Idem: Euphoriant elixirs. *Br. Med. J.* 3: 552, 1973.
10 Lipman, A. G.: Drug therapy in terminally ill patients. *Am. J. Hosp. Pharm.* 32: 270, 1975.
11 Evans, R. J.: Experiences in a pain clinic. *Mod. Med. Can.* 26 (10): 7, 1971.
12 Marks, M. D., Sachar, E. J.: Undertreatment of medical in-patients with narcotic analgesics. *Ann. Intern. Med.* 78: 173, 1973.
13 Jaffe, J.: Drug addiction and drug abuse (chap. 16), in *The Pharmacological Basis of Therapeutics*, op. cit., p. 295.

Chapter 38

The Problem of Caring for the Dying in a General Hospital: The Palliative Care Unit as a Possible Solution

Balfour M. Mount

We emerge deserving of little credit; we who are capable of ignoring the conditions which make muted people suffer. The dissatisfied dead cannot noise abroad the negligence they have experienced.[1]

THE PROBLEM: DEFICIENCIES IN TERMINAL CARE

Approximately 70 percent of Canadians now die in institutions.[2] There is increasing evidence that these patients and their families experience a wide variety of critical problems that usually go unrecognized by those responsible for their care. The terminally ill patient, instead of receiving sympathetic understanding and expertise in meeting his medical and emotional needs, may encounter isolation and depersonalization.[1,3,7]

The hospital staff also find the situation difficult. Lasagna[4] has suggested that the orientation of the medical team may foster a half-hearted approach in seeing to the welfare of the dying. Nurses, for example, do not welcome assignments to dying patients and many are uncomfortable in conversing with them.[8] As death approaches, interaction between patient and staff becomes strained and patient care is affected.[9] This problem is accentuated by the pressures of intrahospital routines that are designed to satisfy efficiency of operation and the needs of the staff.[10] Physicians

Reprinted from CMA Journal, 115:119–121, July 17, 1976.

visit with decreasing frequency the longer a patient is hospitalized,[7,11] and nursing care decreases as a patient's death becomes imminent.[5] It takes longer for a nurse to answer the bell rung by a dying patient than by a patient expected to recover.[12] Isolation, suspicion and distrust develop owing to the lack of communication between patients, family members, nurses and physicians. This is fostered by physicians' reluctance to inform the patient of the diagnosis and prognosis,[6] a natural preference to treat disease rather than to deal with personal and social problems,[6] and an endemic denial of death.[6,13]

These deficiencies in our approach to the terminally ill were confirmed in a recent study of attitudes to dying at the Royal Victoria Hospital in Montreal.[14] The data obtained indicated the patients' desire for complete openness and honesty in discussion of diagnosis and prognosis, the physicians' reluctance to be that candid, the residents' relative lack of concern for the patients' emotional needs, and the social workers' tendency to minimize the problem. The physician's attitude towards his own death was found to be an important variable in determining how he perceived his patients' needs: 84 percent of physicians who felt they would want to know their own prognosis if they were fatally ill thought that their patients also desired direct communication of prognosis, while only 45 percent of physicians not wanting to know their own prognosis thought their patients desired honesty of communication. One physician stated that he would not tell a patient that he had cancer unless he asked and that no patient had ever asked him; this tells us more about the physician's inability to hear what his patients are saying than about his patients' fears.

If terminal care is so poor, why is the problem not more generally recognized? The Royal Victoria Hospital study[14] suggested two important factors that limit our perception. First, there is a general tendency to see ourselves as sensitive individuals and consequently we do not recognize our insensitivity to the needs of those around us. In each professional group the proportion who recognized deficiencies in the way in which their colleagues met the needs of the terminally ill was larger than the proportion who recognized that they themselves had deficiencies. Similarly, the proportion who felt that they personally avoided discussions with patients regarding dying was smaller than the proportion who felt that their colleagues avoided such discussions. Second, patients are reluctant to criticize those who care for them.[7,14]

Why has this deficit in terminal care developed? The isolation and the lack of sensitivity, caring and expertise that these patients encounter cannot be explained on the basis of indifference of the medical team. There are other factors. As individuals we reflect the attitudes of our death-denying society.[15] It is of utmost importance to recognize the misalignment between the needs of the terminally ill and the four goals of the general hospital: to investigate, to diagnose, to cure and to prolong life. As the rate of accumulating medical knowledge increases, so does the pressure on the medical team to concentrate its efforts in the direction of the four goals. The problem arises when we introduce into this general hospital environment patients for whom the hard-won expertise of the health care team is no longer appropriate. In the management of the dying, skills of investigating, diagnosing, curing and prolonging life are irrelevant. The appropriate goal is treatment aimed at producing the optimal quality of life for the patient and his family. The expertise of the staff and the needs of the patient are therefore mismatched. From the perspective of traditional hospital goals "nothing can be done" for the dying patient. Thus, the medical team feels impotent and may become angry or indifferent. Far from there being an absence of caring and concern, these very qualities often magnify the feelings of guilt and anxiety of members of the hospital staff. To cope with the situation the staff increasingly isolate the patient and family, and so the problem is reinforced.

With respect to malignant disease, there are three admissible goals: to cure, to prolong life and to palliate. Until now, interest, concern and financial resources have been applied towards improving the effectiveness of our action in curing patients and, if this is not possible, prolonging life. We must now seek ways to improve the lot of those for whom treatment aimed at improving the quality of life is the only appropriate goal.

THE OPTIONS

Given the significance of the problem and the economic constraints affecting the delivery of health care, we must consider our options carefully.[16]

To Continue Management of the Dying as in the Past

Having recognized the existing deficiencies and the potential for improving the lot of the terminally ill, we can no longer consider this a morally acceptable option.

To Educate Medical and Paramedical Teams
Concerning the Problems of Death and Dying

More and more medical education programs are offering lectures and courses on death and dying. These measures, together with the increased coverage by the scientific press and by mass media, have increased our awareness of the needs of the terminally ill and their families. But much yet needs to be done. The basic problem remains: the difference between the needs of these patients and the aims of the acute treatment ward of a general hospital.

To Develop Separate Institutions with Special Expertise
in Treating Terminally Ill Patients

St. Christopher's Hospice and St. Joseph's Hospice, both in London, England, St. Luke's Hospice in Sheffield, England, Calvary Hospital in the Bronx, New York, and a number of other separate institutions have been established to provide improved care for the dying and their families.

The approach taken at St. Christopher's Hospice illustrates the operation of separate institutions. Founded 8 years ago, St. Christopher's Hospice is a caring community of 54 inpatient beds, with a domiciliary service, a day-care centre for the children of personnel, a number of bed-sitting rooms for the elderly and a vigorous research and teaching program. Most of the patients have advanced malignant disease or a progressing neurologic disorder. The common selection factor is the irrelevance of therapy attempting to modify the natural history of their diseases. Saunders and others[17-21] have described the functioning of this remarkable institution. It provides a high standard of medical care, with close attention to detail in meeting the needs of the patient-family unit in all dimensions: medical, social, psychological and spiritual. Analysis of the economics of maintaining such institutions, however, suggests that society cannot afford to support an adequate number to meet the need.

To Integrate Within the General Hospital a Palliative Care Unit (PCU)

The PCU is a specialized unit within the general hospital, staffed by an interdisciplinary team and designed with goals aligned to the specific needs of the dying.

The results of the Royal Victoria Hospital study[14] and an examination of related matters led to the recommendation that the Royal Victoria Hospital open a PCU as a 2-year pilot project. The aim of the project has been to establish the feasibility of a unit within the general hospital offering services similar to those provided by St. Christopher's Hospice. The premises[7,16,17] on which this project is based are the following:

1   The medical, emotional and spiritual needs of the terminally ill and their families are, in general, neglected in the delivery of health care.

2   Suffering is greatly intensified by the isolation resulting from our present methods of dealing with the terminally ill.

3   The presence of terminally ill patients in a general hospital ward and the type of treatment they receive are demoralizing for the patient, his family, the ward staff and other patients.

4   Terminally ill patients must always be helped toward a positive outlook based on reality, confidence and trust, not dishonesty.

5   The health care system should support, facilitate and assist the terminally ill in their desire to be at home while that is feasible, and to die at home if that is possible.

6   It is important for the patient and his family not to be deserted by the hospital in which they have confidence.

7   A PCU would enable a general hospital to better meet the needs of the community it serves.

8   A highly motivated, trained team of nurses backed by physician, psychiatrist, social worker, physical and occupational therapists, dietitian, chaplain, music therapist, volunteers, receptionist and secretary can meet the multidimensional needs of the terminally ill and their families.

9   A PCU for the terminally ill may be effectively integrated into a general hospital.

10   It is possible for a PCU to provide a positive atmosphere of welcome and confidence rather than the negative one of "a home for the dying."

11   The challenges and rewards of PCU work are sufficient to sustain the nursing, physician and support staff involved in such work.

12   The PCU will allow observations regarding (1) the late effects of treatment; (2) the medical, social, psychological and spiritual needs of the terminally ill and their families; and (3) the means of meeting these needs.

13   With attention to detail and careful regulation of medication according to the patient's needs it is possible to achieve, with few exceptions, a pain-free state without excessive sedation, the medical management of bowel obstruction (without nasogastric tube, intravenous fluid and colostomy) and the satisfactory control of other symptoms.

14 It is possible for the period of terminal illness to be one of achievement, reconciliation and fulfilment for patient and family, facilitating the return of the family to a normal life after bereavement.

15 The supportive relationship with the family should be continued, when necessary, following the patient's death.

16 A PCU should be a monument not to the incurability of some disease but to the dignity of man.

THE PALLIATIVE CARE SERVICE

The palliative care service, opened in January 1975, comprises three areas of care as well as research, teaching and administrative functions: the PCU itself, a domiciliary service and a consultation service.

The PCU

The 12-bed unit is staffed by a multidisciplinary team. Because of the size of the unit during the pilot project phase, the patient pool has been limited to Royal Victoria Hospital patients with malignant disease for whom care aimed at improving the quality of life is the only appropriate therapy. The "team approach" is emphasized in the quest for an improved quality of life. Family members are encouraged to participate in patient care. When necessary to meet the individual needs of the patient-family unit, hospital regulations are relaxed to allow relatives to stay overnight and children—and even pets—to visit. Care is individualized. Blood pressure, pulse and temperature are not taken routinely. The only investigations and treatments performed are those directly related to the alleviation of problematic symptoms.

Family members particularly close to the patient are assessed prospectively for their risk of impairment of health and psychosocial adjustment. Minimum follow-up of relatives after the patient's death includes a visit with the bereaved at 2 and 4 weeks and a letter at 1 year. More extensive follow-up is available when indicated.

The Domiciliary Service

The domiciliary service, staffed by nurse practitioners, facilitates comprehensive home care, with emphasis again placed on the total needs of the patient and the family. Care includes controlling pain and symptoms as well as seeking a resolution of emotional, interpersonal, spiritual and financial difficulties. The domiciliary team works with available visiting nurses and persons from other community resources. Such support assists the patient in remaining at home as long as possible and, if feasible, dying at home.

The Consultation Service

The palliative-care-service physician and consultation nurse visit patients in other parts of the hospital for evaluation regarding PCU admission or domiciliary care. When these goals are not possible or advisable the patient may be followed on his original service by members of the PCU team.

Evaluation

We are currently evaluating the palliative care service to assess the impact of this approach on the needs of the patients and their families and on the palliative-care-service staff itself.

CONCLUSION

The PCU has resulted less from the discovery of new techniques for treating the dying patient than from the assertion of a positive, creative attitude to death and bereavement. The changes in the health care system that such a unit embodies may have significant implications for the majority of Canadians—the 70 percent who will die in institutions.

REFERENCES

1   Hinton, J.: *Dying*, 2d ed., Harmondsworth, England, Penguin, 1972, p. 159.
2   Statistics Canada: *Vital Statistics Bull.* 3: 61, 1973.
3   Kübler-Ross, E.: *On Death and Dying*, New York, Macmillan, 1969.
4   Lasagna, L.: Physicians' behaviour toward the dying patient, in *The Dying Patient*, Brim, O. G., Freeman, H. E., Levine, S., et al. (eds.), New York, Russell Sage, 1970.
5   Mervyn, F.: The plight of dying patients in hospitals. *Am. J. Nurs.* 71: 1988, 1971.
6   Duff, R. S., Hollingshead, A. B.: Dying and death (chap. 15), in *Sickness and Society*, New York, Har-Row, 1968.
7   Mount, B. M.: Part III, case studies, in unpublished report to medical advisory board of Royal Victoria Hospital by ad hoc committee on thanatology, 1973.
8   Quint, J. C.: Obstacles to helping the dying. *Am. J. Nurs.* 66: 1568, 1966.
9   Hinton, J.: *Dying*, op. cit., p. 158.
10   Sudnow, D.: *Passing On*, Englewood Cliffs, N.J., Prentice-Hall, 1967, p. 61.
11   The blocked bed. *Lancet* 2: 221, 1972.
12   Bowers, M. K., Jackson, E. N., Knight, J. A., et al.: *Counselling the Dying*, New York, Nelson, 1964.
13   Caldwell, D., Mishara, B. L.: Research on attitudes of medical doctors toward the dying patient: a methodological problem. *Omega* 3: 341, 1972.
14   Mount, B. M., Jones, A., Patterson, A.: Death and dying: attitudes in a teaching hospital. *Urology* 4: 741, 1974.
15   Feifel, H.: The taboo on death. *Am. Behav. Sci.* 6: 66, 1963.
16   Mount, B. M.: Improving the Canadian way of dying. *Ont. Psychol.* 7: 19, 1975.
17   Saunders, C.: The need for in-patient care for the patient with terminal cancer. *Middlesex Hosp. J.* 72: 3, 1973.
18   Idem: A place to die. *Crux* 12: 24, 1974.
19   McNulty, B.: Discharge of the terminally-ill patient. *Nurs. Times* 66: 1160, 1970.
20   Idem: Care of the dying. *Nurs. Times* 68: 1505, 1972.
21   Idem: St. Christopher's out-patients. *Am. J. Nurs.* 71: 2328, 1971.

Chapter 39

Death and Dying:
A Course for
Medical Students

David Barton
John M. Flexner
Jan van EYS
Charles E. Scott

In an earlier paper Barton (1) discussed the need for including instruction on death and dying in the medical school curriculum. In spite of the physician's close proximity to the psychosocial events surrounding death and dying, the medical literature contains little material related to student instruction designed specifically to teach about this important area of medical practice. There is a growing need for training in this important area of medical practice created by rapidly advancing technical skills and their accompanying ability to prolong life, the increasing numbers of terminally ill patients treated in institutional settings, a growing awareness of psychosocial processes surrounding the death situation, and the expressed need from within and without the medical profession for a more humanistic approach to illness. It is the purpose of this paper to present the format, content, and goals of a course for medical students designed specifically to provide such training.

During the 1971–72 academic year, Vanderbilt University School of Medicine offered an elective course for 14 third- and fourth-year medical students entitled, "Psychosocial Aspects of Life-Threatening Illness." The size of the class was limited in order to ensure group discussion. A psychiatrist, a hematologist, a pediatric hematologist, and a philosophy professor conducted the class, which met once a week throughout a semester (16 sessions). Although the sessions were initially intended to be

Reprinted from *Journal of Medical Education,* **47**:945–951, December 1972.

limited to one hour, the discussion generally lengthened the class to an hour and a half. The course was uniformly well received by students and is being offered during the 1972–73 academic year.

Instruction in this area requires a course format which allows each student to begin to "work through" and synthesize his attitudes toward death and dying, thereby achieving a more therapeutic approach to patient care. In addition, student attention needs to be directed toward the many psychosocial dimensions of life-threatening illness and the death situation—dimensions which involve the patient, the patient's interpersonal and cultural environment, and transactions within the care-giving milieu. For each session a focal topic or patient presentation, described below in the order in which they were given, was provided, and this was followed by extensive group discussion.

Introduction and Patient Presentation   Prior to the class, each student was asked to read Pattison's paper, "The Experience of Dying" (2). A 44-year-old married woman with acute myelogenous leukemia was interviewed by one of the instructors, and the students were encouraged to ask additional questions. She gave a history of long-standing self-sufficiency and said that a major task in adapting to her illness was the acceptance of a dependent role. She spoke at length of the strength she had derived from her religion and, accepting immortality as a certainty, maintained that she had no fear of death. In the discussion the students were encouraged to consider the numerous areas which require attention in the treatment of such patients. Adaptation to acute illness was emphasized.

Death in Literature   Each student read Tolstoy's short story, "The Death of Ivan Ilych" (3), before the class met. The short story was then used as a focal point for the class discussion.

Patient Presentation   A 45-year-old married woman with Hodgkin's Disease was interviewed by the class. Her husband accompanied her to the session and spoke of his adaptation to her illness and the effect of her illness on their interactions and their children's lives.

Patient Presentation   A 39-year-old minister with chronic myelogenous leukemia discussed his adaptation to his illness with the class. He related that he had directed his attention away from death and had turned his interests toward what he considered to be a more constructive and meaningful life. As this patient's illness was of a more chronic nature, adaptation to chronic illnesses was contrasted with adaptation to acute illnesses.

Death Symbolism and the Fear of Death   Lifton's paper, "On Death and Death Symbolism: The Hiroshima Disaster" (4), and Wahl's paper, "The Fear of Death" (5), were assigned as reading. The emphasis of the discussion was on the class participants' consideration of their own perceptions of dying and death and the feelings evoked by the previous sessions.

The Theological Dimension The focal topic for this session was presented by a rabbi. He discussed the theological conceptualizations of death and dying in Judaism and other religions and spoke of his care of dying persons and their families.

The Perspective of the Pastoral Counselor A pastoral counselor illustrated the dimensions of his care of patients with life-threatening illness through discussing the pastoral care of a counselee during an extended illness. He presented the funeral eulogy which he had delivered after the person's death. He discussed the techniques afforded him by his training in counseling and his identification as a clergyman.

Patient Presentation A 37-year-old divorced man with chronic myelogenous leukemia spoke with the class. The patient was involved in psychotherapy for severe depression accompanied by suicidal ideation. Shortly before his speaking with the class, the chronic leukemic process had progressed to an acute stage, and he was rapidly deteriorating physically. He was experiencing a striking absence of inter-personal support from his environment.

The Perspective of a Philosopher The professor of philosophy provided the focal presentation of this session. He spoke of his own considerations of the recognition of finiteness and transientness, contrasting the feeling of concern and caring about the recognition, acceptance, and affirmation of death with stoical acceptance.

The Perspective of the Nurse A nurse from an adult ward, a pediatric nurse, and a clinical nurse specialist in psychiatric nursing told of their perspective in caring for the dying and described the problems involved in this care from their respective points of view. Interpersonal transactions within the care-giving milieu were emphasized.

Survival through Medical Progress and Technology The case of a patient who was a candidate for the employment of a number of newly developed life-prolonging pro-cedures was described, and the multiple determinants of the decisions made were presented for discussion. This provided a focal point for a discussion of ethical con-siderations in prolonging life.

Grief and Bereavement Lindemann's paper, "Symptomatology and Management of Acute Grief" (6), was utilized as a means of focusing the attention of the group on the phenomenon of grief. Some members of the class spoke of their personal experi-ences with loss and grief. The class in general utilized their recollections of the feelings which had been associated with the assassination of President Kennedy as a theme for exploring the topic.

Role-Playing Utilizing role-playing methods, students enacted some of the diffi-cult situations which emerge in the care of patients with life-threatening illness. For example, while one student assumed the role of the attending physician, another assumed the role of a patient dying of leukemia who requested that the physician stop all treatment and let him die. One vignette had the patient confront the physician regarding his religious views. Another dealt with the matter of obtaining permission for a postmortum examination.

Problems of Palliation   During this session, the psychosocial difficulties involved in the treatment of patients receiving palliative forms of treatment over long periods of time were emphasized. A 42-year-old-man who had received radiotherapy, multiple courses of varying kinds of chemotherapy, and surgical treatment for reticulum cell sarcoma was interviewed by the class.

Life-Threatening Illness in Children, 1   A two-month-old infant born with hydrocephalus, multiple meningomyelocoeles, and other physical deformities was shown to the class. The discussion centered on individual attitudes toward available treatment postures and the physician's involvement in ethical matters.

Life-Threatening Illness in Children, 2   The 22-year-old mother of a three-year-old child with acute lymphocytic leukemia spoke with the group of her inability to hear information which would indicate a poor prognosis. She related a dream in which she helplessly was forced to stand by and watch the child die and stated that at times she also had this feeling in reality.

DISCUSSION

This course was designed to fulfill the following specific instructional goals:

1   To facilitate gradual desensitization to the topic through the process of group interaction and discussion in order to promote the students' understanding and management of their personal feelings about death and dying.

2   To focus the students' attention on the numerous and important psychological and sociocultural issues involved in order that they, as physicians, might help the patient, the family, and the interpersonal milieu in which the patient's care takes place to reach a reasonable level of adaptation in the face of death. By focusing on these issues, the need for the physician to develop a flexible therapeutic approach based on an appreciation of the subtle and often unique adaptive means employed by patients, family, and care-giving personnel was emphasized.

3   To present to and discuss with the students the perspectives of medical personnel and others who are involved in providing care for patients with life-threatening illnesses, thereby imparting insights into the transactions which occur between the physicians and these individuals in the context of the death situation.

4   To encourage active consideration and discussion of ethical issues which, though often encountered in medical practice, are rarely discussed with medical students in a way which allows them to begin to formulate and express their own positions and ideas.

Personal Feelings

Influenced by personal anxieties about death, the complexity of conceptualizing death, the absence of formal instruction in the area, the technical emphasis of medical education, and the often incomprehensible feelings evoked in members of the care-giving milieu in the face of death, medical students often find the area of life-threatening illness painfully sensitive. To manage this, the student may resort to a form of avoidance which may obscure many of the important facets of patient care. The student may, for instance, find comfort in a purely "biological" approach to medical care at the expense of failing to appreciate the psychosocial dimensions of the illness. Gradual desensitization through recognition and management of personal feelings about death and dying thus becomes a primary goal of instruction.

In the early part of the course, students perceived the "protective" manner in which some of the patients were interviewed. For example, in one interview the physician asked the patient, "How do you feel about the possible outcome of your illness?" When the patient asked for clarification of the word "outcome," the words "dying" and "death" were not used. Students asked whether this was "protective" for the patient or the physician. It was concluded that it was partly the latter but that the patient's level of adaptation had the potential to exclude discussion of some areas. As the course progressed, however, it became apparent that some patients were able to verbalize their feelings about dying and death and that this was to some extent dependent on the interviewer's ability to deal with the topic with the patient. The level of approach was thus recognized as growing out of the transaction—the attitudes of both the physician and his patient. In order to be in a position to determine the needs of the patient and overcome the avoidance phenomena that may be related to such issues, however, the student must begin to be able to manage his own anxieties about death.

Increasing ability on the part of the class to manage these anxieties occurred through the group process as the course progressed. At the beginning the discussion occurred at a superficial level. There was a paucity of expression of personal feelings by the class participants. Gradually, though, the discussion moved toward deeper levels of expression. The recognition of feelings evoked by presentations and the discussion of these feelings in the group context served as an effective means for facilitating this expression. Students recognized that just as each patient conceptualized matters pertaining to death in an individualized manner, so does each physician.

Individual approaches of the class members ranged from the purely technical to the more purely humanistic. Group interaction allowed the presentation and sharing of these positions and attitudes; achieving uniformity of attitudes, however, was not a goal of the course. Through this interactive process, attention gradually turned away from personal anxieties about death toward the many facets of management of the patient and his family.

The importance of allowing ample time for group discussion was borne out by the fact that the group interaction allowed increasingly closer scrutiny of highly charged areas. Didactic presentations or patient interviews without group discussion do not effectively accomplish the overcoming of the avoidance of the subject of death and dying. On the contrary, it may be expected that when the student is presented with a firmly organized set of generalized rules for managing life-threatening illness, while at the same time experiencing the anxieties growing out of his own uncertainty, his avoidance and frustration is reinforced. It is, therefore, important that the instructors share in the discussion, communicating their attitudes and feelings in such a way that the students view the exploration process as appropriate. In this manner the "working through" and synthesis of personal attitudes toward the area becomes viewed as an ongoing process rather than an event where one instantaneously develops a set of iron-clad attitudes that remain unquestioned.

Psychosocial Issues

A number of issues outlined in the literature as important in caring for dying patients were also brought to the attention of the class, and the discussions included the integration of this material. Selected papers were utilized throughout the course, and the instructors presented additional material where appropriate. When relevant issues arose in the patient interviews, attention was focused on these issues to ensure that didactic material achieved clinical relevance. Included were the numerous psychological and sociocultural adaptive mechanisms employed by the patient, family, and the caregiving personnel in the face of death. In this category are such topics as the derivatives of the fear of death, the symbolic attributes of dying and death, attempts at conceptualization of death, knowledge about the psychological adaptive mechanisms employed by dying patients, interpersonal response in the therapeutic milieu, and concepts pertaining to grief and bereavement.

Psychosocial issues such as the changes brought about by life-threatening illness (for example, the shift from an independent, self-sufficient status to a position of dependency) were brought into bold relief by the patient interviews. Patients who illustrated various aspects of adaptations growing out of different forms of illnesses, life circumstances, and belief systems were chosen for these interviews. Stages of such adaptation as outlined by Kübler-Ross (7) were discussed. The alignments that occur in the family constellation as a result of illness, financial strain, and the grief and bereavement of the surviving persons in the environment were among the many areas identified as requiring attention by the physician.

Medical Personnel

The presence of instructors who themselves often deal with these matters is a vital contribution to the discussion. During the early stages of the course, the students urgently asked for guidance from the instructors; however, they were encouraged then and throughout the course to develop approaches to patients which best suited their individual experiences and personality structures.

An awareness of the importance of the numerous interactions between physicians and other care-giving individuals in the environment of dying patients was brought to the students' attention through the sessions given by the nurses and the clergymen. Left to operate as separate individuals without benefit of constructive communication, the many persons caring for these patients become limited in providing effective care. The nurses told of their difficulties in managing patients with life-threatening illnesses when they do not know how much information has been imparted to the patient by the physician. Similar difficulties may arise from a physician's lack of knowledge about a particular patient's religious views.

Through student dialogue with some of these nonphysician care-giving individuals, the students not only gained an awareness of the perspective of these individuals but also recognized their role in caring for the dying; and so they will be able to utilize their services and techniques in a more effective manner. They saw, for example, that the clergyman and pastoral counselor have functions in caring for the dying and the family aside from purely theological ones. This knowledge begins to overcome prejudices which in the past have often seriously impaired communication, data-gathering, and collaborative effort.

Ethical Issues

Medical progress has enabled the physician to prolong life in the case of a number of illnesses which in the past were associated with extremely poor prognoses. Many of these treatment methods, however, raise issues which fall into the realm of ethics; and they provide new uncertainties and dilemmas for the patient, the family, and the physician. Decision-making and implementation of these treatments often involve considerations which have been outside the sphere of the medical students' education. Unless he happens to be assigned a patient such as one undergoing chronic hemodialysis or provides care for a child born with multiple birth defects, the student may fail to appreciate many of the subtle difficulties associated with these areas of medical practice. Even when the student is working with such patients, the length of rotations often obscures the issues raised by these treatments. Student participants in the class frequently voiced their sense of frustration in being excluded from these ethical considerations in their work with patients. They welcomed the chance to explore and begin to formulate their approach to these problems. They saw that many of the questions involved in these problems and their management have no one answer and are dependent upon the subtleties of the individual situation and the current societal attitudes. However, the students and instructors felt that discussion of these vital areas of medical practice is necessary.

CONCLUSION

It should be noted that additional focal presentations or emphases could easily be incorporated in this type of course or the course could be flexibly changed to emphasize one or another aspect of life-threatening illness. Topics such as the legal aspects of death, matters related to intensive care units, or interviews of patients and families of patients who illustrate other aspects of life-threatening illness could provide additional dimensions and perspective.

It is anticipated that this course will help students to continue to develop more effective approaches to the problems in caring for dying patients. Importantly they came to recognize the individual variations in adaptation to life-threatening illness. The importance of the course in providing a working knowledge of many of the areas which have been delineated but in the past not presented to the student in a way which promotes self-understanding, learning, and continued inquiry was highlighted by one student who, in evaluating his experience in the course, wrote:

Although the course, through dealing with life-threatening illness, concerned itself with death and dying, it became clear in the end that we dealt with life all along, and this clarified a significant aspect of death, i.e., death and dying as an integral part of life that should and must be faced and hopefully, bravely and honestly discussed by us all.

SUMMARY

The format, content, and goals of an elective course designed specifically to teach medical students about the psychosocial aspects of life-threatening illness are described. The course, a semester in length, was held each week and was conducted by a psychiatrist, a hematologist, a pediatric hematologist, and a professor of philosophy. The size of the class was limited to ensure extensive group discussion. Instructional goals included desensitization to the topic, consideration of related psychosocial and ethical matters, and the presentation of the perspectives and roles of other care-giving personnel involved in providing care for patients with life-threatening illness. To accomplish these goals, a format combining a number of focal presentations (patient interviews, selections from the literature, and dialogue with care-giving personnel) with extensive group discussion was utilized. Using this format, students were aided in beginning to synthesize their own feelings about death and dying, thereby better attending the numerous individualized needs of patients with life-threatening illnesses.

REFERENCES

1 Barton, D. The Need for Including Instruction on Death and Dying in the Medical Curriculum. *J. Med. Educ.*, **47**:169–175, 1972.
2 Pattison, E. M. The Experience of Dying. *Am. J. Psychother.*, **21**:32–43, 1967.
3 Tolstoy, L. The Death of Ivan Ilych. In *The Death of Ivan Ilych and Other Stories*. New York: New American Library, 1960.
4 Lifton, R. J. On Death and Death Symbolism: The Hiroshima Disaster. *Psychiatry*, **27**:191–210, 1964.
5 Wahl, C. W. The Fear of Death. *Bull. Menninger Clin.*, **22**:214–223, 1958.
6 Lindemann, E. Symptomatology and Management of Acute Grief. *Amer. J. Psychiat.*, **101**:141–148, 1944.
7 Kübler-Ross, E. *On Death and Dying*. London: MacMillan, 1969.

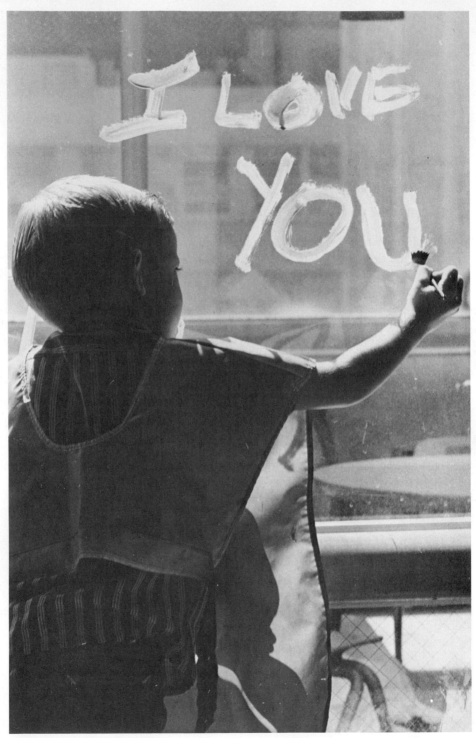

Courtesy of Arlene Bernstein

Epilogue

It is hard to imagine what it meant for a 48-year-old man to be placed in the middle of the technocracy of a modern hospital. It must have been like coming to another planet where the people dress, behave, talk and act in a frightfully strange way. The white nurses, with their efficient way of washing, feeding, and dressing patients; the doctors with their charts, making notes and giving orders in an utterly strange language; the many unidentifiable machines with bottles and tubes; and all the strange odors, noises, and foods must have made Mr. Harrison feel like a little child who had lost his way in a fearful forest. For him nothing was familiar, nothing understandable, nothing even approachable. . . . He had lost control of himself.

The Wounded Healer, Henri J. M. Nouwen

Where do we go from here? This book was compiled specifically for the purpose of affecting people's lives—the lives of physicians, and dying patients and their families. To the extent that the ideas and approaches are utilized in the clinical arena toward more compassionate care of dying people, then our efforts will have been successful.

We learn best through a dialectical process of acting and reflecting, doing and analyzing (and intuiting!). For physicians, nurses, and allied personnel to use this text as a springboard to more effective care of patients and families facing life-threatening illness would constitute a gift to us all. As in any field things change, and new techniques, approaches, theories, and philosophies develop. It will remain the responsibility of the competent practitioner to stay abreast of these developments. I would encourage anyone in search of information related to the psychosocial care of the dying patient to use the SHANTI Project, 1137 Colusa Avenue, Berkeley, California 94707, as a resource center. We will endeavor to supply the most up-to-date information available or to make suggestions about where to obtain such material.

For most of us, the death of a patient to whom we have been deeply committed is a bitter pill to swallow. We are often reluctant to let go of striving toward cure and the preservation of life and acknowledge the inevitability of death. The pill becomes even more bitter for those of us who have not shared ourselves along with our medicines and procedures. We fear for our patients as we fear for ourselves, that we have not given and shared enough and that death always comes too soon. To the extent that we have given too little too late to those who are dying, we may come to realize that although the primary crisis is the patient's, the last crisis is the physician's. With determination, experience, and luck we may discover—as did Albert Camus—that:

In the midst of winter, I finally learned that there was in me an invincible summer.

Index

NAME INDEX

SUBJECT INDEX